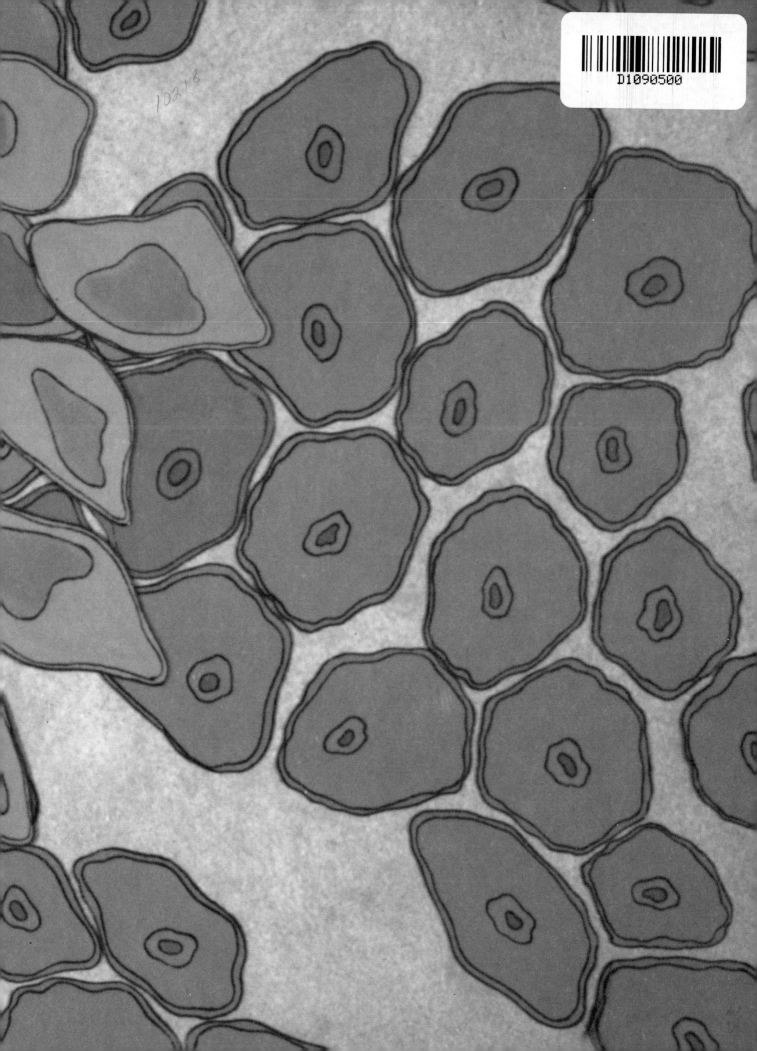

CONTRARY TO

Being an illustrated commentary on some persons and events of historical importance in the development of knowledge concerning • •

DHEW Publication No. (NIH) 76-720

U.S. DEPARTMENT OF HEALTH, EDUCATION, AND WELFARE
Public Health Service National Institutes of Health

For Sale By Superintendent Of Documents, United States Government Printing Office
Washington D.C. 20401

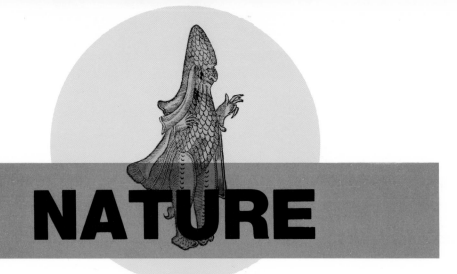

NATURE

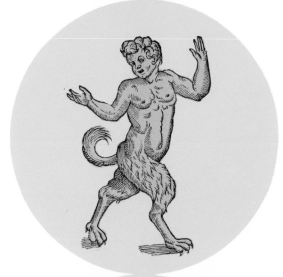

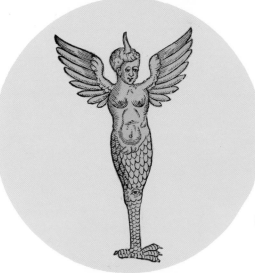

... CANCER

by

Michael B. Shimkin

1977

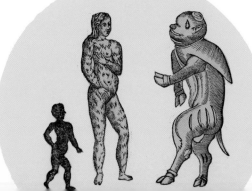

Paré, Oeuvres 1585.

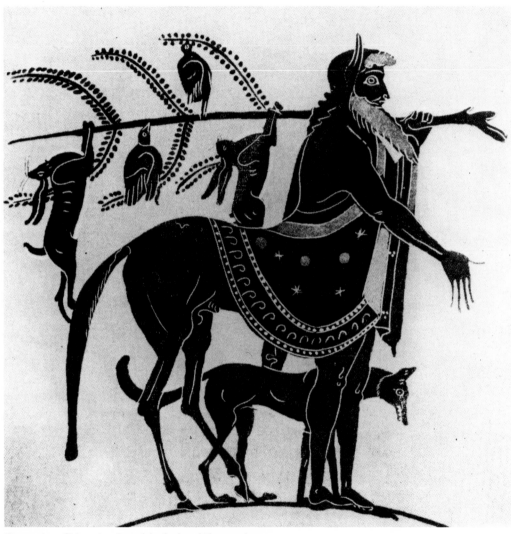

The centaur *Chiron,* teacher of Asclepios. Attica amphora, ca
520 BC (K. Kerenyi, *Der gottliche Arzt*. Basel: Ciba 1948)

Dedicated to the
Eventual
Prevention and Cure of Cancer

Table of Contents

VI   18TH CENTURY: THE AGE OF REASON

VII   19TH CENTURY: INVENTION AND INDUSTRY   101

VII 19TH CENTURY: INVENTION AND INDUSTRY

VIII 20TH CENTURY: TO WORLD WAR II

VIII 20TH CENTURY: TO WORLD WAR II

IX 20TH CENTURY: POST WORLD WAR II

IX 20TH CENTURY: POST WORLD WAR II

IX   20TH CENTURY: POST WORLD WAR II

Prologue

This is the story of one of mankind's ruthless enemies, a group of fatal afflictions called cancer. The villain is the central character. The hero, its conqueror, still waits in the wings.

The **time** of the story reaches back some 5 thousand years, to the earliest written records of Western man.

The **stage** is Europe and its civilization, especially since the Renaissance, and its extensions to America and elsewhere.

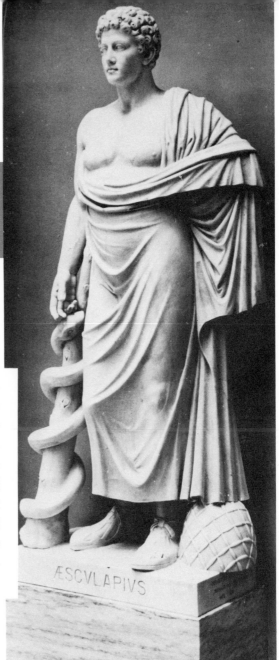

Asklepios, or Aesculapius, statue at the College of Physicians of Philadelphia.

The presentation of the story is through events, persons, and written records. These are organized chronologically and by topics.

The story of cancer is grim and incomplete. Man recognized cancer and named it over 2 thousand years ago, but for all but the last hundred years he could do little against it. Now he stands at the threshold of understanding and of mastering this enemy.

Today cancer is among the diseases aptly called by the ancients as Tumors Contrary to Nature. Tomorrow it will be among the horrors of the past. Its conquest will be by man's intellect, using a disciplined yet unbridled method of imagining and thinking called scientific research.

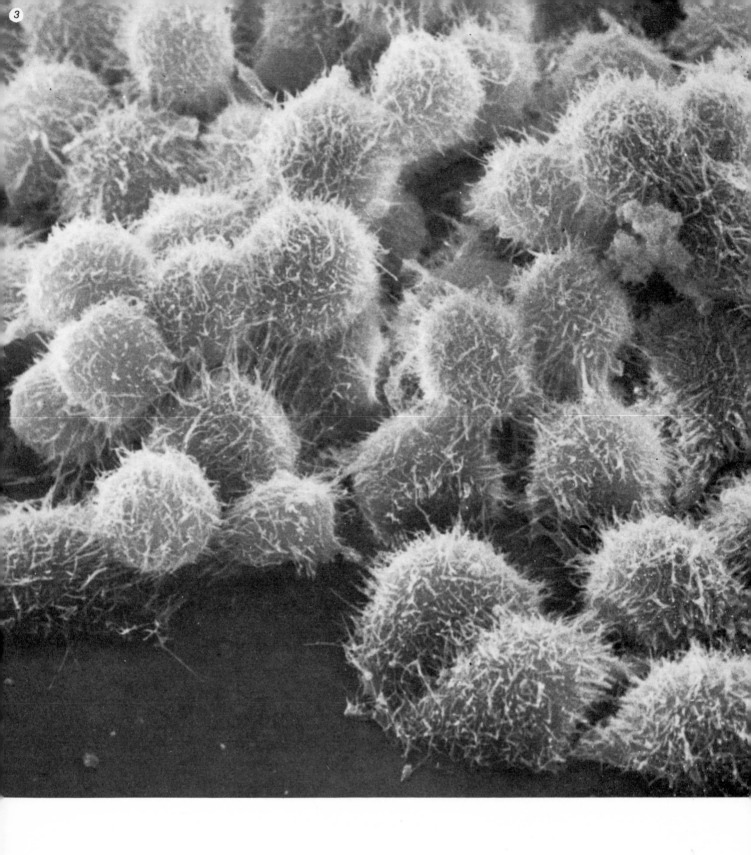

Scanning micrograph of HeLa cancer cells (x 2000) (K.R.
Porter, Virginia Fonte and Gary Weiss, A scanning
microscope study of the topography of HeLa cells. Cancer
Research 34: 1385-94, 1974).

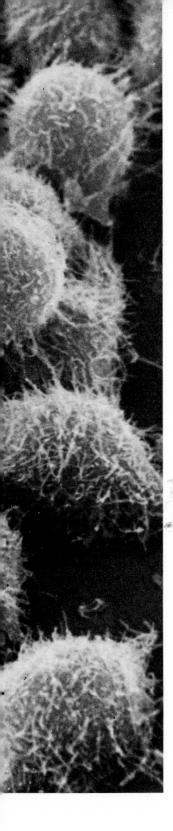

". . . Cancer the Crab lies so still that you
might think he was asleep if you did not
see the ceaseless play and winnowing
motion of the feathery branches round
his mouth. That movement never
ceases. It is like the eating of a smother-
ing fire into rotten timber in that it is noise-
less and without haste."

—Rudyard Kipling,
The Children of the Zodiac, 1893.

I. Introductions

I-A. What is Cancer?

Cancer is a word in the English language, derived from the Greek word for crab, Karkinos. Among its many synonyms are malignant tumor and malignant neoplasm (from the Greek for new growth). Subgroups of cancer, describing the body tissues of origin, include carcinoma, sarcoma, melanoma, lymphoma and many other related or combined terms. The systematic classification of cancers, based upon microscopic appearance, replaced older, more colorful names such as scirrhus (hard, or a scar), and nolimitangere (do not touch me).

Cancer is a word that stands for a great group of diseases that afflicts man and animals. Cancer can arise in any organ or tissue of which the body is composed. Its main characteristics include a seemingly unrestricted or uncontrolled growth of abnormal body cells, with the resultant mass compressing, invading and destroying contiguous normal tissue.

Cancer cells then break off or leave the original mass and are carried by the blood or lymph to distant sites of the body. There they set up secondary colonies, or metastases, further invading and destroying the organs that are involved.

Cancer kills. Unless it can be successfully treated, cancer kills inexorably, slowly, and unpleasantly. Death is the basic fact about cancer. That is what makes cancer a dread disease. All other features of cancer are secondary to its deadliness.

Two important characteristics of cancer are **anaplasia** and **autonomy.** Anaplasia is the loss of normal appearance under the microscope, with the cells comprising the cancer being disorganized in arrangement and varying in size and shape. Autonomy is the loss of inhibition of cell growth, with resultant semi-independent behavior and function. The diseases grouped under cancer are

now second only to diseases of the heart and blood vessels as killers of the people of the Western world. In the United States of 1970, among its 210 million people, approximately 660,000 developed cancer during the year, and approximately 330,000 died of cancer during the year.

There has been a steady, striking increase in the number of cancer deaths in the United States and in Europe during the past century. Some of this rise is due to better diagnosis of cancer and better reporting of cancer cases. But a much more important factor has been the increasingly older population, saved from earlier death from infectious diseases and other causes. Although cancer does not spare the young, its main impact is reserved for the elderly. This is perhaps the only merciful aspect of cancer.

I-B.

An Overview of Oncology

Oncology, the study and knowledge about tumors, can be divided into a number of periods for convenience of presentation.

The first period, extending from 500 B.C. to 500 A.D., is typified by Hippocrates and by Galen. Cancer was recognized, named, and its grave prognosis defined. An excess of black bile, one of the four humors of the body, was stated as its cause. Treatment by excision or cautery was used for superficial lesions, with caution against such treatment for more advanced disease.

The second period, from 500 to 1500 A.D., was one of scientific sleep. Galen's authority was dogma, followed by Arabic as well as by European physicians. The knife and the cautery were used for accessible cancers, and escharotic and soothing ointments for ulcerated, more extensive lesions. Cancer of the skin and mouth, and the female breast were mentioned in surgical treatises. Cancer of the stomach, rectum and the womb were recognized but were untreatable. The humoral theory of causation prevailed.

The 16th Century heralded the Renaissance and the Reformation. Surgery was revolutionized by Paré, and pathology was added to the new anatomy of Vesalius. With the discovery of blood circulation and the lymphatics, the cause of cancer was related to stasis and abnormalities in lymph. John Hunter in the 18th Century made surgery into a science. The diagnosis and treatment of cancer improved as a result. Percivall Pott described scrotal cancer among chimney sweeps, the first occupational cancer with an environmental cause.

The 19th Century was a century of discovery in biomedical sciences. Quantitative methods began to be introduced. In 1837 Johannes Müller looked at cancers through an achromatic microscope, and ushered in the histologic period of oncology. The introduction of anesthesia in 1846 and of antisepsis in 1867 allowed Theodor Billroth and other surgeons to develop operative procedures for internal cancers.

The 20th Century marked the emergence of oncology as a scientific discipline in its own right. The discovery of transplantable and of induced tumors in animals opened the period of experimental cancer research. Radiotherapy was added to surgery as an effective modality of treatment for some cancers by 1930, and chemotherapy by 1960. Oncology now began to make major contributions to biomedical sciences, whereas previously it had applied the discoveries of other sciences to its own particular problems. Cancer was now conceived as an alteration in the basic chemical structure of the cell, perhaps due to a symbiosis with a virus.

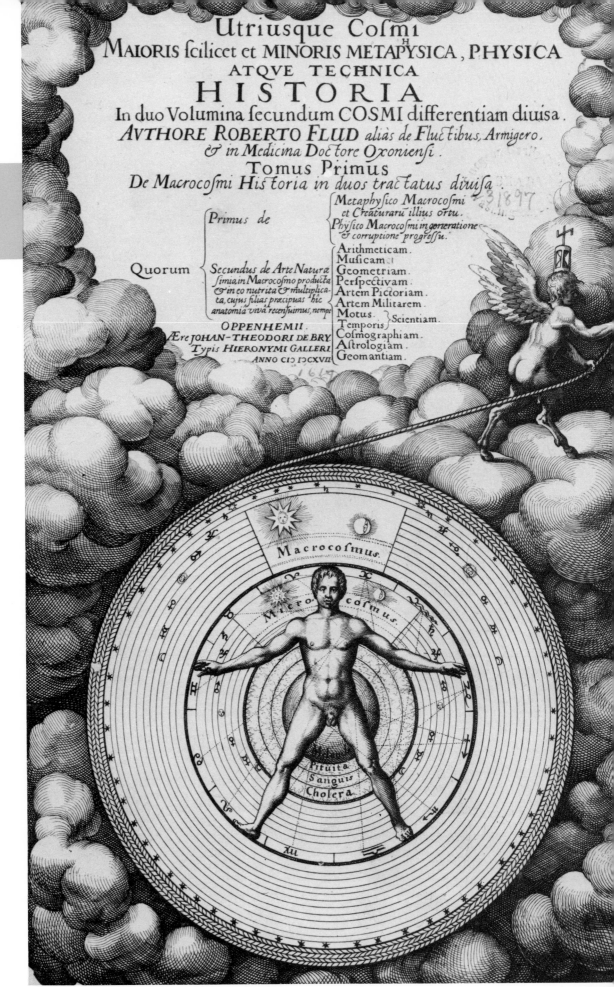

Robert Flud, *Utriusque Cosmi* . . . Oppenheim, 1617, A
historical synthesis

I-C.

Expectations and Limitations

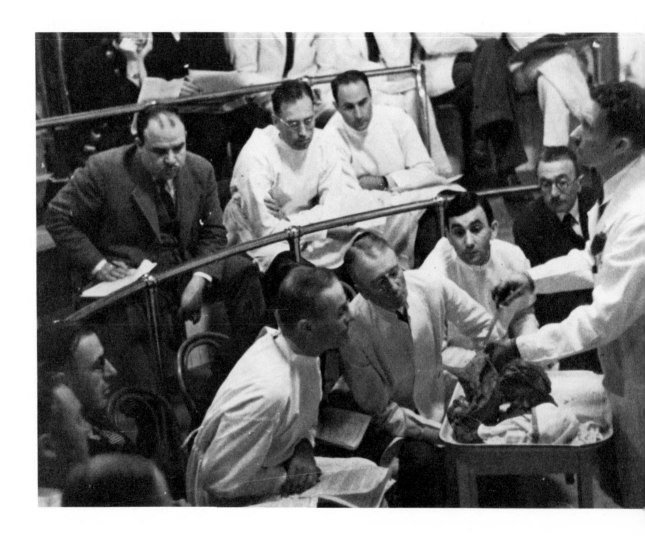

Clinical-pathologic Conference, San Francisco, 1935.

He who writes history has truth at his mercy.

History is written by historians, who are humanly susceptible to errors of misinterpretation, rationalization, and misinformation. The sources of such errors are many, external and internal. They are not rectified by the cloak of learning.

We have learned to be wary of histories of Roman emperors written by medieval Christians, or of Catholic popes written by Reformation protestants. Let us also be wary of histories of science written by historians wedded to a thesis of history, be it one of limitless progress or the decline of the West. It remains unresolved whether history is the gradual climb of man toward enlightenment or his search for lost and forgotten wisdom, or neither. For one thing, the time encompassed by written history is miniscule: some 5000 years on a planet that measures its changes on a scale of millions of years.

Were history limited to the recitation of dates and places, selection still would be inevitable. Selection leads to its own particular errors, especially if such selection is made with a thesis in mind, consciously or unconsciously. In specialized topics such as the history of science and medicine, divorcing such topics from the general background of the time produces further distortions.

Man can look at the world through his own eyes alone, and the clarity of his vision is reduced by time and by distance. It is probably impossible, until a time-machine is invented, for the twentieth-century man to truly understand medieval man or, more accurately, the records and other artifacts left by him.

We must beware of interpreting our forebears as ignorant. But we also must not imbue them with knowledge they can not have possessed. In interpreting the past, we must rely on what is left to interpret. Written records have to be written. Those who wrote profusely are over-represented in history, and those who did not may be lost to history. One polemicist with access to a printing press may loom much larger in history than his role deserves. Publish or perish is an admonition not restricted to academicians.

Records may also be found after being lost for centuries. The glittering role of Leonardo da Vinci in European scientific history, as an example, is of recent vintage, and followed rediscovery of his notebooks several centuries after his death.

The telling of history through accounts of persons has additional pitfalls. In human events, and certainly in science, the chief ingredients for discovery are the state of the art at the time, plus the prepared mind that can exploit an unpredicted occurrence. Man must stand on the shoulders of his predecessors. For even the greatest heroes of science and medicine, there are persons and events that were essential preludes for their discoveries. It is not simply chauvinism that often leads to the claims for a discovery from more than one candidate from more than one country. The fact is that the same stage is often set in more than one location, and as often equally talented men are considering the same problem and the same sets of accumulated data.

Searches for Firsts in discovery are fragile endeavors. It seems almost irrelevant to acknowledge that Columbus was not the first European to discover America; his place in history is assured without such absolutes. In biomedical sciences, no name is greater than that of Pasteur. Yet spontaneous generation was disproved by Redi long before, and the microbial cause of silkworm disease was discovered by Bassi several decades before Pasteur applied his magic touch to the problem.

Nevertheless, there are heroes in science. They may not have been the first, but they often were the best at a given point in history. The release of medicine from the dead hand of authority is dated to Vesalius and his magnificently illustrated **De humani corporis fabrica** of 1543. Vesalius certainly was not the first to resume dissection of cadavers, nor even the first to write about and to teach his findings. Yet his place is entirely se-

cure as long as our European culture persists on this planet.

But it is not my intent to establish my niche as a historiographer by profundities that have been stated before and often by others. Rather it is to set the stage for an explanation of how this material was prepared and its limitations.

The genesis of this book was thus.

In 1964, I became editor of **Cancer Research**, the monthly journal of the American Association for Cancer Research. The staid, drab cover of this prestigious periodical seemed to need a freshening. An experimental design, to include illustrations of historical events in cancer research, was initiated. The January 1966 issue featured Percivall Pott and the chimney sweep, to commemorate the first clear description of an environmental carcinogen.

The historical covers received a favorable reaction from the readers, and were continued when Sidney Weinhouse succeeded me as editor in 1969. By the tenth year, suggestions were made to reproduce the covers as a volume, but this idea had obvious drawbacks. Instead, I was commissioned by the National Cancer Institute to prepare an illustrated history of cancer, using the **Cancer Research** covers as one of the sources, under Contract NIH-74-C-934.

The result is this collection, arranged in a chronological order and with continuity. The **Cancer Research** cover material was used, but revised in almost all instances.

During the preparation of the **Cancer Research** covers, many individuals submitted or were asked to submit specific themes. The contributions are acknowledged in the legends of the covers. For 3 years, Victor A. Triolo designed some and helped with other issues, without individual credits being indicated. There were many others who pitched in and helped. The managing editor of **Cancer Research**, Margaret Foti and her staff; the artists and printers of the publishers provided many inputs. The National Library of Medicine was a primary source of materials; I am particularly indebted to Mrs. Lucinda Keister for her assistance. The medical library staff at the University of California at San Diego was uniformly helpful. Mr. Roland Wussow, my "project officer" of the National Cancer Institute, was invaluable in many ways. The labor of typing the manuscript fell on Mrs. Eileen Innis. My wife, Mary, provided encouragement and remained tolerant of my preoccupation with a hobby.

The collection presented here is not a scholarly, in-depth study. Rather it is a once-over-lightly collection, fitting cancer into the broader arena of medicine and biomedical science. In spite of the forboding subject, I hope that the collection is sufficiently provocative to encourage interest in the reader to pursue further various aspects of medicine and medical research.

This collection was not intended to draw cosmic conclusions, even about cancer, nor to support any particular thesis. Nevertheless, it is heartening to reconstruct a slow but steady movement forward that may well reach its goal of the prevention and cure of cancer within the not too distant future.

In this movement, the limitations and prejudices of the compiler are obvious and are intentionally not disguised. The chauvinism that favors events at the National Cancer Institute of the United States and of the past 40 years reflects my knowledge and is not an intended slight of contributions from other institutions, other countries and from other times. There is ample credit for all in this international biomedical adventure. Perhaps a more balanced version of the events will be forthcoming from some future international collaborative effort in the history of cancer.

Finally, all my professional life I have received generous support from the people of the United States, via their allocations to the National Cancer Institute. **Cancer Research** is heavily subsidized by funds from the same source. The National Library of Medicine is a governmental agency, the property of the people of the United States. Thus, all I have done, and all the materials herein, are in the public domain.

Feel free to use and to copy, please. You might wish to indicate the source, for the convenience of your audience.

I-D.

Sources and Leads

Good books are rewritten rather than written.

The basic source for the early history of cancer is the exhaustive compilation published between 1907 and 1928 by Wolff. He is the acknowledged guide for all subsequent historical reviews, including this one. A thoughtful selection for an exhibit was made in 1932 by Haagensen; his suggestions were carefully considered and often followed. Further compilations of historical cancer events, in the form of exhibits or of periodic vignettes, were added to the **Cancer Research** cover material. These were: the front covers and "Annals of Cancer History" appearing on the back covers of **The Cancer Bulletin** published since 1949 by the Medical Arts Publishing Foundation of Houston, Texas; frontispieces in **Cancer** appearing 1948-1961; and an exhibit assembled by Olch and Leikind in 1962.

Four books on medical history were used throughout, so that no specific citations are considered necessary for each item selected for inclusion here. These references are: Castiglioni (1958), Garrison (1929), Major (1954) and Singer and Underwood (1962). Meade (1968) for surgery, Buschke (1958) for radiotherapy and Long (1965) for pathology were employed as extensions into these specialties. For the history of science, Bernal (1965) was an important source.

In 1974, I published a starter reading list and guide in the history of cancer, limiting the references to those in English and those of more recent vintage.

In this compilation of some 225 items (events or persons) the bibliographic plan is to indicate the primary source of each item, with an English translation when such is available, plus a few key articles dealing with the subject from which further references and leads can be obtained. Thus, the minimum of references is the aim. The references are given at the end of each item.

The sources of the illustrations are the pictorial collection of the National Library of Medicine and of **Cancer Research** unless otherwise specified.

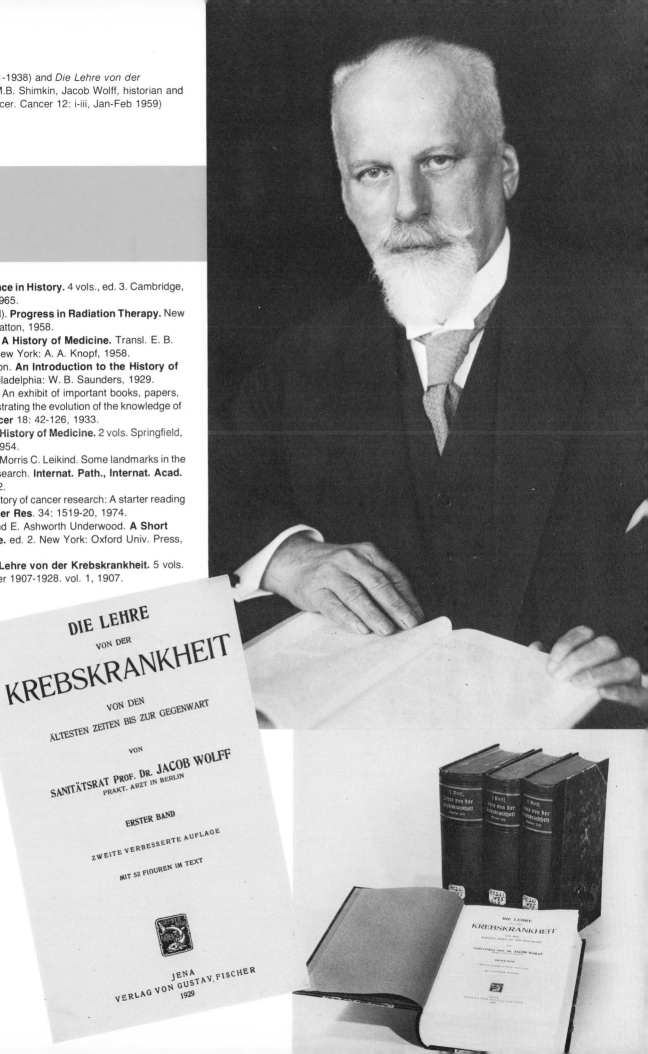

Jacob Wolff (1861-1938) and *Die Lehre von der Krebskrankheit* (M.B. Shimkin, Jacob Wolff, historian and biographer of cancer. Cancer 12: i-iii, Jan-Feb 1959)

J. D. Bernal. **Science in History.** 4 vols., ed. 3. Cambridge, Mass.: MIT Press, 1965.

Franz Buschke (ed). **Progress in Radiation Therapy.** New York: Grune and Stratton, 1958.

Arturo Castiglioni. **A History of Medicine.** Transl. E. B. Krumbhaar, ed. 2. New York: A. A. Knopf, 1958.

Fielding H. Garrison. **An Introduction to the History of Medicine,** ed. 4. Philadelphia: W. B. Saunders, 1929.

C. D. Haagensen. An exhibit of important books, papers, and memorabilia illustrating the evolution of the knowledge of cancer. **Am. J. Cancer** 18: 42-126, 1933.

Ralph H. Major. **A History of Medicine.** 2 vols. Springfield, Ill.: C. C. Thomas, 1954.

Peter D. Olch and Morris C. Leikind. Some landmarks in the history of cancer research. **Internat. Path., Internat. Acad. Path.** 3: 36-38, 1962.

M. B. Shimkin. History of cancer research: A starter reading list and guide. **Cancer Res.** 34: 1519-20, 1974.

Charles Singer and E. Ashworth Underwood. **A Short History of Medicine.** ed. 2. New York: Oxford Univ. Press, 1962.

Jacob Wolff. **Die Lehre von der Krebskrankheit.** 5 vols. Jena: Gustav Fischer 1907-1928. vol. 1, 1907.

DIE LEHRE
VON DER
KREBSKRANKHEIT

VON DEN
ÄLTESTEN ZEITEN BIS ZUR GEGENWART

VON

SANITÄTSRAT PROF. DR. JACOB WOLFF
PRAKT. ARZT IN BERLIN

ERSTER BAND

ZWEITE VERBESSERTE AUFLAGE

MIT 52 FIGUREN IM TEXT

JENA
VERLAG VON GUSTAV FISCHER
1929

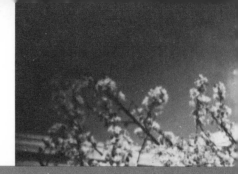

Research Should Begin and

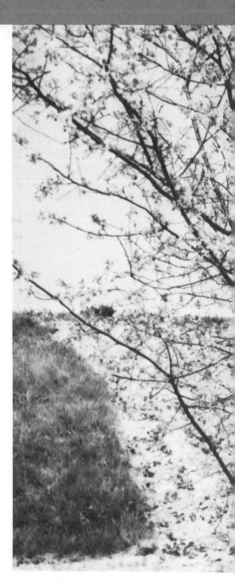

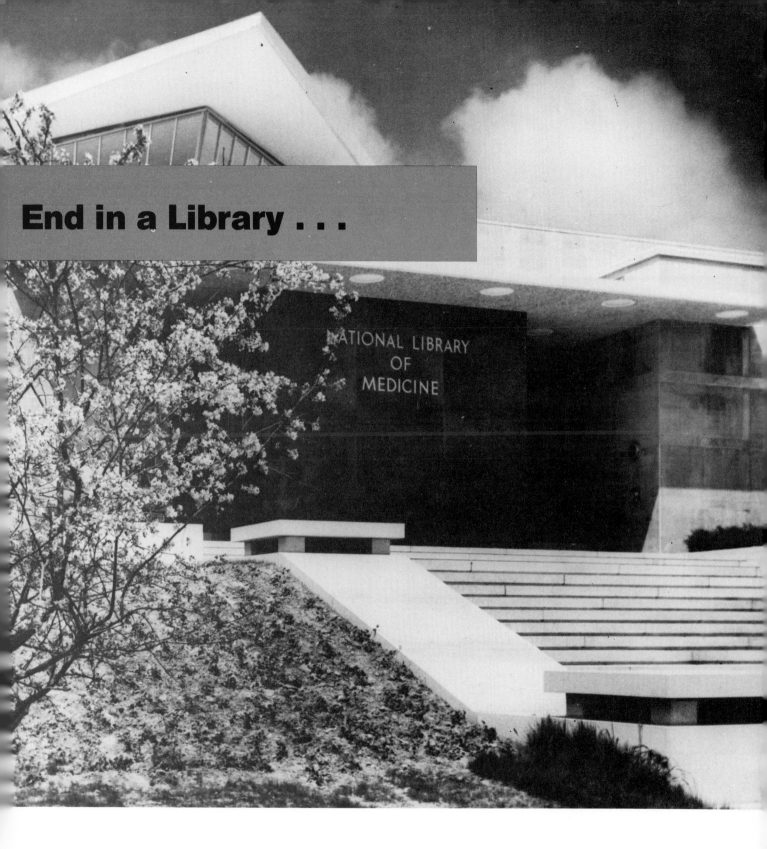

End in a Library . . .

National Library of Medicine,
Bethesda, Maryland

II. Greco-Roman Period (500 B.C.-500 A.D.)

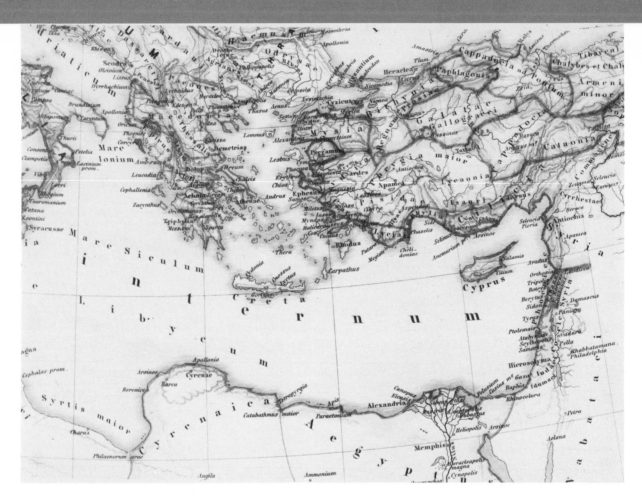

Ancient Greece is the fountainhead of western European civilization. Around the Aegean Sea, on its western and eastern coastlines and its innumerable islands, arose a people of fierce independence of thought and deed, unsurpassed bravery and suicidal combativeness. They annealed the older cultures of the east and reached heights in art, drama and philosophy that have been seldom equalled and never surpassed. The golden age of Athens, under Pericles, is a permanent pinnacle in European history.

Western medicine begins in Greece during the fifth century before the Christian era. It is here that medicine became clearly dissociated from religion and philosophy, albeit it retained its roots in

Eastern Mediterranean, ca 100 BC (from Spruner-Menke, *Atlas Antiquus* Gothae: J. Perthes, 1865.)

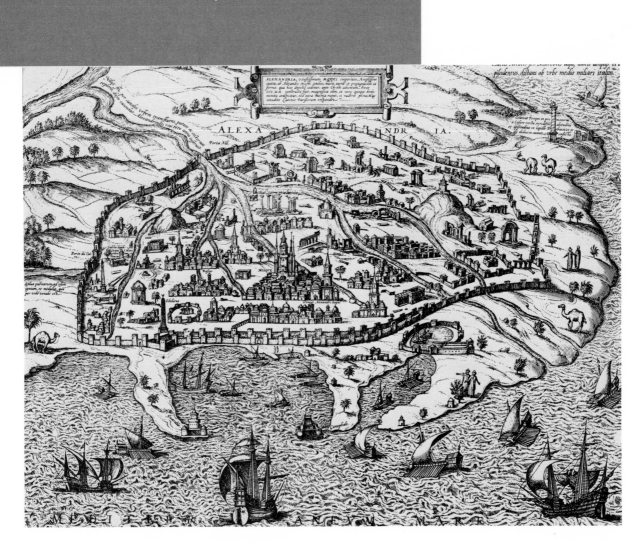

both. It is here that arose observational medicine, and treatment based on prognosis as indicated by the natural history of disease.

Greek learning shifted to Alexandria by 300 B.C., and lasted there until the final destruction of its library 600 years later. At the medical school, dissections of the human body were performed. Greek be-

came the language of science and medicine, and Greek physicians diffused throughout the civilized western world.

Greece became part of the Roman Empire in 146 B.C. Roman talents lay in organization and administration, and environmental and personal hygiene became well developed. Medicine emerged as a recognized segment of the social structure.

Alexandria, Egypt, 1575 (from Historic Urban Plans, Ithaca, New York)

II-A.

Antiquity of cancer: Fossils and mummies

It is more than probable that cancer afflicted animals long before man appeared on earth. This assumption is based upon extrapolation of rather recent evidence. All animals that have been thoroughly studied at older age groups develop some types of cancer. Therefore, the ability to develop cancer must extend to the early history of the species. Cancer in animals, as in man, is essentially a disease of older age. In the natural wild state few animals survive to old age, and cancers are rarely detected in free-living animals. Animals in protected environments, allowing observations of older individuals, reveal occurrences of neoplastic disease that are characteristic for the species.

Early age at death, and the limitation of fossil remains essentially to bones limit factual proof of prehistoric cancers in animals. In the paleopathology literature summarized by Brothwell and by Janssens, references are found to two tumors in Cretaceous dinosaurs and one in a Pleistocene cave bear. The dinosaur tumors are said to be an osteoma and a

hemangioma of vertebras. Neither is a malignant tumor, even if the diagnoses be accepted. The cave bear tumor was stated to be an osteogenic sarcoma of the femur, but an alternate diagnosis of an exuberant post-traumatic callus also has been proffered. In any case, the hard evidence is thin.

Malignant neoplasms in man have been described among mummies from the Egyptian Third to Fifth Dynasties, or some 5000 years ago. The number of cases is small, considering that tens of thousands of Early Egyptian bodies have been examined. The best documented cases include some 3 osteogenic sarcomas and some 3 carcinomas of the nasopharynx.

Calvin Wells recorded one well-studied skull of a young adult male, with extensive destruction of the base of the skull and multiple circular holes of the outer table of the cranial vault. Radiography revealed some 26 rarifications, as pictured. As Wells says, "The overall picture leaves little doubt that this is a case of carcinoma of the naso-pharynx with pri-

D. Brothwell. The evidence for neoplasms. In D. Brothwell and A. T. Sandison (eds), **Diseases of Antiquity.** Springfield, Ill.: C. C. Thomas, 1967 (p. 320-45).

P. A. Janssens. Palaeopathology. **Diseases and Injuries of Prehistoric Man.** London: John Baker, 1970.

O. Urteaga and G. T. Pack. On the antiquity of melanoma. **Cancer** 19: 607-10, 1966.

Calvin Wells. Ancient Egyptian pathology. **J. Laryngol. Otol.** 77: 261-65, 1963.

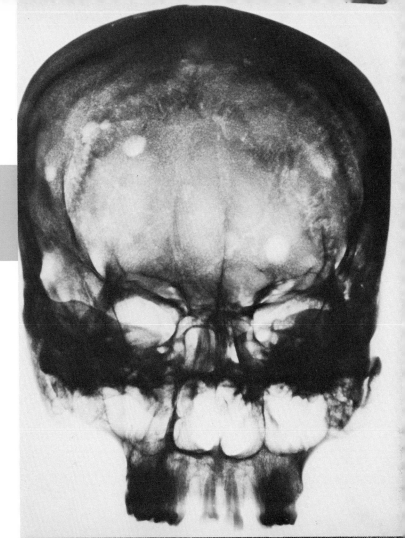

Radiograph of skull of a young Egyptian male, ca 3000 BC, showing metastases from probable nasopharyngeal cancer (from Wells).

mary destruction of the maxillary, palatal and pterygoid elements and secondary deposits widely scattered in the skull." It is of interest, and supportive of the conclusion of the antiquity of cancer that nasopharyngeal carcinoma is still rather common in East Africa.

Evidence of cancer also exists among mummies of pre-Columbian Incas of Peru, determined by radioactive carbon dating to be approximately 2400 years old. In addition to an osteogenic sarcoma, some cases of disseminated malignant melanoma have been recorded. Urteaga and Pack, in a poetic mood, described 2 cases, with the unmistakable black metastases involving the skull and the bones of the extremities. One of these skulls is illustrated.

The totality of evidence, therefore, indicates that cancer is a very old affliction that existed before written history. New methods in the young field of paleopathology will add interesting information in the future.

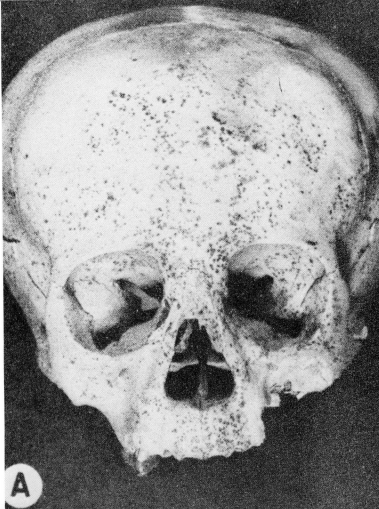

Pre-Columbian Inca skull containing metastatic melanoma in bone. (from Urteaga and Pack).

II-B.

Early writings: Egyptian papyruses

Egyptian papyruses are among the oldest written records of man that have survived for our inspection. Two are concerned with disease. The Edwin Smith Papyrus is a surgical treatise, and the Ebers Papyrus is a medical one. Both were written approximately 1600 B.C. and are, thus, approximately 3500 years old. Both are based on even older sources.

The Edwin Smith Papyrus was translated by Breasted, and the Ebers Papyrus by Ebbell. Various portions of these translations have been reproduced and commented upon by Bryan and by Butterfield. The commentaries demonstrate some frustration at being unable to penetrate clearly the distances of time, language and cultural differences. Uneasy assumptions are inevitable, buttressed by well-selected but not necessarily representative passages.

The Edwin Smith Papyrus contains the oft-quoted Case 45, of "Bulging Tumors of the Breast," recorded in lines 9 to 20 of the reproduction:

"If thou examinest a man having bulging tumors on his breast, (and) thou findest that [swellings] have spread over the breast; if thou puttest thy hand upon his breast upon these tumors, (and) thou findest them very cool, there being no fever at all therein when thy hand touches him; they have no granulation, they form no fluid, they do not generate secretions of fluid, and they are bulging to thy hand, thou should say concerning him 'One having bulging tumors. An ailment with which I will attend. There is no [treatment]'."

From the Ebers Papyrus there is the following case description:

"When thou meetest a large tumor of the god Xensu in any part of the limb of a person, it is loathsome and suffers many pustules to come forth; something arises therein as though wind were in it, causing irritation. The tumor calls with a loud voice to thee, 'It is a tumor of the god Xensu. Do thou nothing there against'."

This could well be a flowery description of tropical ulcer or gas gangrene, but could also fit a neoplastic entity endemic in the area, Kaposi's sarcoma.

Both papyruses, as well as more fragmentary additional writings, are filled primarily by complex recipes and incantations. Bryan, for example, after recording 4 remedies to stop diarrhea, includes the instructions to sing "O, Hotu!" and again, "O, Hotu!" He cannot resist the comment, "Which in the circumstances appears to be a very appropriate word to chant."

Nevertheless, these two papyruses, and the half-dozen more fragmentary ones, reconstruct a practical, empirical medical practice. Tumors that are described as fitting our present categories of benign, such as lipomas and polyps, are cut out with the knife or a red-hot iron. Palliative treatment of a possible cancer of the stomach is with boiled barley mixed with dates, and of cancer of the uterus by a concoction of fresh dates and pig's brain, introduced into the vagina.

Fragment of the Edwin Smith papyrus, reproduced and translated by Breasted.

Cyril P. Bryan. (trans.) **The Papyrus Ebers.** London: Geoffrey Bles, 1930.

W. C. Butterfield. Tumor treatment, 3000 B.C. **Surgery** 60: 476-79, 1966.

J. H. Breasted. **The Edwin Smith Surgical Papyrus.** Chicago: Univ. of Chicago Press, 1930.

B. Ebbell. (trans.) **The Papyrus Ebers: The Greatest Egyptian Medical Document.** Copenhagen: Levin and Munksgaard, 1937.

The School at Cos: Hippocrates

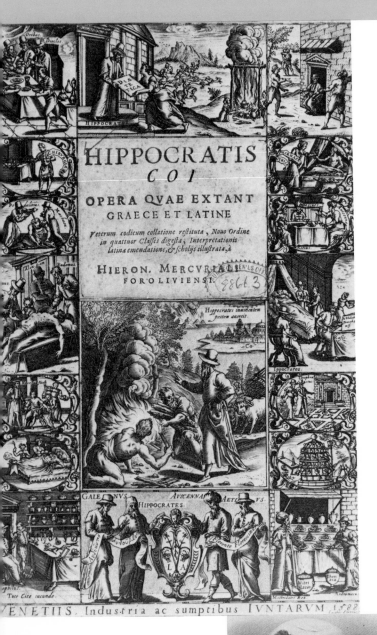

Title page of a collection of the works of Hippocrates, printed in Venice in 1588.

Bust found near Ostia in 1940, with circumstantial evidence that it is a true representation of Hippocrates. (From Barrow)

Hippocrates (c. 460-c. 370) is the most venerated name in medicine, the epitome of the wise, tolerant, honest physician. He was born on the island of Cos, and his whole life was closely associated with the temples of healing dedicated to Asclepios, the Greek semideity of healing.

The name of Hippocrates is given to the many books that were probably written by many people. Hippocrates is still a lively subject for medical writings, not only as the Father of Medicine, but as the Father of Proctology, Rhinology, and any other specialty an author espouses. Thus the statement that he is the Father of Oncology should be expected and there is no question but that he and his school knew cancer. Indeed, he named it carcinos and carcinoma. A full dissertation on the development of these words has been published by Keil.

Hippocrates could not do much for cancer, and applied to it one of his cardinal rules, "Primum non nocere," first do no harm. Among his Aphorisms, number 38 states, "It is better not to apply any treatment in cases of occult cancer; for, if treated, the patients die quickly; but if not treated, they hold out for a long time." Modern commentators insist that by "occult" Hippocrates meant not ulcerated or deep seated, an interpretation of disputative correctness. In any case, Hippocrates knew cancer of the breast, uterus and stomach as well as of the skin and mouth.

The Hippocratic approach to medicine was observational and empirical. His theoretical framework was elaborated by Aristotle and subsequent commentators, but is well summarized by Osler in the Hippocratic "Nature of Man:"

"The body of man contains in itself blood and phlegm and yellow bile and black bile, which things are in the natural constitution of his body, and the cause of sickness and of health. He is healthy when they are in proper proportion between one another as regards mixture and force and quantity, and when they are all well mingled together; he becomes sick when one of these is diminished or increased in amount, or separated in the body from its proper mixture, and not properly mingled with all the others."

This is a statement of the Four Humors. Cancer was a disease of an excess of black bile, which was manufactured by the spleen and stomach (not the liver). These were biological counterparts of the Four Elements, Air, Fire, Earth and Water of Empedocles, which in combinations produced the qualities of heat, cold, wetness and dryness. Black bile, or melanchole, or atrabilis, as the cause of cancer remained the predominant theory for two thousand years. Cancer is, indeed, a melancholy disease.

Hippocrates was a real man who lived to an advanced age. He wore a beard, and became bald. His visage was recorded in statuary, and many Roman copies of his purported appearance are available. A damaged bust found near Ostia in 1940 seems to be the leading current candidate of the true representation, according to Barrow.

Mark V. Barrow. Portraits of Hippocrates. **Med. Hist.** 16: 85-88, 1972.

S. Glaser. Hippocrates and proctology. **Proc. Roy. Soc. Med.** 62: 380-81, 1969.

The Genuine Works of Hippocrates. Translated by Francis Adams. 2 vols. London: Sydenham Society, 1849.

Harry Keil. The historical relationship between the concept of tumor and the ending -oma. **Bull. Hist. Med.** 24: 352-77, 1950.

William Osler. **The Evolution of Modern Medicine.** New Haven: Yale Univ. Press, 1921.

II-D.

Roman medical encyclopedist: Celsus

Aulus Cornelius Celsus lived in Rome during the first Christian century. He wrote an encyclopedia of which a part was on medicine. **De medicina** is considered to be the greatest Latin work on the subject.

The place of Celsus' compilation in history is obscured by the fact that it apparently was either lost or neglected for 1400 years. Pope Nicholas V rediscovered the work and had it issued in Florence in 1478. It was one of the earlier books to be published by the new movable type. The first page of the book is reproduced here.

Celsus represents a summary of Greek and Alexandrian medicine, and is a valuable historical benchmark between Hippocrates and Galen. The interval of 3 centuries between Hippocrates and Celsus saw the rise of the Roman empire, with Rome now the center of western civilization. Alexandria, however, remained for a long time a center for scientific and medical studies. A diversity of medical sects sprang up, of which only some followed the humoralistic approaches of Hippocrates. Of particular significance was the school of Erasistratus and Asclepiades, the Methodists, who explained disease as mechanical disturbance of the move-

ments of atoms through the pores of the body. Although the Methodists opposed the passive observational approach to Hippocratic medicine, they also were against bleeding and purging.

The views about cancer as summarized by Celsus appeared in Book V, chapter 28 of **De medicina**.

"A carcinoma does not give rise to the same danger (as a carbuncle) unless it is irritated by imprudent treatment. This disease occurs mostly in the upper parts of the body, in the region of the face, nose, ears, lips, and in the breasts of women, but it may also arise in an ulceration, or in the spleen. Around the spot is felt a sort of pricking; there is a fixed, irregular swelling, sometimes there is also numbness. Around it are dilated tortuous veins, pallid or livid in hue, sometimes in certain cases they are even hidden from view; and in some the part is painful to the touch, in others there is no feeling. And at times the part becomes harder or softer than natural, yet without ulcerating; and sometimes ulceration supervenes on all the above signs. The ulceration at times has no special characteristic; at times it resembles what the Greeks call condylomata, both in a sort of roughness and in size; its colour is either

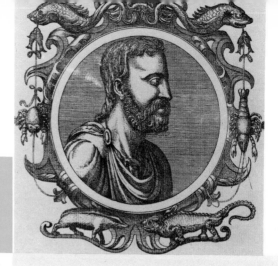

Imaginary portrait of Celsus (from I. Sambucus, Icones Veterum . . . Antwerp, 1574)

red or like that of lentils. The first stage is what the Greeks call cacoethes; then from that follows a carcinoma without ulceration; then ulceration, and from that a kind of wart. It is only the cacoethes which can be removed; the other stages are irritated by treatment; and the more so the more vigorous it is. Some have used caustic medicaments, some the cautery, some excision with a scalpel; but no medicament has ever given relief; the parts cauterized are excited immediately to an increase until they cause death. After excision, even when a scar has formed, none the less the disease has returned, and caused death; while at the same time the majority of patients, though no violent measures are applied in the attempt to remove the tumour, but only mild applications in order to soothe it, attain to a ripe old age in spite of it. No one, however, except by time and experiment, can have the skill to distinguish a cacoethes which admits of being treated from a carcinoma which does not. Therefore, as soon as the lesion is first noted, caustic medicaments should be applied. If the disease is relieved, if its indications are lessened, the treatment can be advanced to the use of the knife and of the cautery."

CORNELII CELSI DE MEDICINA LIBER INCIPIT

T alimēta sanis corporibus agricultura: sic sa
nitatem aegris medicina promittit. Haec nusq̄
quidem nō est. Siquidem etiam imperitissimæ
gētes herbas / alia que prōpta in auxiliū uulne
rū/morborū que nouerūt. Verūtamē apud græ
cos aliquanto magis q̄ in cæteris nationibus ex
culta est, ac ne apud hos quidē a prima origine: sed paucis ante
nos saeculis: ut pote cum uetustissimus auctor Aesculapius cele
bretur. Qui quoniam adhuc rudem & uulgarem hanc scientiam
paulo subtilius excoluit: indeorum numerum receptus est. Huius
deide duo filii Podalirius & Machaō bello troiano ducem Aga
memnonē secuti non mediocrem opem commilitonibus suis attu
lerunt. Quos tamen Homerus nō inpestilentia: neq̄ inuariis ge
neribus morborum aliquid attulisse auxilii: sed uulneribus tantū
modo ferro & medicamentis mederi solitos esse proposuit. Ex
quo apparet has partes medicinæ solas ab his esse tentatas: easq̄
esse uetustissimas. Eodem uero auctore disci potest morbos tum
adiram deorum immortalium relatos esse: & ab iisdem opem po
sci solitam. Veri que simil e est inter non nulla auxilia aduersæ
ualitudinis plerūq̄ tamē eam bonam cōtigisse ob bonos mores:
quos neq̄ desidia /neque luxuria uitiarant. Siquidem hæc duo /
corpora prius ingræcia: deinde apad nos afflixerunt. Ideo que
multiplex ista medicina /neq̄ olim /neq̄ apud alias gentes neces
saria /uix aliquos exbonis ad senectutis pricipia perducit. Ergo
etiā post eos /dequibus rettuli nō nulli clari uiri medicinam ex
ercuerunt: donec maiore studio litterarum disciplina agitari coe
pit.quæ ut animo præcipue ōnium necessaria /sic corpori inimi
ca est. Primoq̄ medendi scientia / sapientiæ pars habebatur: ut &
morborum curatio & rerum naturæ contemplatio sub iisdem
auctoribus nata sit. Scilicet iis hanc maxime requirentibus: qui

First page of *De Medicina,* printed in Florence in 1478.

Arturo Castiglioni. Aulus Cornelius Celsus as a historian of medicine. **Bull. Hist. Med.** 8: 857-873, 1940.

Celsus. **De Medicina.** With an English translation by W. G. Spencer, 3 vol. Cambridge, Mass.: Harvard Univ. Press, 1935-8.

I. Sambucus. **Icones Veterum**. . . . Antwerp, 1574.

II-E.

The Alexandrian School: Aretaeus the Cappadocian

Aretaeus, from a province of eastern Asia Minor, Cappadocia, lived in Alexandria during the Second or Third Century, and was a member of the Pneumatic School of medicine. His writings were not mentioned by Galen, and remained in oblivion until his manuscript was discovered and published in the 16th Century.

His descriptions of many infectious diseases are considered classic, and he is credited with the first clear account of diabetes. He is evaluated by Garrison as being nearer than any other Greek to the spirit and method of Hippocrates. He was also a stylist in his medical writings, which were translated into English in 1858 by the indefatigable Francis Adams (1796-1861), physician and classical scholar of Aberdeen, Scotland.

Aretaeus describes cancer of the uterus as follows:

"Ulcers, too, are formed in the womb; some broad and attended with tingling, which, being close together, are, as it were, a superficial excoriation; pus thick, without smell, scanty. These ulcers are mild. But there are others deeper and worse than these, in which the pains are slight, pus somewhat more abundant, much more fetid, and yet, notwithstanding, these also are mild. But if they become deeper, and the lips of the sores hard or rough, if there is a fetid ichor, and pain stronger than in the former case, the ulcer corrodes the uterus; but sometimes a small piece of flesh is cast off and discharged, and this sore not coming to cicatrization, either proves fatal after a long time, or becomes very chronic. This sore gets the appelation of phagedaena. The sores are also dangerous if in these cases the pain gets exacerbated, and the woman becomes uneasy. From the sore there is discharged a putrid matter, intolerable even to themselves; it is exasperated by touching and by medicines, and irritated by almost any mode of treatment. The veins in the uterus are swelled up with distension of the surrounding parts. To the skilled it is not difficult to recognise by the touch, for it is not otherwise obvious. Febrile heat, general restlessness, and hardness is present, as in malignant diseases; the ulcers, being of a fatal nature, obtain also the appellation of cancers. Another cancer: no ulceration anywhere, swelling hard and untractable, which distends the whole uterus; but there are pains also in the other parts which it drags to it. Both these carcinomatous sores are chronic and deadly; but the ulcerated is worse than the unulcerated, both in smell and pains, in life and in death."

Aretaeus, *De morbis acutis*, Paris, 1554

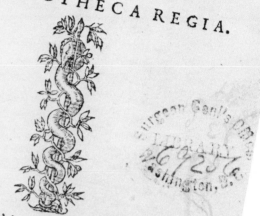

The Extant Works of Aretaeus, the Cappadocian. Edited
and translated by Francis Adams. London: Sydenham
Society, 1856.

E. J. Leopold. Aretaeus the Cappadocian. **Ann. Med. Hist.**
n.s. 2: 424-35, 1930.

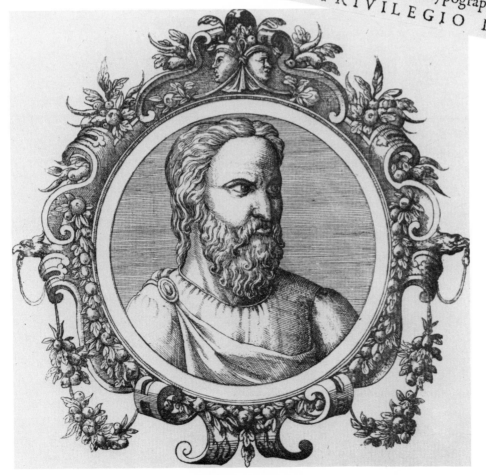

Imaginary portrait of Aretaeus the
Cappadocian (from I. Sambucus,
Icones Veterum . . Antwerp, 1574)

Authority for a millenium: Galen

94 CL. GALENI PERGA

MENI DE TVMORIBVS PRAETER
NATVRAM LIBER,

IO. GVINTERIO ANDERNACO INTERP.

QVAE RES tumoris uocabulo fignificatur, unum aliquod eorum eft, quae corporibus accidunt. Sic enim diftentionem in longum, latum, & profundū nominant. Eft quum incrementum naturalē ftatum excedens, tumorem appellemus: qui non modo ægris, in qualibet particula, fed etiā fanis adeft. Siquidem craffi ultra naturæ habitum in latum & profundū aucti funt, nō tamen iam præter naturam fefe habent. Nam, ficut plerunq; diximus, corporum quæ non pro naturæ modo affecta funt, tertia quædam eft conftitutio, medio inter eos qui fecundū naturam, & præter eam habent, ordine cōfiftens: ita craffus & gracilis non egreffi funt naturæ limites, uerum fimplici fermone tantū hic fupra naturalē habitum, ille infra ipfūm deuenit: uterq; autem naturaliter nō habet. Porrò qui ex aqua inter cutem intumefcit, uel ex tabe tenuior euafit, naturalem uterq; difpofitionē reliquit. Cæterum in præfenti hoc libro, de tumoribus præter naturam, corpus totum & quamlibet eius particulā occupantibus cōfiderare propofuimus, tantū diftinguentes uidelicet, cōftitutionum à natura declinantiū exceffus præter naturam exiftere: quorū finis eft, actionis læ fio. Atqui de his tumoribus plura dicere nō opus eft: quippe à carnis & pinguedinis immoderatione illos generari cōftat uniuerfis hominibus, non tantū medicis, Reliquos tumores, qui pro corporū ipforū ftatu, non qualitate duntaxat primaria à naturali modo recefferunt, iam infpiciemus, ab inflammatione exorfi: quod nomen Græcis dici confueuit de carnofis particulis tumidioribus, fimul & tenfione, renixu, dolore pulfatili, caliditate & rubore infeftatis. At quæ horū fymptomatum caufa exiftat, ne ipfis quidem medicis uniuerfis, tantū abeft ut uulgo comperta fit. Neq; enim uia quadam pleriq; ipforum inquifitionē eius moliuntur, fed quicquid uifum ipfis fuerit, fimpliciter pronunciant. Quod fi ratione ac uia procedas, confideratio talis effe queat. Maior tumor in nullo unquam corpore contigerit, nifi horum alterutrū fubftantiæ eius accidat, uel ut à copiofo calore ceu inferuefcens fundatur, uel extrinfecus recentiorem aliquam fubftantiam conquirat. Fufa nanq; in fpiritum abit, difflaturq;, & refrigerata eadem priftinum tumorem facile recuperat. Sed neq; fpiritus contentus in ipfis phlegmone laborantibus particulis confpicitur, quemadmodū in multis aliis tumoribus: & refrigeratæ ad priorē ftatum neq; ftatim neq; ex integro reuertuntur. Quod autē fpiritus non cōtinetur, ex fectione innotefcit. Apparet enim, fi pars inflammatione laborans fecta fuerit, fanguis permultus effluere, & locus uniuerfus abunde fanguinis plenus, ficut fpōgiæ madentes: fpiritus autem neq; ftatim excidere, neq; poftea. Cæterū folus color fanguinis proprius fimul & infeparabilis eft: fiquidem nulla corporis particula, nullus ue humor rubet, quàm caro & fanguis. Attamen inflāmationis affectus, corpulētia non eft, quam Græci πολυζαρκιαν appellant. Et fi quando corpulētia fola in corpore citra fanguinis copia confiftat, tumor naturæ ftatum exuperat, color intra fanitatis fines permanet, nec à priftina natura recedit. Quippe nulli, quod fecundū fubftantiam augefcit, color primus intenditur: fic enim nix candidior, pix nigrior, aurū flauum magis euaderet. Quamobrē fubftantiæ incrementū ab alteratione diuerfum eft. Augefcit enim fecundū quantitatē, alteratur fecundū qualitatem. Eft fanè & color

Galen was the medical authority of the western world for over 1300 years, between the final sack of Rome and into the Renaissance. During that long stretch of history the choice was between the axe of the barbarian and the cross of the authoritarian. The latter preserved what could be preserved from the past, at the price of dogmatic authority from which deviation was heresy. In religious matters, the Church; in philosophy, Aristotle; in medicine, Galen.

Clarissimus (or Claudius) Galen (138-201) was a real person, born in Pergamon in Asia Minor, who devoted his life to medicine. He studied at Alexandria, traveled widely, became the most respected physician in Rome, and managed to write some 400 works on anatomy, physiology, pathology, surgery, treatment, and seemingly all other topics of medicine. His tone was didactic and confident, well suited for a final authority.

Galen's views on cancer were similar to those of Hippocrates. Cancer was due to excess of black bile (atrabilis), and was best left alone. Cancers were classified among Tumors Contrary to Nature (Tumores Praeter Naturam), which included phlegmonic inflammations, sinuses, ulcers, fistules, gangrene and carbuncles, erysipelas and edema.

Galeni Librorum, Title page

ΓΑΛΗΝΟΥ· Α:

GALENI LIBRORVM
PARS PRIMA, QVORVM IN·
DICEM VI· PAGINA
CONTINET·

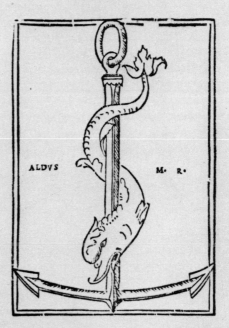

ALDVS   M· R·

Ne quis alius impune, aut Venetiis aut usquam locorum hos Galeni libros imprimat, & Clementis VII· Pont· Max· & Senatus Veneti decreto cau-
tum est·

Thomas Gale, in his 1567 treatise on surgery, summarized Galen's view on cancer in a two-sentence chapter 7:

"Of blacke cholor, without boylying (that is to say melancholic) cometh cancers, and if the humor be sharpe, it maketh ulceration, and for this cause, these tumors are more blacker in colour, then those that cometh of inflamation, and these be not hote, but the veines in these, are both more fuller, and more distended forth then those whiche be in inflamations. For lesse matter goeth out of the veines, into the fleshy partes, whiche compasseth them about, through the grosseness of the humor, whiche breadeth the Cancers, neither yet are the veines so reade as they be in inflamations, but sheweth themselves accordyng to the humor, that they be filed with."

No reliable representations of Galen exist. Five imaginary portrayals gathered by Walsh are presented. The Latin translation of Galen on tumors is from the **Opera Omnium** published in Basle in 1536.

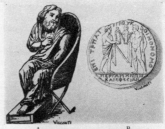

Five imaginary portraits of Galen (from Walsh, 1926)

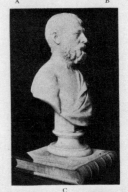

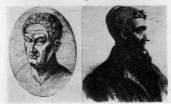

Thomas Gaille. **The Institucion of Chyrurgerie.** Chapter 7, p. 367. London: Henry Denham, 1567.

Clavdii Galeni. **Opera Omnia**, ed. C.G. Kühn, 20 vols. Hildesheim: George Olms Verlagsbuchhandlung, 1964-65. (Leipzig, 1821-33). Greek and Latin text.

Owsei Temkin. **Galenism. Rise and Decline of a Medical Philosophy.** Ithaca, N.Y.: Cornell Univ. Press, 1973.

Joseph Walsh. Galen's discovery and promulgation of the function of the recurrent laryngeal nerve. **Ann. Med. Hist.** 8: 176-184, 1926.

III. Medieval Period (500-1500 A.D.)

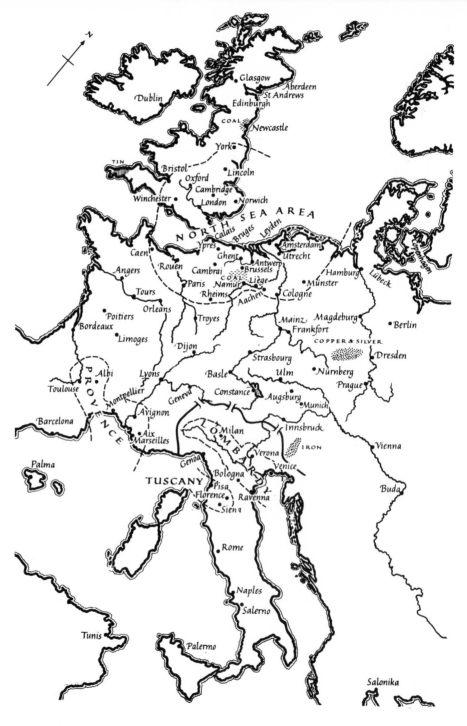

Medieval Europe, showing centers of learning. (from J.D.
Bernal, *Science in History*, ed 3, p 338. London: CA Watts &
Co. Reproduced by permission).

Rome died in 476 A.D. Constantinople became the center of European civilization for a thousand years.

There is little to indicate that the thousand years of the Byzantine Empire (395-1453 A.D.) were marked by prog-

ress in science or in medicine. Byzantine history is primarily political and religious. Its medical history is represented by industrious compilations of, and commentaries on earlier Greek teachers.

During the 7th Century, Mohammed and his followers spread the religion of Islam from the Indus to the Pyrenees. In the many contributions of Islamic culture, medicine was poorly represented. Galen and Aristotle were embraced as ultimate authorities, and religious prohibitions against dissection precluded advances in anatomy. Greek texts were translated and expanded in Arabic, from which they were translated into Latin and diffused back into western Europe.

Learning and medicine during the Dark Ages were preserved in monasteries. In retreats such as the Benedictine order at Monte Cassino, the remnants of the past were studied and laboriously copied by hand. Slowly, there developed centers of learning that were not entirely scholastic. Medical schools began around the earlier universities, perhaps first in Salerno in the 10th Century. During the next century medical schools came into existence in Bologna, Paris, Montpellier and Oxford.

In the 12th Century surgery became separated from medicine, a schism stimulated by decrees against shedding of blood by ecclesiastics. The most effective medical art of the time was thus relegated to barbers, whose duties included bleeding as well as shaving. The cautery and "laudable pus" in surgery won out over the knife and cleanliness until the 16th Century. Medicine, practiced by learned physicians in long gowns, was a concoction of astrology, herbal potions, purgation and blood-letting.

The history of oncology during this millenium is monotonously unfortunate. Cancer remained one of the tumors against nature, caused by excessive or abnormal black bile. Its treatment, limited to superficial ulcers and tumors, remained wide excision by cautery if it could be removed with its roots. Caution was expressed against surgical treatment for cancers beyond such excision. Caustic pastes, usually containing arsenic, were used for the palliative control of more extensive cancers. And this treatment was combined with phlebotomy, diet, a wide variety of herbal medicines, as well as powder of crab and other symbolic charms.

The recommendations of the physicians who wrote treatises remain available to us for review. Traveling mountebanks and secret practices that remained unrecorded also abounded. The results of treatment, and the actual practice of medicine in the population, have to be inferred. Hospitals were founded in the Middle Ages, but most practice was conducted in private homes. For patients with cancer, the intercession of a surgeon could have been important only if they had cancers of the skin, mouth or breast that could be readily excised.

There are no statistics regarding cancer for the medieval period, but cancers of most internal organs as well as external ones are mentioned. Cancer of the uterus seems to have been the most frequently encountered neoplasm. The breast is included most often in surgical treatises, since it was approachable. Cancers that were cured must have been few indeed, and most cancers that were reported as cured probably were not cancers.

III-A.

Physician of Byzantium: Aetios of Amida

Aetios of Amida was court physician to Justinian I, emperor of Byzantium from 527 to 565 A.D. He wrote an encyclopedia of medicine, the **Tetrabiblion**, in which many sections are attributed to Archigenes of Apamea and to Leonides, Greek physicians of the 1st Century.

The following sections are from Ricci's translation of the Latin edition of Cornarius, printed in 1542, and are revealing of the practices recommended for cancer of the breast and uterus.

"Chapter XLV. **Operative Treatment of Breast Cancer, According to Leonides**.

"I personally am in the habit of operating for cancer arising in the breast thusly: I make the patient lie down; then I incise the healthy part of the breast beyond the cancerous area and I cauterize the incised parts, until the loss of blood ceases by the formation of a coating. Then I again incise and excise the breast from its depth and I again cauterize the incised areas. And I repeat this procedure often, first cutting then cauterizing until bleeding stops. Thus the danger of a severe haemorrhage is avoided. Following amputation of the entire breast, I cauterize again all the areas until all bleeding has ceased. The initial cauterizations are made to staunch the blood; the last ones to destroy the remaining parts of the disease. Often I performed my task without cauterization, where there was an indurated tumor which was threatening a cancerous degeneration. In such a form of the disease, it is sufficient to amputate up to the healthy tissue, since no danger of haemorrhage threatens."

"Chapter XCIV. **Concerning Cancers of the Uterus, According to Archigenes.**

"Of the cancerous tumors of the uterus, some are ulcerated; some are not ulcerated, much in the same way as we have mentioned above about breast tumors. Thus in the non-ulcerated ones, the tumor about the cervix appears hard, resistant, irregular, prominent, of a dirty reddish to grayish color and giving rise to severe pain. The pain radiates to the groin, to the upper and lower abdomen and the sides, and these tumors are irritated by touching with the hand and by a variety of drugs. But if the ulcerated tumor is cancerous, in addition to the pain, the induration and the mass, the ulcerated areas appear corroded and irregular; and the majority of these ulcers appear dirty, whitish and elevated. And those which in truth are considered to be clean, are in reality dirty, grayish, reddish and bloody. At the same time, there oozes out a discharge from these ulcers which is thin, watery, black or yellowish and foul smelling. Sometimes there is frank bleeding. And there are other signs which have been described above and which occur with inflamation of the uterus. This is, as Hippocrates thought, an incurable disease. . . ."

James V. Ricci. **Aetios of Amida.** Philadelphia: Blakiston Co., 1950.

Aetios, *Medici Graeci Contractae*. . . Basle, 1542. Title page and page 884.

Following this are formulas for sitz baths, ointments and suppositories for alleviative treatment. The last sentence reads: "The Philosopher's remedy for cancer of the uterus: burn either three or five river crabs, an uneven number, over live coals, powder in Cyprian oil and apply to the ulcerated part with a feather."

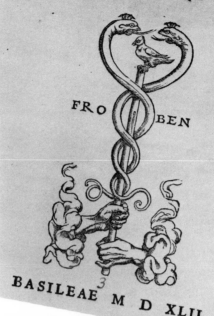

AETII MEDICI GRAECI CONTRACTAE EX VETE=RIBVS MEDICINÆ TETRABIBLOS, HOC EST QVA-ternio, id est libri uniuersales quatuor, singuli quatuor sermones complectêtes, ut sint in summa quatuor sermonum quaterniones, id est sermones XVI. per Ia-num Cornarium Medicum Physi-cum Latinè conscripti.

FRO BEN

BASILEAE M D XLII

---

884   AETII TETRABIBLI

De exedentibus mammarum ulceribus.   Cap. XLII

Phagedænicum & exedens ulcus à cancerato differt, eo quod circumsitas partes non ita duras, neque uenas uaricosas habet, neque ita ad fundum perre ptat. Sed & omnis phagedæna medicamentis cedit. Maligna uero & esferata ulcera medicamentis magis exacerbantur. Ad exedentia itaque ulcera com-pendiariam curam adhibere oportet, callosorum uidelicet labiorum excisio-nem, ita ut eadem labia ignitis cauterijs inurantur. Nam sic & sanguinis eru-ptionem coërcebimus, & tutiorem medicationem peragemus. Postea uero medicamenta ad mammarum putrefactiones commoda adhibeantur, infrà ad cancros descripta.

De cancris mammarũ. Archigenis & Leonidæ.   Cap. XLIII

Cancerati tumores circa mammas frequentissimè generantur, & mulieres magis quàm uiros inuadunt, & ex illis eas quæ amplas ac carnosas mammas habent. Veteres autem ulcus canceratũ, malignũ ac ferum appellabant, & can cerati sanè appellatio à cancro animante transumpta est: sunt enim ea animan tia aspera & dura, & si quid forcipibus suis ceperint, haud facilè auelluntur. his itaqp canceratus tumor similis est. Nam & prominet, & ad tactum renititur, & difficulter tractabilis est. Maleficum autem & ferum ulcus à feris ac malignis animalibus cognominatur. Est enim proteruum, & curatione esferatur, & manuum tractatione exacerbatur. Duæ uero sunt supremæ cancrorum diffe-rentiæ. Quidam enim sine ulcere, quidam cum ulcere consistunt. Qui sine ul cere sunt ab omnibus fermè ueteribus Occulti appellantur. Philoxenus tamen cancrum occultũ priuatim nominauit, qui in utero ac intestinis esset. Cancro itaqp non ulcerato in mamma existente, tumor apparet ingens, ad tactum reni tens inæqualis, instar feræ sæuus, penitissimè pertinaciter insertus, radices lon gè latéqp extendens, & uenis circumsitus uelut illigatus, quas circum circa ua ricosas habet, colore cinericius ad ruborê uergens, & aliquando subliuidus, & uidentibus quidem mollis apparet, tangentibus autem durissimus est, ut uisui hac parte non sit credendum: dolorem autem inducit pungentem latè se exten dentem, ut sæpe per consensum, glandularũ malignas inflammationes sub alis excitet. Pertingunt etiam dolores usqp ad clauiculam & scapulas. At uero exul ceratus cancer assiduè erodit, & ad profundum perfodit, nec sisti potest, & sa niem emittit omni ferarum ueneno deteriorem, copia & odore abominabi-lem. Adsunt & huic dolores pungentes. Atque hic præcipuè medicamentis ac manuum tractatione exacerbatur.

Qui cancri curatu faciles, & qui difficiles.   Cap. XLIIII

Cancros in pectore obortos omnino deploratos esse scito, quemadmodũ & eos qui in capite, collo, humeris, sub alis, & in inguinib. generantur: sunt enim & hi incurabiles. Nam præterquã quod perfectè tolli non possunt, sanguinis eruptionis timor incumbit, ne ex ea æger inter manus pereat, Eos uero qui pa pillæ summitatem occupant, affectæ partis amputatione facilè curaueris.

Cancri chirurgia. Leonidæ.   Cap. XLV

Ego quidem in cancris in pectore obortis chirurgia uti soleo, quæ sic fit. Ae gram supinam decumbere facio. Deinde supra cancrum partem mammæ sa nam incido, & incisam cauterijs inuro, donec crusta inducta sanguinis eruptio sistatur. Mox iterum incido & profundũ mammæ disseco, ac rursus partes inci sas uro, sæpéqp idem repeto, & secans, & sistendi sanguinis gratia inurens. Ita enim sanguinis eruptionis periculum euitatur: post amputatione uero integrè pera

III-B.

Byzantine synthesis: Paul of Aegina

Paul of Aegina lived during the 7th Century and practiced in Alexandria. He is representative of the Greek Byzantine physicians during the decline of the western Roman empire, among whom can also be listed Oribasius (325-403) and Alexander of Tralles (525-605).

Paul's Seven Books, translated by Francis Adams in 1844, are an attempt to reduce medical teaching to a compendium similar to the legal synopses of the lawyers. "On this account," he wrote, "I have compiled this brief collection from the works of the ancients, and have set down a little of my own, except a few things which I have seen and tried in the practice of the art."

In Book VI, on Surgery, Cancer is dealt with in Section 45, as follows:

"Cancer is an uneven swelling, rough, unseemly, darkish, painful, and sometimes without ulceration (which Hippocrates called also concealed cancer), and if operated upon, it becomes worse, and sometimes with ulceration, for it derives its origin from black bile, and spreads by erosion; forming in most parts of the body, but more especially in the female uterus and breasts. It has the veins stretched on all sides as the animal the crab (cancer) has its feet, whence it derives its name. Since putrid parts and such as are simply altered from their natural state require amputation, cancers in the womb, indeed, it is neither possible nor expedient to operate upon; but of those of the external parts, and espe-cially of the breasts, we have now to ex-plain the surgical treatment. Some, then, have consumed the whole redundant matter by cauteries; but others first make an excision of the whole breast, and then burn the place. But Galen approves only of the excision, writing thus of the opera-tion: 'If ever you attempt to cure cancer by an operation, begin your evacuations by purging the melancholic humour, and having cut away the whole affected part, so that not a root of it be left, permit the blood to be discharged, and do not speedily restrain it, but squeeze the sur-rounding veins so as to force out the thick part of the blood, and then cure the wound like other ulcers.' "

There follows commentary on Hippoc-rates and some 8 other authorities. In Book IV, Section 26, are given directions for incipient cancer that suggest some doubt: "It may be possible to prevent in-cipient cancer from increasing, by evacuation of the melancholic humour before it becomes fixed in that part" by venesection and purgation. Then are in-dicated constituents of soothing and es-charotic pastes, and, finally, "From Ar-chigenes, for carcinomatous and malig-nant ulcers. Levigate equal parts of burnt river crabs and calamine, and sprinkle or apply the ashes of crabs with cerate; or apply the seed of hedge mustard tritu-rated with honey."

The Seven Books of Paulus Aegineta. Translated from the Greek with a Commentary by Francis Adams. 3 vol. London: Sydenham Society, 1844-47.

Constantinople, 1493 (from Historic Urban Plans, Ithaca, New York)

Imaginary portrait of Paul of Aegina (from I. Sambucus, *Icones Veterum*... Antwerp 1574)

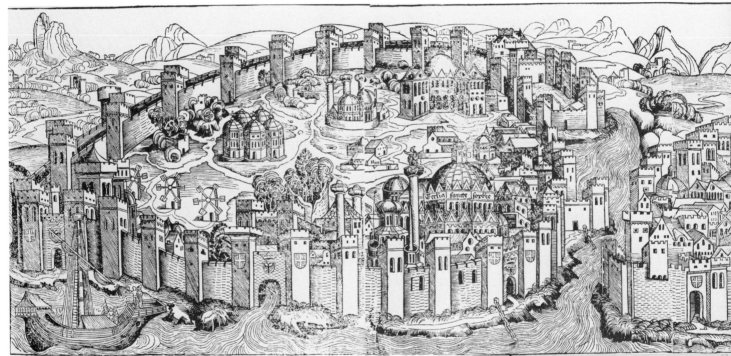

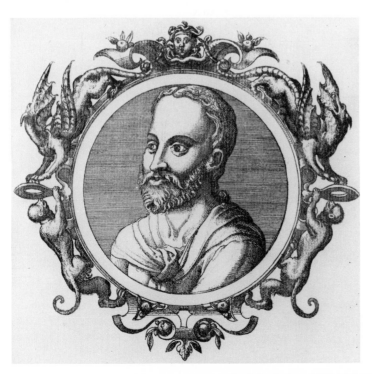

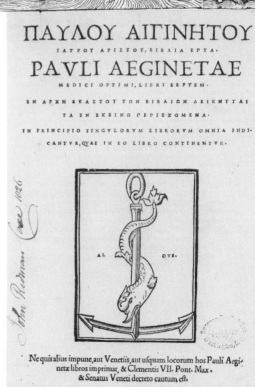

ΠΑΥΛΟΥ ΑΙΓΙΝΗΤΟΥ
ΙΑΤΡΟΥ ΑΡΙΣΤΟΥ, ΒΙΒΛΙΑ ΕΠΤΑ.
PAVLI AEGINETAE
MEDICI OPTIMI, LIBRI SEPTEM.
ΕΝ ΑΡΧΗ ΕΚΑΣΤΟΥ ΤΩΝ ΒΙΒΛΙΩΝ ΔΕΙΚΝΥΤΑΙ
ΤΑ ΕΝ ΕΚΕΙΝΩ ΠΕΡΙΕΧΟΜΕΝΑ.
IN PRINCIPIO SINGVLORVM LIBRORVM OMNIA INDI-
CANTVR, QVAE IN EO LIBRO CONTINENTVR.

Ne quis alius impune, aut Venetiis, aut usquam locorum hos Pauli Aegi-
netæ libros imprimat, & Clementis VII. Pont. Max.
& Senatus Veneti decreto cautum est.

Pauli Aeginetae, 1528, Title page.

III-C.

Prince of Arabic physicians: Avicenna

Islamic medicine was essentially a re-statement of Galen as transmitted from Alexandria and Constantinople. Arab physicians were prohibited from human dissection, and preferred the cautery to the knife in surgery.

The most influential Islamic writer was Ibn Sina or Avicenna (980-1037), who lived a life of opulence in Bagdad and wrote profusely and beautifully on medicine.

Avicenna's **Canon of Medicine** was "a statement of authoritative, scholastic dogmatism" that was founded on the humoral theory. Thus, cancer was due to black bile:

"**The difference between cancerous swelling and induration.** The latter is a slumbering silent mass which destroys the sensation (so that the part is numb), and is painless, and stationary. It may produce weakness of the part. A cancerous swelling progressively increases in size, is destructive, and spreads roots which insinuate themselves amongst the tissue-elements. It does not necessarily destroy sensation unless it has existed for a long time, and then it kills the tissues and destroys the sensation in the part. It would seem that indurations and cancerous swellings differ less as to substance than in the inseparable accidental qualities.

"The hard swellings arising from at-rabilious humours are usually hard from the outset. They are often autumnal. They often become 'indurations,' especially if there be sanguinous humour present.—The same sort of change may take place in the swellings arising out of serous humour."

O. Cameran Gruner. **A Treatise on the Canon of Medicine of Avicenna.** London: Luzac and Co., 1930.
David Riesman. **The Story of Medicine in the Middle Ages.** New York: Paul B. Hoeber, 1935. (p. 52-54.)

كتب القانون في الطب

لابو علي الشيخ الرئيس

ابن سينا

مع بعض تاليفه وهو علم المنطق وعلم الطبيعي

وعلم الكلام

ROMAE,
In Typographia Medicea.
M.D.XCIII.
Cum licentia Superiorum.

Avicenna, 1593, Title page.

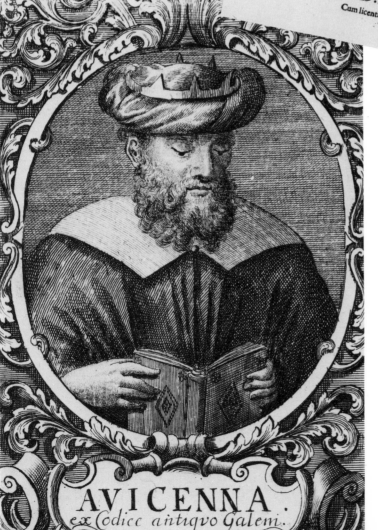

AVICENNA.
ex Codice antiquo Galeni

Imaginary portrait of Avicenna,
from the Renaissance Period

V-D.

Physicians of Cordova: Albucasis and Avenzoar

Abul Qasim (1013-1106 A.D.), known as Abulcasim or Albucasis, was one of the Islamic physicians of the western lands conquered by the Arabs. He practiced in Cordova, and wrote a book on surgery and surgical instruments.

The teachings reflect Greek writers and contribute little evidence of practical or theoretical progress. He did add passages indicating personal experiences.

Chapters 50 and 53 have the following to say about cancer:

"When the cancer is in its initial stage and you wish to arrest it, burn all around the circumference of the cancer with the circular cautery. Some doctors have said that it may be cauterized with one extensive cauterization in the middle. This hardly seems right to me, for I should expect it to ulcerate out; which I have several times seen. So it is correct to burn around the circumference with a circular cautery as we have said, or with multiple cauterizations."

"The Ancients said that when a cancer is in a site where total eradication is possible, such as a cancer of the breast or of the thigh, and in similar parts where complete removal is possible, and especially when in the early stage and small, then surgery was to be tried. But when it is of long standing and large you should leave it alone. For I myself have never been able to cure any such, nor have I seen anyone else succeed before me. The procedure in a case amenable to treatment, as we have said, is first for him to be purged several times from black bile; then bleed him if his veins seem full. Then put the patient in the most convenient position for operating. Then attach to the tumour hooks suited to it; then make a circular incision all round to include the skin with the utmost thoroughness so that not the least root of it remains; let the blood flow and do not stanch it quickly; but put pressure upon the place and squeeze out all the thick blood, either by hand or with any instrument you can. If in operating you get a very severe haemorrhage from cutting an artery or vein, cauterize the vessel until the bleeding stops; then dress in the usual way until healed."

Another Cordovan physician, Abu-Marwan' Abd-al Malik ibn Zuler or Avenzoar (1070-1162) described the clinical signs and symptoms of cancer of the stomach and of the esophagus. Avenzoar used esophageal sounds made of silver or tin in the diagnosis and treatment of cancer of the esophagus.

M. S. Spink and G. L. Lewis. **Abulcasis on Surgery and Instruments.** Berkeley: Univ. of California Press, 1973.
David Riesman. **The Story of Medicine in the Middle Ages.** New York: Paul B. Hoeber, 1935. (p. 59-60.)

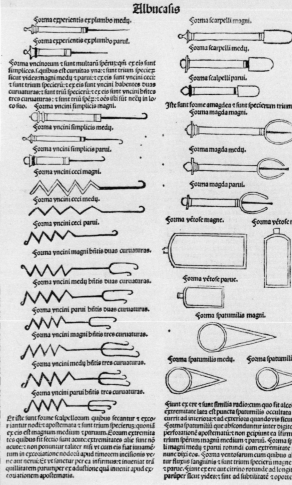

Forma experientis ex plumbo medy.

Forma experientis ex plumbo parui.

Forma vncinorum ⁊ sunt multaru sperus:qn ex eis sunt simplices.f.quibus est curuitas vna:⁊ sunt trium specie: sicut vides:magni medy ⁊ parui:⁊ ex eis sunt vncini ceci: ⁊ sunt trium specieru:⁊ ex eis sunt vncini habentes duas curuaturas:⁊ sunt triu specieru:⁊ ex eis sunt vncini brites tres curuaturas:⁊ sunt triu spe:⁊ oes isti sut necg in lo= co suo.

Forma vncini simplicis magni.

Forma vncini simplicis medy.

Forma vncini simplicis parui.

Forma vncini ceci magni.

Forma vncini ceci medy.

Forma vncini ceci parui.

Forma vncini magni britis duas curuaturas.

Forma vncini medy britis duas curuaturas.

Forma vncini parui britis duas curuaturas.

Forma vncini magni britis tres curuaturas.

Forma vncini medy britis tres curuaturas.

Forma vncini parui britis tres curuaturas.

Et iste sunt forme scalpellozum quibus secantur ⁊ exco= riantur nodi:apostemata ⁊ sunt trium specierum:quonia ex eis est magnum medium ⁊ paruum.Eozum extremita= tes quibus fit sectio sunt acute:extremitates alie sunt nõ acute:⁊ non ponuntur taliter nisi vt cum eis fiat inuame= tum in excoriatione nodozu apud timozem incisionis ve= ne aut nerui:Et vt sanetur per ea infirmus:⁊ inueniat tra quillizatem parumper ex adustione quam inuenit apud ex= coriationem apostematis.

Forma scarpelli magni.

Forma scarpelli medy.

Forma scalpelli parui.

Iste sunt forme amagdea ⁊ sunt specierum trium.

Forma magda magni.

Forma magda medy.

Forma magda parui.

Forma ventose magne.

Forma ventose medie.

Forma ventose paruc.

Forma spatumilis magni.

Forma spatumilis medy. Forma spatumilis parui.

Fiunt ex ere ⁊ sunt similia radio:cum quo sit alcobol:⁊ in extremitate lata est puncta spatumilis occultata:⁊ in ea currit ad interioza:⁊ ad exteriora quandovis sicut vides. Forma spatumilii que absconduntur inter digitos apud perfozatione apostematu:⁊ non gcipiunt ea ifirmi:⁊ sunt trium sperum magnu medium ⁊ parui.Forma spatumi= li magni medy ⁊ parui rotundi cum extremitate puncte nunc dixi eos.Forma ventosarum cum quibus abscindi= tur fluxus sanguinis ⁊ sunt trium specieru magne medie ⁊ paruc.fiant ex ere aut citrino rotunde ad longitudines parúper sicut vides:⁊ sunt ad subtilitate ⁊ opoztet yt sint

Primus

etiã dicta raucedo ex apostemate facto i neruo retrogra= do.Et cura ei° est cura pdicta:subtiliãdo regime.Et si su= perius noiaui olea piura ⁊ diuersa:⁊ in vnu collecta buic egritudini conferentia nõ credas me fecisse illud abscg premisione ⁊ cautela:qn oes medicine que operant itrin secus vel extrisecus si fuerit plures vnius gplonis ⁊ vni= nãe:⁊ in vno gradu sil´mixte:regiunt maiozis vtutis ⁊ ef ficacie in oib° egritudinib°:quã si dederis vnã solã illius gplonis ⁊ nãe:⁊ illi° gradus in vno eodé podere.vbi gra: qn si recipies medicinã vnã simplicé ⁊ sit calida vel fri gida:sicca vel bu.in pn° scõi gradus.⁊ decoposita sùperi in eadé quãtitate q in illo codé gradu fuerit gplonata.i uenies gposità longe maiozis efficacie gg simplicé in tan tus g.⁊.⁊. vna de composita plus operatur gg.⁊.l. de sim plici:⁊ hoc nõ recipit solu in vtutib° pmis.veru etiã in se cundis ⁊ tertus.certissime istud idem inuenitur.⁊ gguis causa bõ sit manifesta:tñ ipsas ad psens obimitto i tedes breuitate seruare:sicut in pncipio buius libzi pmisi.ni= bilomin° lj ⁊ alia in sequetib° vtilia ero rememozat° deo cõcedéte:⁊ ia supius memozaui gg opilatio fieri põt i ner uo retrogrado:sicut in alys neruis fieri cõsueuit.⁊ qua raucedo ozit ⁊ gñat.Et etiã in duob° neruis opticis g= bus lux oculis delegat fit opilatio:⁊ in tãtu gg qn claudi= tur oculus:vn° nullaten° pupilla alterius dilatã.Et qn sic est:medici sút despati de cura bui° egritudinis:hoc ia declaratú est i tractatu oculoz.Sed de hoc gg medici di= cunt gg cura aliqua nõ pdest in illo casu nullaten° suz cu eis:nec eis assentio vllo mõ.Et sicut dico de ista opilatio= ne:ita dico de opilatiõe facta in neruo retrogrado gg cura nõ est ipolis oino:imo medicine p certo se debét valere ⁊ eos iuuare si debite exhibeant.Quare iniungere debes locú cu pdictis oleis simul mixtis:non omittédo purga= tione vlcm toti° cozpis.⁊ et particularé capitis:sciédo gg ma egritudinis nõ trahit a capite nisi medicine ⁊ virtus ipsaru illuc deferant.vñ ofulo vt alie a dictis medicinis ppareñt g deferat vtutes ipsaru ipsi capiti velociter ppi nando eas distéperatas cu aqua mellis.⁊ bácviã ⁊ doctri nã adiuuit pr meus:⁊ fuit valde bona.⁊ postgg ipe obyt ego posui aliu núciú delatozé medicinaru ad caput:gguis de hoc cu eo minime fuisse locutus.Et non diffidas oino quãdo beneficiu ⁊ iuuamé istaruz medicinaruz nõ appa= ruerit velociter ⁊ subito:quonia aliquãdo excitado ipfas nõ tñ signu aliquod beneficy ⁊ iuuaminis apparebit:sed interdum liberabitur subito deo dante.

¶ La.XVI.Qd est de pustulis i meri seu in ysofago.

Ozium pustule in meri ex comestiõe reru acutaru:sicut est sinapis ⁊ silia.vel ex assum ptiõe medicinaru foztiu ⁊ acutaru g recipiu tur a medicis ad occidédu sanguisugas exi= stétes in gula.Et fiut bac de causa ibidé pu= stule rubee paruc ⁊ minute.Et cura b°est succus reglitie cu mucillagie seiuz cittoniog cu ag rosacea dissolutoz: retét° in oze ⁊ paulatine suggédo ⁊ lãbédo deglutire.

¶ La.XVII.Qd é de corruptiõe ⁊ putrefactiõe in gula ⁊ meri:⁊ eoz ptib° adiacétib° in tpe epidimie.

Rit ét in istis mébzis ⁊ in suis partib° adia= centibus putrefactio tpe magne epidimie ⁊ pessime moztalitl:sic in alys mébzis fieri gsueuit.gre ptes gule cozrupunt.Et hoc nõ accidit nisi qn est epidimia pestifera pessima ⁊ maligna.⁊ nõ est miru:qn aliqn in tali tpe cozrupunt nerui pedu qui sunt mébza solida ⁊ cadunt.Et qn tracta bo de epidimia:⁊ de egritudinib° que fiút in ipsa:⁊ de su is accidétib° túc cura oium ponã cu adiutorio dei.

¶ Cap.XVIII.Quod est de priuatione sensus ⁊ motus ⁊ relaxatione meri i ysofago.

A Lcidit ét aliqn in neruo deglutiédi spes relaxatio sus ⁊ mot°.⁊ põt etiã hoc in ipso neruo a quo dict° entiã ⁊ vtuté sensus ⁊ mo re põt ppter frigiditaté gplonis sue. dictã lesioné.Et hoc ei cõtingere põt. coticaru medicinaru:aut ex potatiõe gna gstitate:⁊ spãliter illis g nõ sut as test aliqñ hec egritudo subito euenire efficit.Et qñ fit ex potatiõe aque mul bito.Et qñ cõtinue ⁊ paulatine vsus l successiue ⁊ paulatine hs egritudo es pit cu dolore leui:⁊ cu difficultate deg tine ⁊ successiue augmentat donec de onem deglutiédi perfectã.Et hoc acci pessimú valde.qñ infirmus nõ põt v medicinas deglutire.quare opoztet cu ne pperare ad eius sanitaté recuperãda:aut in breui mo rietur.Et quãdo ad hoc deuenit:curatur plurib°modis. primus modus est vt apponas cánulas argenti vel stan ni in gulam.Et sit cánula habens caput gd ponitur intus in oze strictum:⁊ illud gd remanct in manu a parte exte= riozi sit latú valde.Et scias qn appones cánulá in gulam: monebit stõachus ad subuersioné ⁊ vomitú náliter.gre eaz túc subtrahere debes:⁊ stare donec cesset vomitus.⁊ iterú cã int° ponere:⁊ cu subuersio ⁊ vomitus vel motus supueniet subtrahere.⁊ sic facies donec ex psuetudine re= moueat subuersio ⁊ mot°.⁊ g sit absg abbominatõe in= firmus ex appositione ipsi°cánule.Et túc sicut dictuz est pone latus strictú itus in gula:tenédo latus amplú i ma= nu:⁊ ide lac piice recéter mulctú:aut pultes ex farina tri tici.tñ ex aliquo istoz gg ide possit infirm° nutriri.stude= do semp in remouédo cãm egritudis cu gb° tibi videbit cõuenire.cognoscédo gg tali cura segtur nõ modicum nocumétú.f.gg inde debilitant vtutes mébzoz gule oes. Secúdus modus curatiõis bui° egritudis é ponere ifir= mu nudú i tina lactis:gd sit tepidú ⁊ recéter mulctú:aut in tina plena ex pultib°farine tritici g sint ligde cocti.qñ opinio quozúdã medicoz é vt illud nutrimétú igrediat per ptes inferiozes cozpozis.⁊ ét p pozos toti°cozpis ipi. sed hec opinio debilissima valde existit atg friuola.Ter= tius gdé modus est.⁊ est rectus cert°:atg verax.f.gg tali modo nutriri ifirmum absg dubio.⁊ est talis.f.vt recipias lac vel pultes ex farina tritici liquide decoctas:in vesica vna capre:vel ei° simili.⁊ sit in collo ipsius ligata vna cã= nula argéti ad modú clisteris:⁊ facta mundificatiõe inte= stino pfecta cu clisteribus abstersiuis ⁊ mundificatiuis. pone dictã cánulá intus in ano:⁊ exprime dictã vesicam diligéter cu manu:donec totú lac vel pultes in intestino recto ab ifirmo recipiat:⁊ sic ide dictú itestinú sugendo recipit nutrimétú.⁊ ab ipso aliud itestinú sibi gtiguu ra= piédo sugit:⁊ ab illo aliud donec sic successiue ad funduz stomaci dictú nutrimétú bz deuenire.ide stomacus reci= pit gd sibi gueniere ⁊ ab eo nutrit.Et iam gdã repiunt medici g nitunt pbare gg nutrimétú nullaten° recipi põt p clistere i itestinis vt ad stõm possit deuenire.⁊ hec per dicta.H.g dicit gg clistere iniectú p inferioza in itestinis nõ põt vllo mõ ad stõm pringere ⁊ ueriuare.Et sic argue do affirmant gg nec nutrimentú inde iniectú vllo modo ad stomachú poterit peruenire.sed isti tales decipiunt ⁊ errãt cõparãdo ⁊ egparãdo medicamia iniecta p clistere nutriméto predicto iniecto fm modú determinatú:qñ certú est gg violétia ⁊ ipulsio gg é in clisteri nõ é táta neg ita foztis:gg possit medicamina iniecta p ipm vsg ad stõ= machú pyicere ⁊ delegare:eo gg virt° attractiua itestioz

Surgical instruments, by Albucasis
(from Cyrurgia, 1500)

Avenzoar's description of esophageal
and gastric cancer.
(*Liber theiser*... Venetis, 1496).

III-E.

School of Salerno: Theodoric and Rolando

Rolandi

lidatu3 vulnus extrinfecus eu3 futura τ alijs curetur vt
dictum est superius. ℂ Oe si vulnus fuerit magnu3 hoc
super addimus :vt petia fatis longa in vulnere mittaτ:
in longu3 ab vna extremitate ad alia3 existens:τ supra
ipfam petia3 vulneris interio2 pars caute suatur:τ puluis rubens, superponatur . petia vo que remansit interius omni die versus pendente3 partem trahatur vt pá-
nus in vulnere quottidie renouetur . Cu3 aute3 vulnus
videris confolidatu3:petia3 totam abftrahas:τ in extre-
mitatibus nondu3 confolidatis vt in alijs vulncrib9 cura adhibeas.dieta quoq3 fit multü tenuis τ digeftibilis.

ℂ De cancris τ fiftulis τ apoftematib9 in his locis nafcen-
tibus,f.inteftino2 τ ventris. CAP. XXVII.

D E cancris τ fiftulis τ apoftemati-
bus in his locis nafcé-
tibus ide3 dicimus; qó superius:q2 cü i carno
fis locis sint incifiones τ vnguenta violenta
τ incenfiones facere poffumus.hoc aüt super
addimus; q9 si fistula ventrem penetrauerit : nec pulue-
rem nec vnguenta immittere debem9; ne ledere poffint
interio2a. Sed si meatus fuerit ftrictus cum tenta mali
terre elargetur:τ supra difcus se inclinet:vt putredo que
interius est poffit exire.poftea immittatur fiuellü in vn-
guentum de vnguento ruptozio τ caute intromittatur:
τ deinde cura vt dictü est fupis.   ℂ Itë de cancro.

Cancer est apoftema melancolicum ex melanco-
lia adufta a materia colerica:ficut di-
cit Auicenna:τ quandoq3 accidit i incipiendo ; quándoq3
poft apoftemata calida cu3 indurantur τ in principio fi
fuccurratur ei:quandoq3 ftat τ fanatur:τ figna eius funt
q9 incipit apoftema fimile auellane τ minus:deinde pau
latim augmentatur cum duritie vehementi τ tenebzofi
tate colozis ; τ rotunditate figure:τ aliq3tulo caliditatis
in tactu; τ quádo incipit magnificari apparét in eo vene
virides:τ habet radices penetrantes in cozpoze.Et cura
eius est sicut dicit Auicéna cura dicta in capitulo de le-
p2a ex flobotomia τ affiduatione eo2 que educunt me-
lancolia3;τ permutatione3 fanguinis totius cozpozis cü
fanguine nouo fubtili:aquofo:temperato:per cibos hu-
mectantes laudabilis humozis τ boni. Et cancer nafciτ
in qualibet parte cozpozis:sed pzecipue in mámillis mu
lieru3;que non purgantur naturaliter: τ tempoze folito
menftrui3;na3 omnes mulieres:que tépoze folito τ con-
gruo ex moze purganτ:fane funt:τ raro huiufmodi egri
tudines illis contingunt . Heneraliter autë sicut dictum
est:cancer ex melácolico humoze nafcitur; q2 ex nigra fe
ce fanguinis τ fpiffa sicut dicit Auicéna.S.admixto felle
ruffo.hoc cü abundauerit τ excreuerit:miro modo vitia
in cozpoze generanτ:nó solum cartimáta vex τ varices.
τ elephantias.aliquotiens etiam hic talis humoz p emo
roydas purgatur:q2 fplen non poteft triñ qtu3 mozis et
ad se pertrahere atq3 confumere:τ infunditur in venis τ
in cute totius cozpozis:τ maxime in extremitatib9 ficut
in vultu.manibus.τ pedibus:τ diciτ elephantia. aliquo-
tiens etia3 in quibufda3 partibus cozpozis eiufdem na-
fcitur:ficut in mámillis:in quibufda3 occultis: vt in ma
trice:τ dicitur cancer. videntur etiá vene loco2:vbi con-
federit hic talis humoz: plene atq3 tenfe fanguine co2ru-
pto nigro τ fpiffo ; q3to nigrioz τ fpiffioz fuerit:tanto pe-
ioz τ periculofioz credendus est τ grauioz τ infanabilioz
caufa si cü cancro pedis ac si vene tenfe ex vtraq3 parte
cernuntur:quá quidem caufam ait.S.Scias a nobis in

principio mox incipiëntur medicamine nullo vnq3 fine
fanari.Quippe si excreuerit:τ totam mámillam occupa-
uerit:dubium est de mozte:q2 emozofagia verenda est:τ
flegmon:ex quo folen ...
nus fozdidant τ peri ...
medicos:Non aucto ...
bium quippe si incid ...
quo febzes folent ac ...
τ periculum moztis ...
si hec oía nó ante pz ...
mox in principio pu ...
melancolicü purgat ...
donec caufa penitus ...
tozia:ad hoc vltima ...
bil obftet vel pzohib ...
tomia de bzachio vt ...
purgabit. τ si mulier ...
hementer pzonocab ...
patitur:minime hoc ...
fuerit:fucco ftringi ...
di mozbis cögruit. ...
cum ipm mifceas m ...
gos: qó dictus est in ...
téperabis:τ in linte ...
cancrum si iam vul ...
caminibus:τ magis ...
Maxime his cönen ...
in aqua de olerib9 ...
fuo cucurbite cocte. ...
xatiles.de volatilib ...
ouo2 fozbiliü τ fimi ...
vaccinum:ftatim ex ...
folutionem ventris ...
libet vice quattuo2 ...
si fuerit fo2tis:detur ...

ℂ Et hoc cap ...
ℂ De cancro mámille ...

D E ca ...
q2 si tota ...
q2 incura ...
euellatur ...
fit dura:τ in alijs loc ...
uere affodillo2 τ vn ...
vt dixim9:vel fiat pu ...
terficit τ deficcat:qu ...
tramentum.falgéma ...
ftercus humanum c ...
fanguinis dzaconis. ...
cancrum fluuialé vf ...
ficcam.piper nigrum ...
tru3.puluerem fole ...
pzimo abluatur cu3 ...
tur puluis abundan ...

ℂ De duritie mámille ...

M Amm ...
attrahit ad ... fanguin ...
conuertitur in lac:q3 cum in partu m ...
tur:remanens ibi membzum indura ...
doloz magnus fit:cui sic fubueniu ...
ratia apponantur:vt malua.bzanca vzfina:τ al ...

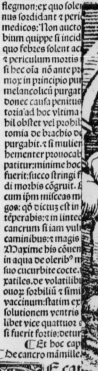
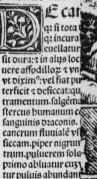

Interior scene at the School of Salerno. (from *De Conservanda bona valetudina*, Frankfurt, 1553).

Description of cancer according to Rolando Capelluti of Parma (c 1230) (from *Libellus de Cyrurgia editus suie compilatus a Magistro Rolando feliciter incipit*. Venice, 1498).

The School at Salerno, in legend founded in the 10th Century by a Greek, a Latin, a Jew and a Saracen, was one of the earliest revivals of medical learning in western Europe.

The Schools at Salerno and, later, at Bologna were notable for the use of sleeping draughts for anesthesia, and for a number of sturdy physicians who contradicted the dogmas of laudable pus and healing of wounds by second intention. The soporific sponge dates to the Alexandrian school, and contained a herbal mixture including opium.

The advocates of dry, clean wound treatment included Ugo Borgognoni (1160-1257), known as Hugo of Lucca, and his son, Teodorico Borgognoni (1205-1296), known as Theodoric.

The Surgery of Theodoric includes consideration of cancer in 3 chapters of Book III. He divides cancer into those "arising from a hot abscess or wound" and "the melancholic abscess." The first is a wide round ulcer of shell-like hardness, "proceeding from external causes, i.e., a wound, or an ulcer improperly treated." "Nolimetangere," "Lupus" and "Cancer" are included under this type of cancer. The second type of cancer is produced in any part of the body, but especially in the breasts of women. "The

signs of this are that a hot abscess begins at the size of a hazel nut or smaller, and then increases in size little by little, with notable hardness, darkness of coloring, round shape, and some warmth to the touch. When it begins to grow larger, green veins appear in it, and it has roots penetrating into the body."

As to treatment, Theodoric wrote in Chapter 6:

"The older a cancer is, the worse it is. And the more it is involved with muscles, veins and nutrifying arteries, the worse it is, and the more difficult to treat. For in such places incisions, cauteries and sharp medications are to be feared.

"But if the cancer should be in fleshy places where one need not fear for veins and muscles, incise it as far as the sound flesh and burn it away afterwards, to treat it just as was said in the case of fistulas.

"Or employ the treatment which we ourselves always use, and have proved times without number: Mortify the cancer with arsenic sublimate according to our teaching, for it kills fistula, cancer, herpes estiomenus (or lupus), 'nolimetangere' (or formix), and all similar affections, on the first day. Thereafter see to it that dead flesh is sloughed off, and then treat as has been stated."

Rolando Capelluti of Parma was another member of the Salerno school; a page of his work is pictured.

The Surgery of Theodoric (ca A.D. 1267). Translated from the Latin by Eldridge Campbell. New York: Appleton-Century-Crofts, Inc., 1955.

Libellus de Cyrurgia editus sine compilatus a Magistro Rolando feliciter incipit. Venice, 1498.

III-F.

The School of Montpellier: Mondeville and Chauliac

Henri de Mondeville (c. 1260-1320) and Guy de Chauliac (c. 1300-1370) represent contrasts in surgery of the 13th and 14th Centuries. By then, medical schools of Italy had important counterparts in Montpellier, Paris and Oxford. Henri de Mondeville, surgeon to King Philip the Fair, espoused dry, clean wound management and held that suppuration was not a stage in healing but a complication. His unfinished manuscript remained buried in libraries until 1892-93, when it was printed in Berlin by Pagel and in Paris by Nicaise.

Nicaise analyzed Mondeville's treatise on diseases ("apostemes") in light of his humoral physiology. Scirrhus and cancer were now expressions of combinations of normal and abnormal humors, a far cry from the original simplicity of the humors.

Guy de Chauliac was a papal physician at the court in Avignon, where he remained during successive epidemics of plague. His **La Grande Chirurgie**, written some fifty years after Mondeville, remained important for over 2 centuries.

It is divided into three sections, on anatomy, on description of diseases, and on instruments. Chauliac held that although Nature was the chief healer of wounds, the physician had to assist by a wide variety of salves and plasters. Thus he promoted coction and suppuration, and rejected the dry management of wounds espoused by Theodoric and Henri de Mondeville.

Chauliac's recommendations in regard to cancer followed those of his predecessors. If the growth seemed operable, a wide excision to remove all the rest of the disease was indicated. Along with the surgical approach, a dietary regime, purgation and bleeding were part of the program. With more extensive involvement, recourse was taken to a caustic paste.

Chauliac's work appeared in a printed edition in 1478, and went through seventy editions, translations into 7 languages and abridgements. It is representative of the state of the art of surgery and oncology until Paré.

Henri de Mondeville (from E. Nicaise, 1893)

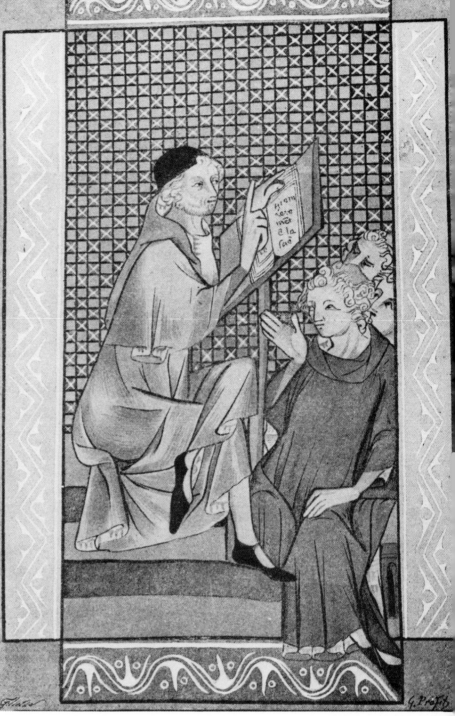

Guy de Chauliac

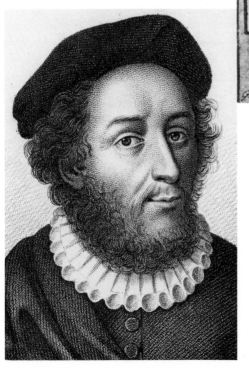

J. F. Pagel. **Leben, Lehre and Leistungen des Heinrich von Mondeville.** Berlin: A. Hirschwald, 1892.

E. Nicaise. **La Grande Chirurgie de Guy de Chauliac.** Paris: Felix Alcan, 1890.

E. Nicaise. **La Chirurgie de Maître Henri de Mondeville.** Paris: Bailliere, 1893.

Clement C. Clarke. Henri de Mondeville. **Yale J. Biol. & Med.** 3: 459-81, 1930-31.

III-G.

English surgery: John of Arderne

John of Arderne (c. 1307-1390) was the first great surgeon of England. He is noted for the revival of successful corrective surgery for ischiorectal abscess and fistula, occupational hazards for knights on horseback.

John is presumed to have been a Saxon who studied at Montpellier and acquired wide surgical experience during the Hundred Years War. He was a Master of Surgery, surgeons of the long robe that distinguished them from the barber surgeons of the short robe, but still below the rank of Doctor of Physic. He finally settled in London, but his first writing of 1349 was prepared while practicing in Newark. His works were written in Latin, and copied and translated into English by scribes. Over 60 manuscripts are still preserved in libraries, and were widely read for some 200 years. The presentation of the work is through personal experience, with details of the patients.

John clearly described carcinoma of the rectum, as indicated by a contemporary English version:

"Of Bubo [Cancer] Within the Rectum and the Impossibility or Great Difficulty of the Cure of It.

"Bubo is an apostem breeding within the anus in the rectum with great hardness but little aching. This I say, before it ulcerates, is nothing else than a hidden cancer, that may not in the beginning of it be known by the sight of the eye, for it is all hidden within the rectum.

"To that also will leeches [physician-surgeon] assure the patient, that he has dysentery, that is, the bloody flux, when truly it is not. Dysentery is always with flux of the intestines, but out of bubo [cancer] goes hard excretions and sometime they may not pass, because of the constriction caused by the bubo, and they are retained firmly within the rectum, so that they may be felt with the finger and drawn out.

"I never saw nor heard of any man that was cured of the bubo of the rectum but I have known many that died of the foresaid sickness."

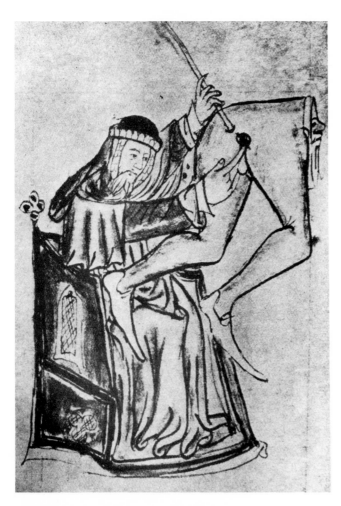

John of Arderne probing an ischiorectal fistula.

De Arte Phisicali et de Cirurgia of Master John Arderne, Surgeon of Newark, dated 1414. Translated by Sir D'Arcy Power. London: John Bale, Sons and Danielsson, Ltd., 1922.

T. McW. Millar. John of Arderne, the father of British proctology. **Proc. Roy. Soc. Med.** 47: 75-84, 1954.

IV. 16th Century: Renaissance and Reformation

The transition from the medieval to the modern period of western European history can be dated at around 1500 A.D.

A number of important antecedent developments are considered to have been important in the history that unfolded in Europe during the 16th Century. The Black Death, between 1347 and 1353 eliminated a quarter of the population, and recurred into the 16th century, with deep consequences on all aspects of life. Constantinople fell to the Turks in 1453, accelerating the mingling that started during the Crusades of Byzantine and eastern cultures with western Europe. Portugal and Spain initiated oceanic explorations, culminating in the discovery of America in 1492. The introduction of that most subversive agent against authority, the printed page, was represented by Gutenberg's Bible of 1454.

The first printed edition of Celsus appeared in Florence in 1478, and of Avicenna a year later. But these were glances backward before a century of change. The century was heralded by Luther nailing his thesis of rebellion against the Church to the door at Wittenberg in 1517. His counterpart in medicine was the bombastic, disturbing, unpredictable physician known best by his pseudonym, Paracelsus (1493-1551), who in 1527 publicly burned the books of Galen and Avicenna to symbolize his break with the past.

In 1543 there appeared two books that will remain permanently among man's greatest creations. One was by Copernicus, **De revolutionibis orbium coelestium**, establishing man's place in his physical universe. The other was by Vesalius, establishing the structure of man's body. If there be any date which modern medicine can indicate as its birthday, it is 1543, the date of publication of **De humani corporis fabrica**.

The blinders of hallowed tradition enforced by absolute authority were finally loosened. Talented, brave men again could see the world with their own eyes and think their own thoughts. In oncology, however, new concepts had to await another century.

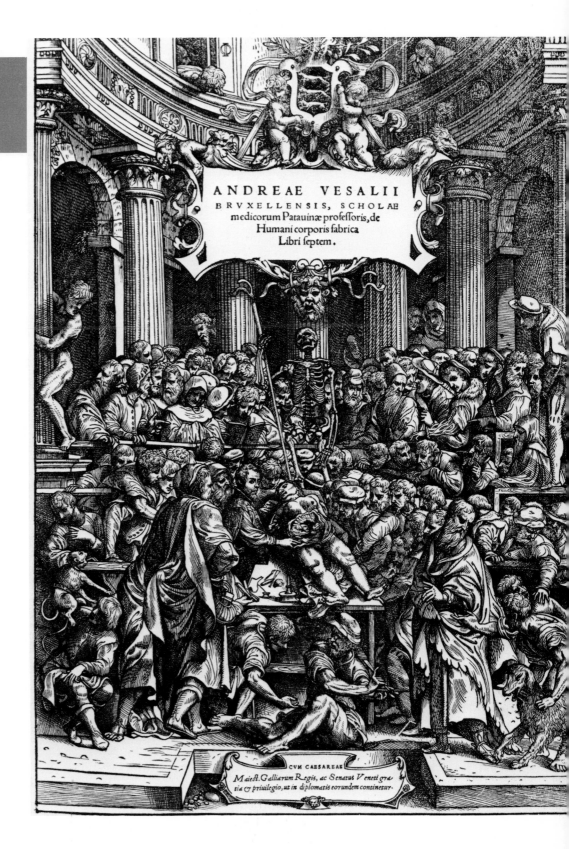

Title-page of Vesalius, *De humani corporis fabrica*, Basle, 1543.

IV-A.

Morbid anatomy begins: Benivieni

Antonio Benivieni (1443-1502), of Florence, collected notes on autopsies, which were published by his brother in 1507.

In chapter 36 of the book on **Hidden Causes of Disease** is described cancer of the stomach, translated by Singer as follows:

"XXXVI. Hardening of the stomach.

"My kinsman, Antonio Bruno, retained the food he had eaten for too short a time, and then threw it up undigested. He was most carefully treated with every kind of remedy for the cure of stomach trouble, but as none was of any use at all, his body wasted away through lack of nourishment till little more than skin and bone remained. At last he was brought to his death.

"The body was cut open for reasons of public welfare. It was found that the opening of his stomach had closed up and it had hardened down to the lowest part with the result that nothing could pass through to the organs beyond, and death inevitably followed."

Benivieni is regarded as a pioneer in morbid anatomy that came to full flower over 2 centuries later with Morgagni.

Antonio Benivieni. **De abditis nonnullis ac mirandis morborum et sanationum causis.** 1507. Translation by Charles Singer. Springfield, Ill.: C. C. Thomas, 1954.

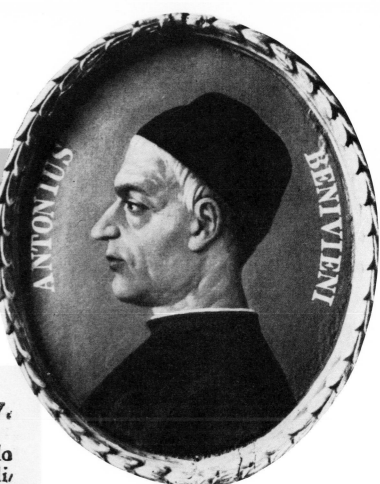

Antonio Benivieni

Tuberculū fupra cordis arteriam. XXXV.

m Vlier Clara nomine & gener cordis do
lore interdum uexabatur : quē medi/
ci a malo ipfi⁹ cordis habitu fieri arbitrabá/
tur. Sed cum plurib⁹ iam annis connubio
iuncta non conciperet, & fterilitatis caufam
quæreret ac tollere conaretur multis præfi/
diis, Ita demum dolor ille cordis increbre/
fcere occepit, ut perpetuus fieret: Ex quo
fæpius etiam mulier ipfa deficiens, recreari
uix poterat, donec eo iam magis magifq̃ in
ualefcente e medio fublata eft. Cætex̃ mor
tuæ corpore incifo & fruftulū nigrioris car
his in finiftro cordis uentriculo fupra arte/
riam, qđ mefpilii formam haberet, & uul
ua a medio infra uerfus imam eius partem
iunctis oris obcalluiffe reperta eft. Quare
ut tuberculum illud mortis, ita hoc fterili
tatis caufam fuiffe cognouimus.

Stomachum obcalluiffe. XXXVI.

a Ntonius Brunus affinis meus, cum
emanducatum cibum breuiori q̃ par
fuerat temporis fpatio contineret : & ita
ut erat incoctum reiiceret, omnibus medi/
camtis, q̃ ftomachi uitiis adhiberi poffūt, di
ligētiffime fot⁹ ē. Vex̃ cū ea nihil oĩo pfice
rēt, & corpori ob inopiā alimēti iā abfūpto

Chapter XXXVI of Benivieni's Hidden Causes of Disease, 1553.

IV-B.

Tumor listing: Ingrassia

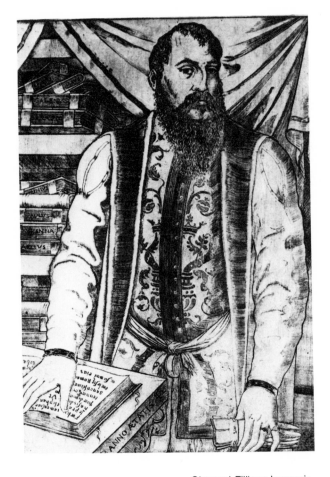

Giovanni Fillippo Ingrassia

Galen's tumors "contrary to nature" were not restricted to what is now called cancer, but included no less than 61 categories of inflammations, swellings and ulcerations.

Giovanni Fillippo Ingrassia (1510-1580) extended the list to 287 varieties of tumors in his treatise of the subject in 1553. This was perhaps the largest conglomerate of diseases due to black bile abnormalities, and included ulcers, gangrene, carbuncles, erysipelas, furuncles, leprosy, scabies, buboes, aneurysms, varices, and hernias. Scirrhus was categorized separately from cancer, which was an ulcerated lesion.

Ingrassia was born in Sicily and studied at Palermo and Padua, receiving his medical degree in 1537. He became professor of medicine and anatomy at Naples in 1544. He returned to Sicily as the Protomedicus and instituted reforms in sanitation there. He was called "the Sicilian Hippocrates," so that his high standing in 16th Century medicine was indisputable.

Ingrassia's list of tumors, 1300 years following Galen's, was an excellent example of the sleep of medicine during that long period. It was an elaboration and confusion, without a conceptual base.

Ingrassia, *De tumoribus praeter naturam,* Naples, 1553. Title page.

IOANNIS PHILIPPI INGRASSIAE

SICVLI RACHALBVTENSIS, DE TVMORIBVS PRAETER
NATVRAM TOMVS PRIMVS. IN QVO GENERATIM TVMO=
rum omnium Præternaturalium ſpecies: præſertimq; earum nomina & definitio=
nes, atq; etiam cauſæ, multaq; generalia declarantur. Græciq;, & Latini,&
Arabes, quatenus ad hæc ipſa pertinet, enucleantur. Occaſione ſum=
pta ab Auicennæ uerbis, Arabum Medicorum Principis, Tertia
Fen Quarti Libri, Tractatu Primo. Cuius interim uni=
uerſum Primum Caput in hoc Tomo elucidatur.
Reliqua in ſex alys Tomis declarabuntur:
quos Elenchus pagina duodeci=
ma demonſtrabit.

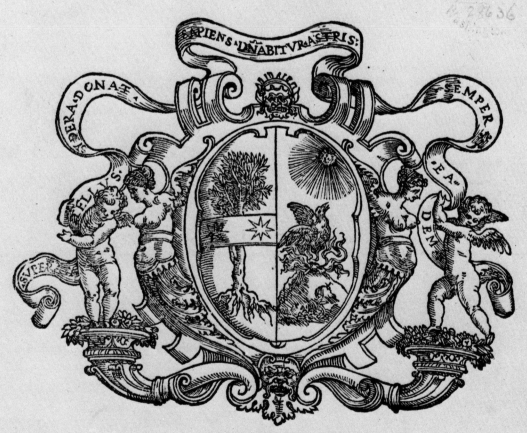

AVTHORIS INSIGNIA.

N E quiuis alius impunè uel hìc, uel uſquam locorum hos ſeptem de tumoribus præter naturam
tomos, uel imprimat, uel impreſſos, uenales afferat: Iulij Tertij Pontificis Maximi, ac Cæſareæ
Maieſtatis Caroli Quinti Priuilegijs cautum eſt per decenium, ut omnia perdat uolumina,& præ=
terea .300. aureos ſoluat, pro quolibet uolumine. quorum duæ partes Apoſtolicæ Cameræ, uel
Regio Fiſco, Tertia Authori, Quartaq; accuſatori debetur.

GABRIELIS
FALLOPPII
MVTINENSIS,
Physici ac Chirurgici præclarissimi,

IN FELICISSIMO GYMNASIO PA-
tauino olim rem Anatomicam & Chirurgicam ad-
mirabili cum laude profitentis,

OPERA QVAE ADHVC EXTANT OMNIA,
in vnum congesta, & in Medicinæ studiosorum gratiam
nunc primum tali ordine excusa:

VOLVMEN TAM EXCELLENS, TANTAQVE DOCTRINA RE-
fertum, vt omnes qui eiusmodi scriptis sese applicuerint, in morbis & dignoscen-
dis & curandis, non paruam gloriam adepturi sint.

Omnia multo accuratius nunc edita, & præter INDICEM capitum in limine positum,
altero etiam INDICE alphabetico adaucta.

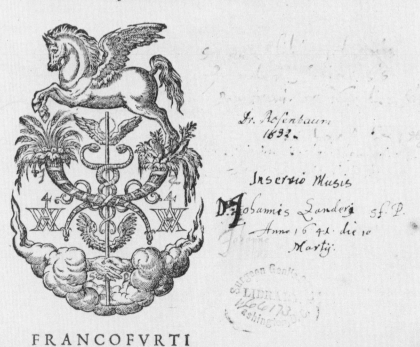

Fallopius, *Opera,* 1584.

FRANCOFVRTI
Apud hæredes Andreæ Wecheli,
MDLXXXIIII.

Gabriele Fallopius

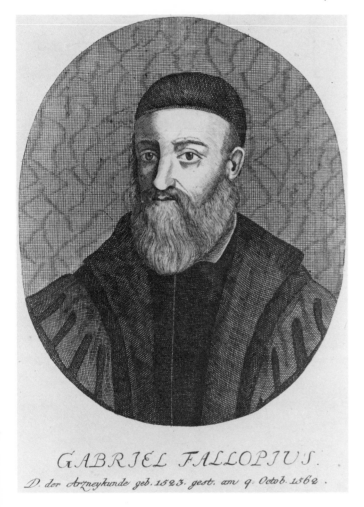

Gabrielis Falloppi. **Omnia quae adhuc extant opera.** . . . Francofurti: Andreae Wecheli, 1584.
Roberto Margotta. **The Story of Medicine.** New York: Golden Press, 1968. (p. 157-166.)

Anatomy was the most important medical development of the 16th Century, and the first significant turn away from the dead hand of classical authority. Anatomy arose in the Italian schools of Padua and Bologna. Had Marco Antonio della Torre (1473-1506) of Padua not died in his early 30's, his anatomy, illustrated by Leonardo da Vinci (1452-1519) might have been an immortal work. The role fell to Andreas Vesalius (1514-1564) a Fleming who studied in Paris and Padua, who at the age of 28 issued his **De humani corporis fabrica**, with illustrations by Stephen Calcar (1500-1546), a pupil of Titian.

Gabriele Fallopius (1523-1562) of Pisa and Padua was a contemporary of Vesalius. He was an illustrious anatomist in his own right, and a doughty opponent of Galenical teachings.

The views of Fallopius in regard to cancer were included in his posthumous **Opera omnia** of 1584. He described tumors under 38 chapters which included abscesses, carbuncles, gangrene, bubo, erysipelas, edema, scirrhus, aneurysm, struma, hernia and hydrocephalus. Along with Vesalius, Fallopius considered scirrhus to be an occult cancer, and cancer was the ulcerated stage of scirrhus. The early form was susceptible to excision and cauterization. Cancer, however, was incurable and treated by a variety of pastes. Fallopius devoted 10 folio pages to the compounding, preparation and use of such pastes, the active ingredient of which was arsenic.

The views of Fallopius in regard to cancer were, thus, classical in concept and in treatment, and representative of the medical thought of the period. "Quiescente cancro, medico quiescendum" was the 16th Century equivalent of the earlier "Noli me tangere."

IV-D.

Brain tumor described: Plater

Felix Plater or Platter (1536-1614) was a professor of medicine at the University of Basle for 43 years. He was an able and brave man, staying at his post during plague epidemics and performing autopsies soon after Vesalius.

Plater described an autopsy on "Casper Benecurtius, a noble knight," who over a two-year period lost his mind until he was completely irrational. "...there was discovered on [the corpus callosum] of the brain a remarkable round fleshy tumor like an acorn. It was hard and full of holes and was as large as a medium-sized apple. It was covered with its own membrane and was entwined with the veins. . . . We perceived that this ball by compressing the brain and its ducts with its mass and by flooding them, had been the occasion of the lethargy and listlessness and finally of death. Although at first some physicians maintained that the application resulted from poisoning and others that it resulted merely from humors... the abstruse and hidden cause subsequently became known to us in this case by opening of the brain."

Netsky and Lapresle state that this account leaves no doubt that Caspar Bonecurtius suffered from a parasagital meningioma, and was the first such account to be found. "It is remarkable that Plater was able to discard poisons and humors as causes of this mental syndrome and to attribute the signs so clearly and unequivocally to the mass which compressed the brain."

Felix Plater

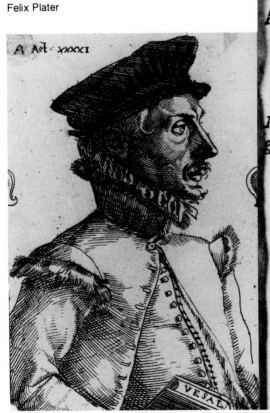

FELICIS
PLATERI
ARCHIATRI ET
PROFES. BASIL.
Obſeruationum,
*In Hominis Affeɛtibus pleriſą̃, corpori &
animo, funɛtionum læſione, dolore,
aliáve moleſtiâ & vitio incommodantibus,*
LIBRI TRES.
*Ad Praxeos illiu s Tractatus tres, quorum
primus Funɛtionum læſiones , ſe-
cundus Dolores, tertius Vitia
continet, accom-
modati.*

*In quibus eo ordine, diuerſorum affeɛtuum ſub
generibus hiſce comprehenſorum, progreſſus,
euentus, curationes, vti ab authore hæc
obſeruata traɛtatá̃ fuerunt Hi-
ſtoricè deſcribun.*

BASILEÆ,
Impenſis LVDOVICI KÖNIG,
Typis CONRADI WALDKIRCHIL.
M DC XIIII.

Plater, *Observationum, 1614*. Title page.

Beloved Son Felix. The Journal of Felix Platter. Translated
and introduced by Sean Jennett. London: F. Muller, 1962.

F. Plater. **Observationum in hominis affectibus
plerisque, corpori et animo, functionum laesione, dolore,
aliave molestia et vitio incommodantibus, libri tres.**
Basilae, Impensis Ludovici König, 1614.

Martin G. Netsky and Jean Lapresle. The first account of a
meningioma. **Bull. Hist. Med.** 30: 465-68, 1956.

IV-E.

Master of Renaissance surgery: Paré

Ambroise Paré (1510-1590) an unlettered French barber surgeon who rose to being surgeon to four French kings, ran out of boiling oil for the treatment of gunshot wounds during a battle in 1536. Next morning the men not so treated were more comfortable than those who had received the oil. "Then I resolved within myself never so cruelly to burn poor wounded men," wrote Paré, interpreting correctly the unpremeditated clinical experiment in an epidemic of war trauma.

Paré also returned to ligature for hemostasis, abandoning the cautery, reintroduced podalic version in obstetrics, and designed artificial limbs. His own personality and example, however, were the greatest contributions to surgery. Withal, his motto was, "Je le pensai; Dieu le guarist" (I dressed him, God cured him).

Paré's conservative surgical approach extended to cancer. The following two cases gathered by Hamby are beautiful examples:

The first concerns cancer of the lip.

"Sometimes one may otherwise and more happily cure cancers of the lip without applying caustics or any similar thing. . . . The way is this: Pass a threaded needle through the cancer so the thread held in the left hand can lift and control the cancer without any of its escaping. One can then cut to good flesh with scissors in the right hand; and cut so that a layer of good flesh of the lip remains to serve as a base and foundation for regeneration of flesh in place of the portion amputated, supposing the cancer has not taken root and spread from top to bottom. This done, having let enough blood flow from within and without, at the right and left of the amputation, make deep enough incisions with the razor so that later, when one would draw together and unite the edges of the sound . . .the flesh would be more obedient to the thread and needle."

The second case deals with cancer of the breast.

"I shall give the history of Mme. de Montigny, a Maid of Honor of the Queen Mother, who had a cancer the size of a nut in the left breast. . . . I presuaded her to go with me to M. Houllier, Regent Physician of the Faculty of Medicine, recognized and known by all as a wise man. When he had examined the Lady he considered the tumor to be cancerous and we decided upon a palliative course, fearing to irritate this Hydra, and cause it to burst in fury from its lair. He ordered his regimen and certain purgations which should be used on alternate days, and on the tumor was placed a sheet of lead covered with quick-silver. Certain unguents were ordered for a period of two months. Finally the Lady became restless . . ." Another physician was consulted and a more aggressive treatment with hot applications, emollients and astringents terminated with ulceration that was treated with a caustic powder. "The heart failed and death followed."

Ambroise Paré. **Les Oeuvres de M. Ambroise Paré**. . . Paris: Gabriel Buon, 1585.

Wallace B. Hamby. **The Case Reports and Autopsy Records of Ambroise Paré**. Springfield, Ill.: C. C. Thomas, 1960.

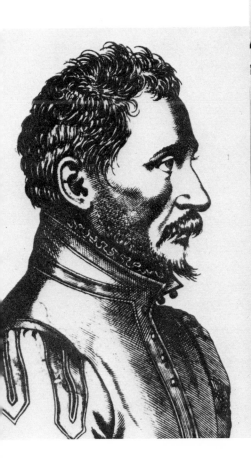

Ambroise Paré

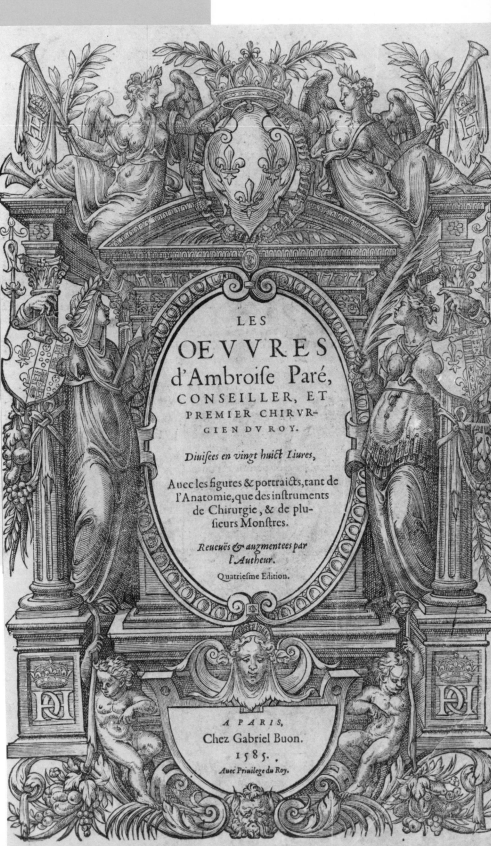

Paré, *Oeuvres*, 1585. Title page.

V. 17th Century: Experimental Medicine Begins

Galen and Aristotle passed into history during the 17th Century. In the physical sciences, Galileo solidified the Copernican concepts, and extended man's vision by his telescope. Newton by 1687 synthesized man's concepts of the physical nature of the universe.

In the biological sciences, Harvey in 1628 published his **De Motu Cordis**, one of the immortal books in the medical field. He laid the foundations of physiology and experimental medicine by his discovery of the circulation of the blood. Leeuwenhoek explored the microscopic world with his magnifying lenses.

During the 17th Century were begun many trends in science and medicine that emerged as important two centuries later. Robert Hooke in 1665 described "little boxes or cells" in plants. Malpighi discovered capillaries in the lung in 1661, and rediscovered embryology in 1673. Redi in 1671 experimentally challenged spontaneous generation. DeGraaf in 1664 created pancreatic fistulas in dogs, extending experimental physiology. Sanctorius, in 1614, introduced thermometry and metabolic measurements. Graunt in 1662 analyzed bills of mortality and initiated medical demography.

The greatest medical practitioner of the period was Sydenham, who revived the Hippocratic methods of observation and personal experience. He contributed many fine descriptions of disease. He was a therapeutic moderate, even in blood-letting, and willing to attribute to Nature the result of recovery. Surgeons began to describe more extensive operations, including the removal of enlarged axillary lymph nodes in cancer of the breast. The first periodic journals in biomedical sciences were initiated in France and in England.

The humoral views of disease were replaced by iatrochemical hypotheses. Cancer was no longer an atrabilious affliction. There appeared opinions that cancer was contagious, but more popular was the attribution of cancer to stasis and abnormalities of lymph.

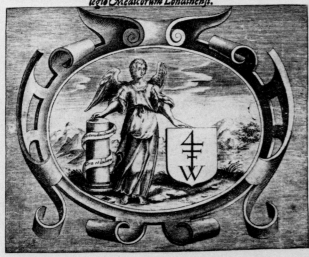

Harvey, *De Motu Cordis,* 1628. Title page.

V-A.

Discovery of lymphatics: Aselli

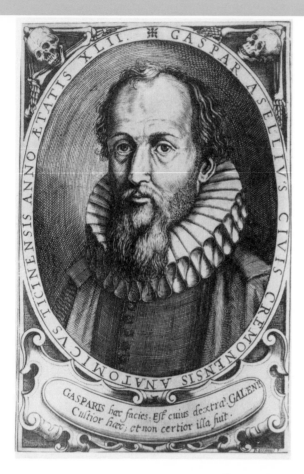

Gaspare Aselli

Gaspare Aselli (1581-1625) of Milan is the acknowledged discoverer of lymphatic vessels. He recorded the precise dissection of a well-fed dog, and his exclamation of "Eureka" as he identified the lacteal fluid in the lymph channels of the mesentery. His book **De Lactibus** appeared in 1627, two years after his death and a year before Harvey's **De Motu Cordis.**

Further clarification of the lymphatic system came through the demonstration of the thoracic duct in 1651 by Jean Pecquet (1622-1674), and the unnecessary disputations for priority between Rudbeck and Bartholinus in Scandinavia in 1653.

Edema and ascites were quickly ascribed to lymphatic occlusion. There soon also arose suggestions of a similar pathogenesis for a wide variety of diseases manifested by swelling of lymph nodes, such as tuberculosis and cancer. In breast cancer, the association of axillary lymph node involvement was known since antiquity, but now the primary disease was attributed to stasis and degeneration of lymph.

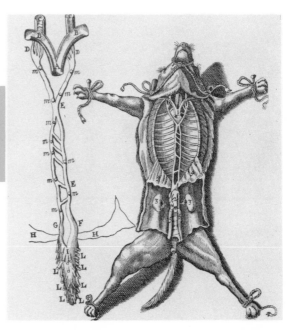

Thoracic duct in a dog, from Pecquet, 1651. (from I. Rusznyak et al., 1967).

The lymph theories of the origin of cancer did have the advantage of pointing attention to lymph nodes, which were then removed more frequently when they were enlarged and located close to the tumor. In this respect the theory was preferable to the humoral explanation and to the speculations of iatrochemists, such as cancer through acidosis. And, of course, the lymphatic drainage became the key consideration in the development of more extensive surgical resections of cancer.

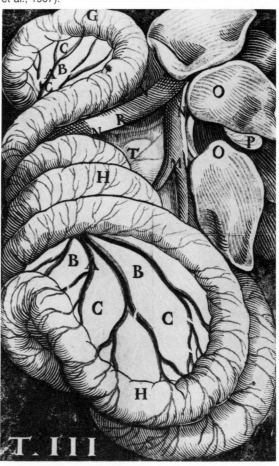

Lacteals in dog's mesentery, from Aselli, *De Lactibus,* 1627.

Gasparis Aselli. **De Lactibus sive Lacteis Venis.** Milan: Bidellium, 1627.

István Rusznyák *et al.* **Lymphatics and Lymph Circulation.** ed. 2. New York: Pergamon Press, 1967. (p. 15-24).

V-B.

Wider surgery espoused: Fabricius Hildanus

Wilhelm Fabry (1560-1624) of Hilden, or Fabricius, is often called the Father of German Surgery. After a good classical education, he became a barber surgeon in Düsseldorf, travelled widely and was accepted by doctors of medicine.

Fabry was a daring surgeon for his time. He recorded a number of operations for cancer of the breast that included excision of enlarged lymph nodes, and amputation at the thigh. Although he devised a tourniquet to control bleeding, he also continued to use the cautery, and believed in the weapon-salve, which was applied to the weapon instead of the wound.

Fabry was the author of some 20 books, most of which were collected in his **Opera**, published in 1646. It included clear descriptions of cases. He developed a special forceps for the amputation of the breast. The instrument constricted the base of the breast while the blade swept the organ off the chest wall. Various modifications of this instrument appear in later contributions, such as those of Helvetius and Bidloo.

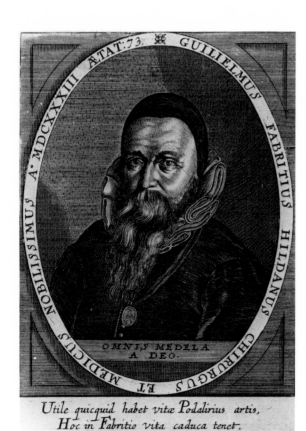

Utile quicquid habet vitæ Podalirius artis,
Hoc in Fabritio vita caduca tenet.

Wilhelm Fabry, or Fabricius Hildanus

William A. Cooper. The history of the radical mastectomy. **Ann. Med. Hist.** 3: 36-54, 1941.

Fabricius Hildanus. **Collected Works** published by Frederick Greift, 1646.

Fabricius Hildanus. **Opera quae extant omnia** . . . Balthas: Christoph Wusti, 1682.

Helvetius. **Lettre sur la Nature et la Guerison du Cancer de monsieur Helvetius.** Paris: Jean Cusson, 1691.

G. Bidloo. **Exercitationem Anatomico-Chirurgicarium.** Luchtmans, 1708. (p. 166).

Obf.78.
& 79.

infantulum lactaffe, qui tamen infantulus vix
fextum menfem ætatis attigerat, cùm circa cinun-
ctoria undique fcirrhofis tumoribus fcatueret :
unde tamen languidè vitam finivit. Materia enim
cancri in mamma concreta atque incuneata, lac
procul dubio acre, malignum & femi veneno-
fum effecerat. Matres itaque fic affectæ, infan-
tulos lactare minimè debent. Sic enim lac in fto-
macho coagulatum, veneni inftar graviffima
fymptomata infert, ut Galenus, Aëtius, & multi
alii teftantur, multò malignius efficietur, fi in
mammis coaguletur ac includatur. Quomodo
autem in præcedenti operatione proceffi, proxi-
mè tibi literis communicabo, nunc non licuit.
Vocor enim Freiburgum ad nobilem matronam,
quæ fimiliter, ut audio, Cancro exulcerato laborat : quicquid autem fit, pofthac ad te fcribam.
Salutant T. Exc. Reverendus Dn. MERULA,
Dn. OECONOMUS, & domeftici mei omnes.
Saluta, quæfo, meo nomine peramanter Dn. D.
PAULUM HEBNERUM. Ille quod me in
tranfitu hác non offenderit, doleo. Vale vir clariffime & feliciter vive diu. Paterniaci Aventi-
corum 25 Januar.1610.

OBSERVATIO LXXIX.

De excifione tumorum axillarum, & abfciffio-
ne mammarum.

Ad eundem
Virum Clariffimum atque doctiffimum D.D.
ANDREAM WEICKIUM.

HEri fub noctem, clariffime Dn. D. WEICKI
Freiburgo redii : Matrona illa, ad quam vocatus fueram, non cancro, fed fteatomate in ulcus aliquomodo malignum degenerato, laborat.
Ante paucos dies puella hic fub plauftrum, lignis
onuftum, cadens, graviffimum affectum cruris
finiftri contraxit. Rota enim non folum mufcu-
los & vafa, verùm etiam ipfa offa dilaceraverit atq;
confregit. Multos mihi parit labores atque mole-
ftias affectus ifte, propter fymptomata quæ fu-
perveniunt: qualifnam verò erit exitus, pofthac
ex me intelliges. Nunc enim reliqua quæ in præcedenti, tibique communicata obfervatione defi-
derantur, addenda funt.

Difficilem autem fimul & periculofum effe
excifionem tumorum axillarum, præcipuè fi magni fuerint, cùm in aliis, tum in primis in illa fœ-
mina, cujus in proxima præcedente Obfervatione mentio facta, obfervavi. Periculofa propter
venarum thoracicarum eo in loco concurfum,
ex quo hæmorrhagia timenda : deinde quoque
eam ob caufam, quòd attrahendo hujufmodi tumores, mufculi pectorales, & refpirationi infervientes, fimul lædantur, hinc fuffocationis periculum. Quamobrem paulatim, modeftè &
clementer hifce in partibus operandum convenit.
Difficilis verò propterea, quòd brachio depen-
dente tumor in profundo delitefcat atq; abfcon-
datur, & brachio tota axilla obtegatur : fin verò elevetur brachium, mufculi, membranæ, vafa,
fimul & tumor ipfe adeò extenduntur, ut dif-
ficillimè feparari poffit, inprimis verò, fi pro-

Gal.lib. de
cibu boni
& mali
fucci. Aë-
tius Te-
trab. 4.
ferm.1.

fundiùs membranis adhæferit. Prudenter itaque
in hujufmodi operationibus agendum eft. Sed
& ante omnia diligenter explorandum, an tumor
ex una in alteram partem vacillari atque moveri,
& radicitùs extirpari poffit? Inanis enim foret
operatio, fi pars aliqua tumoris, quantumvis mi-
nima, imò etiam membrana, quâ ut plurimùm hujufmodi tumores integuntur, remanferit : repul-
lulat enim malum, fitque priori malignius. Nec
fperandum, id quod remanfit, caufticis auferri
poffe: iis enim cancri ita irritantur, ut ad fummam
malignitatem perveniant, ficuti Obf.1. Centur.1.
& alibi demonftravimus.

Hoc autem modo in operatione præce-
dentis Obfervat. proceffi. Brachio mediocriter à
miniftro in altum elevato, cutem in longitudinem
fecundùm tumoris magnitudinem incidi, poftea
tumorem diligenter feparavi, cavique, ne venæ
abrumperentur aut inciderentur, propter hæmorrhagiam, quæ in hac operatione totum negotium
invertiffet. Ab ea itaque ut fecurus effem, ma-
jorem partem iftius tumoris, qui magnitudinem
ovi gallinacei adæquabat, unguibus feparavi.
Deinde tumore fequenti forcipe apprehenfo, mi-
niftrum juffi, ut forcipis hujus beneficio tumorem, quantum (abfque tamen maximo dolore)
fieri poffet, deorfum attraheret. Poftea acu in-
curvatâ, quam in promptu habebam, interim dum
minifter forcipe tumorem ad fe attrahebat, venas,
quæ tumori inferebantur, primò ex fuperiori,
deinde quoque ex inferiori parte tumoris appre-
hendi, ac firmiffimo nodo ligavi. Tandem tumorem audacter feparavi, atque intra ambas li-
gaturas fili, excidi, ita tamen, ut filum extra vulnus propenderet, quò & fuo quoque tempore ex-
trahi poffet. Reliquos quoque binos tumores,
avellanæ magnitudinis, majori adjacentes, parvo
cum negotio avulfi atque extraxi.

Mamma
abfciffio.

Tandem ad fcirrhum cancrofum, totam fe-
rè mammam ad coftas penè ufque occupantem
pervenimus. Incifâ itaque cute circumcirca tumorem (quandoquidem cuti tenaciter adhære-
fcebat) ipfum tum digitis, tum cultellis fepara-
riis, facili negotio feparavi atque extraxi, & poft-
quam aliquid fanguinis effluere permiffem, pul-
verem noftrum ad fanguinem fiftendum, ftupis
albumine ovi madefactis, impofui : Pectus, hu-
merum & brachium oleo rofarum inunxi, & pul-
villum ex ftupis mollibus, vitello & albumine ovi
cum ol. rofar. conquaffato, intinctis, applicui, fa-
fciaque omnia colligavi. Cordi verò epithema ad-
movi, & ad virium lapfus nonnihil aquæ cinamo-
mi abfque vino deftill. in qua confectio Alker-
mes diffoluta erat, ea die, & fequenti nocte fre-
quenter ex cochleari exhibui.

Alterâ die denuò fupradictas partes ol. rofar. inunxi, vulneribus verò fequens digeftivum
cum filamentis impofui, & Emplaftro Bafilicone
obtegi.

Vnguent.
Digefti-
vum.

R. Terebinthinæ lotæ in aq. fcabiofæ ʒij.
Ceræ novæ &
Gummi elemi ana ʒj.
Ol. rofar.
Amygdal. dulc.
de vitell.

Obf.79.

de vitell. ovor. ana ʒß.
Croci ℈j.
Vitellum unius ovi. Mifce, fiat un-
guentum f.a. His & fimilibus vulnus aliorum vul-
nerum more, brevi curavimus, ficque divino folo
favore, fœminam illam fanitati reftituimus, quæ
& poftmodum prolem fanam progenuit, ipfa-
metque lactavit.

In excifione autem atque extractione tumorum axillarium, leniter & paulatim procedendum
eft: dum enim five forcipe, five quovis alio modo
tumorem attrahimus atque feparamus, mufculi
refpirationi infervientes fimul attrahuntur: hinc
factum, ut durante operatione mulier hæc aliquando refpirare non poffet. Id quàm primum
animadvertiffem, paululùm ab operatione remifi,
ne fuffocaretur, fed vires recolligeret, dein denuò
opus aggrediebar. Frigida quoque & valdè
repercutientia, his in locis applicanda minimè
funt, ne materia ad pleuram, aliafq; partes nobiles
repellatur, ibique inflammationes excitet. Ut igi-
tur incommodum hoc evitarem, corpus ante operationem quater aut quinquies per intervalla, &
diebus interpofitis purgavi, apozemata propina-
vi, venam incidi, & optimam atque tenuem victus
rationem præfcripfi. Quod fi verò affluxus aliquis
humorum poft operationem fupervenerit, cu-
curbitulæ fcapulis funt applicandæ, venæ item
malleoli incidendæ, ut fanguis & humores deorfum trahantur. Dolor item ingens fi fequatur, loco Emplaftri bafilici, fequens Cataplafma calidè
applicetur.

R.Micæ panis albi ʒ vj.
Butyri recent. non faliti ʒij.
Pulv. fem. cydonior. &
fœnigræci ana ʒ ij.
Coquantur in lacte vaccino recens emulcto
ad confiftentiam cataplafmatis; tum admifce
Croci pulverifati ℈ j.
Ol. de vitell. ovor. &
Rofar. ana ʒ ß.
Vitellum unius ovi. Mifce, fiat Cataplafma,
quod bis aut ter interdiu calidè applicetur. In
excifione præterea cancri, diligenter obfervanda
eft Galeni doctrina lib.14. meth. med. ubi jubet,
ut excifo cancro cum tota fua radice, finamus aliquid fanguinis ex proximis venis effluere, quod &
ego hactenus in omnibus ftudiofè obfervavi.
In prædictis verò tumoribus fcirrhofis doctri-
nam Galeni fequi non licuit : propter maximam
enim, quæ fequuta fuiffet, hæmorrhagiam, prius
expiraffet ægra, quàm tota abfoluta fuiffet operatio, quandoquidem ex longa hac operatione jam
antea fatis debilitata erat. Quapropter venas fub
axilla conftringere ac ligare coacti fuimus. Sed &
non ufque adeo neceffe fuiffe videbatur fanguinis fluxus, quandoquidem tumores illi, qui fub
axilla latitabant, nondum maligni & cancrofi
erant. Cæterùm quæ promifi, nimirum Scal-
pellum fimul & Anatomiam Vitrioli mitto, tu,
quæfo, omnia æqui bonique confule. Domeftici
mei omnes mecum T. Exc. plurimùm falutant.
Vale, vir clariffime, & me tuum cenfe. Paterniaci
1. Februarii 1610.

T. Guil. Fabricius Hildanus.

Figura Forcipis & cultelli feparatorii.

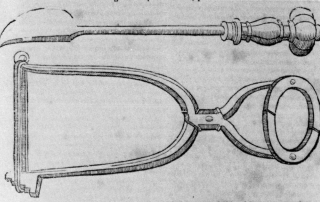

OBSERVATIO LXXX.

*Incipiens Scirrhus ex lacte coagulato, quo-
modo fanatus?*

Matrona quædam juvenis & robufta, Hildenæ
in patriâ dum infantem lactaret, inflammatione finiftræ mammæ correpta fuit. Quâ fe-

datâ, tumor & durities adeò magna remanfit, ut
de fcirrhi generatione non parva effet fufpicio.
Multis licet & variis, præfertim Empiricis, medicamentis, topicis, emollientibus ac difcutientibus
ufa effet, nihilominus tamen tumor & durities
remanfere. Ego tandem vocatus, pulvere Paf-
favanti cum rhabarbaro leviter ipfam purgavi,
infans quoque ut ablactaretur, protinus impera-
vi. Po-

Instruments for mastectomy, from Fabricius Hildanus, *Opera,*

Mastectomy with removal of axillary lymph nodes (Hildanus,
Opera quae extant omnia, Frankfurt am Main, 1682).

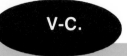

Total mastectomy: Scultetus

Johann Schultes (1595-1645) or Scultetus, graduated in medicine at Padua in 1621 and became city physician of Ulm, his native city. He was the author of the popular **Armamentarium chirurgicum**, published in 1645 and translated into several languages. It contained many illustrations of surgical instruments and procedures. Included was the oft-reproduced series of a mastectomy, combining total slice-removal followed by cauterization. The panels of the plate were arranged in different manners in

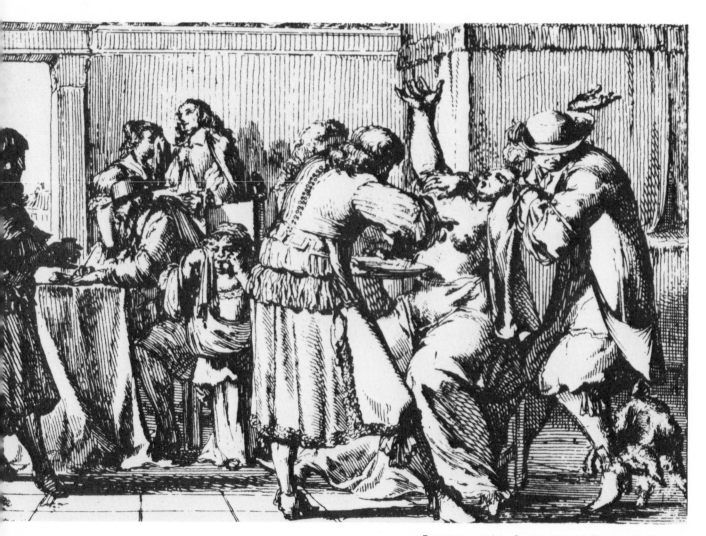

Breast amputation. Copper plate by Romeyn de Hooghe (1645-1708). From De Moulin.

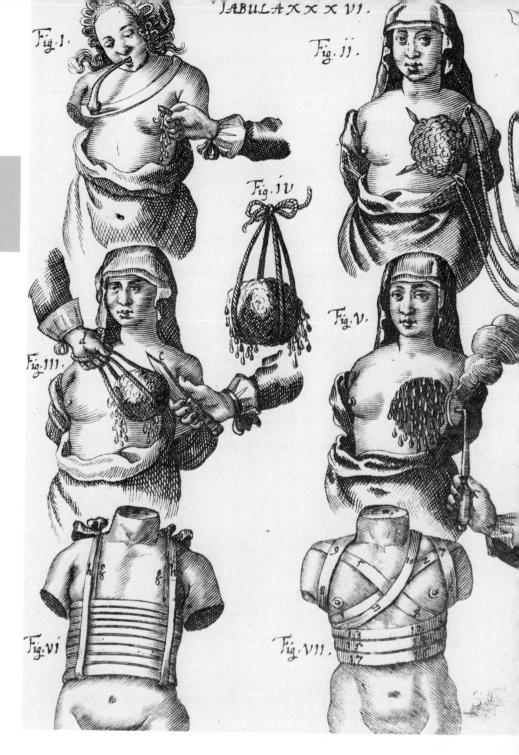

Mastectomy, from Plate 36
of Scultetus *Armamentarium
Chirurgicum,* 1666.

various editions, but were usually combined with a picture of the Scultetus bandage.

The peaceful face in this illustration belies what the procedure must have entailed for the woman, in the pre-anesthesia, pre-antisepsis days. The illustration can be compared with a contemporary copper plate of a breast amputation, by Romeyn de Hooghe (1645-1708). We can only wonder how many women consented to the procedure, and what the post-operative survival rate could have been.

W. A. Cooper. The history of the radical mastectomy. **Ann. Med. Hist.** 3: 36-54, 1941.

Johannes Scultetus. **Armamentarium Chirurgicum.** [XVIII Tabulis aeri elegantissime incisis.] Frankfort: 1666 (plate 36).

Daniel De Moulin. Historical-phenomenological study of bodily pain in Western man. **Bull. Hist. Med.** 48: 540-570, 1974.

V-D.

Surgical pathology: Severinus

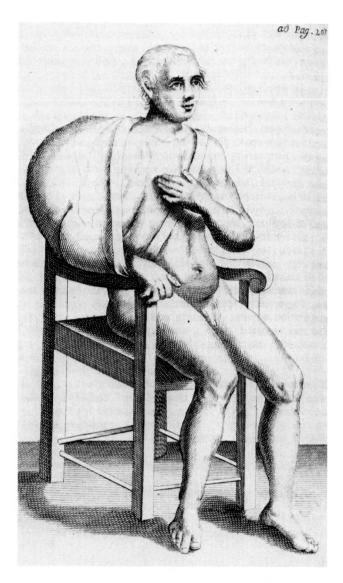

ad Pag. 207

Tumor of right upper extremity, possibly a sarcoma. From Severinus' *De recondita natura,* 1724; opposite p. 207.

Marco Aurelio Severino (1580-1656), or Severinus, was a professor of anatomy and surgery in Naples. He is perhaps best known in history for performing tracheostomies during an epidemic of diphtheria in Naples in 1610. He was the author of several noteworthy books, including a pioneer comparative anatomy, **Zootomia Democritae** of 1642.

De Recondita Abscessuum Natura, first published in 1632, included descriptions of neoplasms, granulomas, bubos, and abscesses, and is an important landmark in surgical pathology. It included illustrations of cases, such as the probable sarcoma of the right arm, taken from the 1724 edition.

Severinus included cancer under one of four major groups of tumors, along with carbuncles and other infections. However, he did divide tumors of the breast into four categories: glandular, stromal, scirrhous and cancerous. Clinically and on the basis of gross pathology he thus could distinguish between benign and malignant tumors of the breast. He believed in removing benign tumors because of the possibility of their becoming malignant.

Marcus Aurelius Severinus. **De Recondita Abscessum Natura.** Libri VIII Editio Secunda. Francofurti ad Moenum: apud Johannem. Beyerum, 1643.

Josiah C. Trent. Five letters of Marcus Arelius Severinus to the very honourable English physician, John Houghton. **Bull. Hist. Med.** 15: 306-23, 1944.

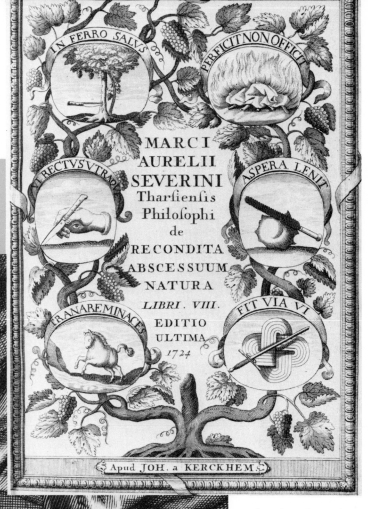

Severinus, *De recondita abscessum natura. . .,*
Title page,

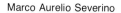

Marco Aurelio Severino

V-E.

Contagiousness of cancer: Zacutus and Tulp

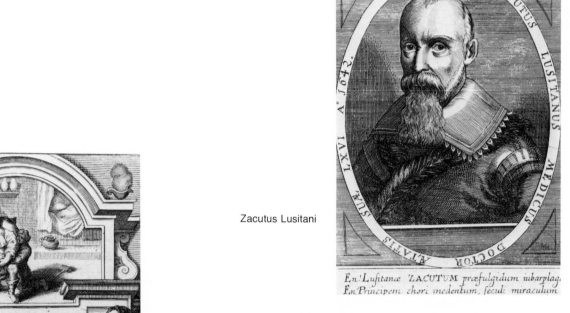

Zacutus Lusitani

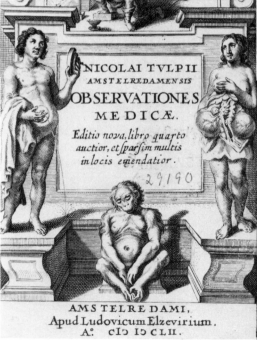

Tulp, *Observationes Medicae*, 1652. Title page.

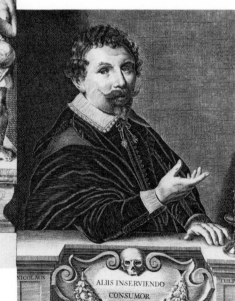

Nicholas Tulp

It is somewhat surprising that the idea of cancer being contagious is practically lacking among the ancient and medieval writings. Perhaps the overwhelming acceptance of cancer as an exteriorization of internal imbalance and excess of black bile inhibited other postulations.

During the 17th Century, however, appeared statements on the contagiousness of cancer. Among the first was from Zacutus Lucitanus (1575-1642), a Jewish physician of Portugal who settled in the Netherlands. "A poor woman who had suffered for many years from an ulcerated cancer of the breast, slept at night on the same couch with her three sons. All three became affected with a like disease. Five years after the death of the mother, two of the sons died; but the third, being more robust, recovered with difficulty after having submitted to excision of the cancer at the hands of a surgeon."

Nicholas Tulp (1593-1674), professor of anatomy at Amsterdam who was immortalized in a painting by Rembrandt, The Anatomy Lesson, also believed that cancer was contagious. He reported the following occurrence: "Adriana Lambert, a woman advanced in years, was afflicted with a cancer of the breast that had advanced to such a putrid condition as to infect by its exhalations her body-servant who attended upon her, living in close contact with the mistress. Some evil spark lighted such a conflagration as to destroy the maid no less than her mistress, for such a foul, irregular ulcer invaded the breast and armpit of each that I am undecided which of these two was tortured with the greater savagery."

Tulp's description of cancer of the urinary bladder, in a merchant who had a vesico-rectal fistula secondary to removal of stone, has been reproduced by Long.

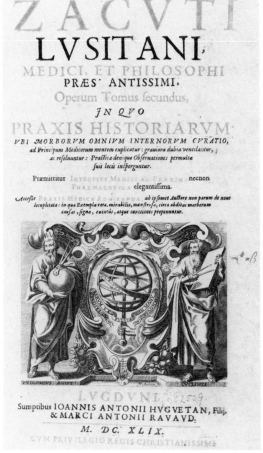

Zacutus Lusitani, Praxis, 1649. Title page.

Contagious diseases were well known to medieval man. Leprosy and plague were primary examples, with complete societal exclusion being practiced for leprosy, and, for plague, the instructions, "Run fast, go far, tarry long." Of course, the reasons for contagiousness were unknown, but involved the concepts of punishment for sin and of magic. Fracastoro, in his 1530 poem on syphilis and his later work on contagion, focused attention on such diseases.

Zacutus Lusitanus. **Praxis Medical Admiranda**, p. 31, obs. 124 (Appendix to **Opera**, tome ii, Lugduni, 1649).

Nicolai Tulp . . . **Observationes Medicae.** Amstelredami: Elzevirium, 1652. (Lib. IV, p. 308-9).

E. R. Long. **Selected Readings in Pathology.** ed. 2. Springfield, Ill.: C. C. Thomas, 1961. p. 42-6.

VI. 18th Century: The Age of Reason

The 18th Century in Europe was the century of Voltaire and of Rousseau, and of the American and French Revolutions. The Encyclopedia of Diderot promised a rational synthesis of human knowledge, and is a symbol of the age.

Leyden and Edinburgh were added to Padua, London and Paris as important medical centers. The school of Boerhaave reestablished clinical teaching in medicine.

Among the important developments in medicine and biomedical sciences were the rise of morbid anatomy and of physiology. Priestly and Lavoisier clarified the chemical physiology of respiration. Lind, in a classical therapeutical trial with controls, established the value of lemon juice in scurvy, over a century before vitamins and vitamin-deficiency diseases were understood. Jenner replaced variolation with vaccination as one of the preventive victories over a frightful human disease. Foxglove (digitalis) was added to Peruvian bark (quinine) in the small list of effective medical remedies.

The 18th Century concept of cancer causation tended toward local interpretations rather than manifestations of a constitutional diathesis. This provided a better base for surgical excision. The first descriptions of environmental cancer were recorded, and the first specialized hospitals for cancer were opened in France and in England. The first experimental approaches were being attempted, and new questions regarding cancer were formulated. Oncology as a discipline was still embryonic, but its patterns were emerging.

Denis Diderot, *Encyclopédie, ou Dictionaire Raisonné de Sciences, des Arts et des Metiers*. 35 vols, 1751-80. Paris. Frontispiece.
(Harrison D. Horblit, *One Hundred Books Famous in Science*. New York: Grolier Club, 1964).

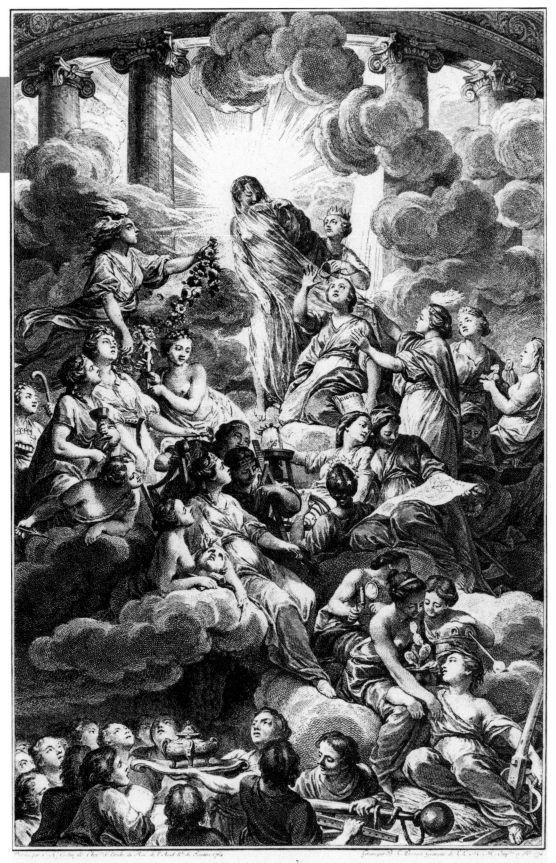

FRONTISPICE DE L'ENCYCLOPEDIE.

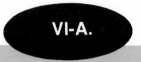

VI-A.

Morbid Anatomy

VI-A-1. Gross pathology emerges: Morgagni.

Necropsies became more acceptable during the 17th Century. Bonet in 1679 published his **Sepulchretum sive Anatomica Practica**, a "well ordered mortuary" of nearly three thousand necropsy protocols. Modern pathology, however, is dated from **De Sedibus et Causis Morborum** of 1761, the achievement recorded in 70 letters by Giovanni Battista Morgagni (1682-1771), professor of anatomy at Padua.

Morgagni's particular contribution was to relate the clinical history to the post-mortem findings. The 700 autopsies, most of them personally performed, range over all pathology. His descriptions of diseases of the vascular system are particularly admirable. Cancers of the breast, stomach, rectum and pancreas are included. Tumor metastases as such were unknown to him although descriptions include what are obviously secondary deposits in lymph nodes and the liver.

An account of a patient with a gastric carcinoma is given in Letter XIII, article 2:

"A man of about fifty-four years of age, had begun, five or six months before, to be somewhat emaciated, in his whole body, when in the beginning of the month of August, of the year 1689, a troublesome vomiting came on, of a fluid which resembl'd water, tinctur'd with soot. And the same kind of fluid was discharg'd by stool, sometimes, when the vomiting was upon the patient, and sometimes, when it was absent, but this discharge was not constant. At length the vomiting being very violent, with a discharge of the same matter, and the pulse growing, by degrees, very languid, death took place of life, on the thirteenth of November.

"In the stomach, towards the pylorus, was an ulcerated cancerous tumour, and this seem'd to be made up of congeries of glands, which, being press'd, discharg'd a kind of humour, like the male semen. And the stomach contain'd three pints of a matter, almost of the same nature with that, which was thrown up by vomiting. Betwixt the stomach and the spleen were two glandular bodies, of the bigness of a bean, and in their colour, and substance, not much unlike that tumour which I have describ'd in the stomach. These were the appearances in the belly."

Morgagni's *De Sedibus et Causis Morborum,* 1761,
Title page.

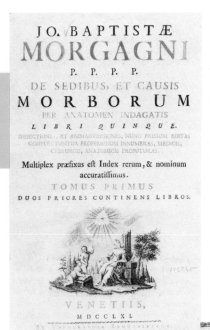

Giovanni Battista Morgagni

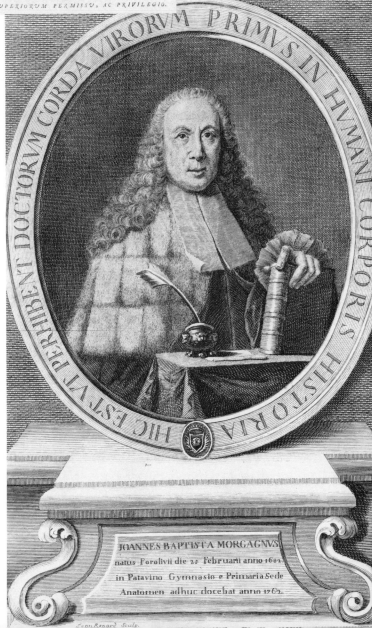

Morgagni's interests included comparative pathology. In Letter L, article 41, "There was at Padua a nun who had begun, thirty years before, first to labor under tubercles within one of her breasts." Finally a walnut-sized tumor was removed by a surgeon who judged it not to be a cancer. "This body consisted of many little pieces of bone," and was probably a calcified fibroadenoma of the breast. In article 43 were described similar findings in a dog: "under the very teat I found a small roundish body, of more than a cartilagenous hardness."

Long evaluates Morgagni as follows: "His inestimable service to the science of pathology was his emphasis on detail and thoroughness. He was never hurried in a description. He introduced nothing new in the way of method and made few out and out discoveries." But he set a new, high standard, and avoided facile systematics popular in his day.

The Seats and Causes of Diseases Investigated by Anatomy. Translated from the Latin of Giovanni Battista Morgagni by Benjamin Alexander, 3 vol. New York: Hafner Publishing Co., 1960.

E. R. Long. **A History of Pathology.** New York: Dover Publications, 1965. (p. 63-75).

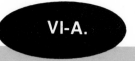

VI-A-2. Progress in pathology: Baillie

Thirty years after Morgagni, a nephew of William and John Hunter produced a systematic, illustrated atlas on gross pathology, using preparations in Hunter's museum.

Matthew Baillie (1761-1823) was one of the talented Scotsmen who settled in London and contributed greatly to medicine. In his middle age he became Physician Extraordinary to King George III.

The Morbid Anatomy of Some of the Most Important Parts of the Human Body appeared in 1793, and was followed, 1799 to 1802, by a series of engravings illustrating the text. Baillie arranged the material by organs, "in the same manner as if we were describing natural structure." His descriptions and engravings included cancer of the esophagus, stomach, bladder, and testes and reached new heights of clarity. Thus, for scirrhus and cancer of the stomach:

"This affliction of the stomach is not very uncommon towards an advanced period of life, and I think is more frequently met with in men than in women. This may probably depend upon the greater intemperance in the one sex than in the other.

"Scirrhus sometimes extends over almost every part of the stomach, but most commonly it attacks one part. The part which is affected with scirrhus has sometimes no very distinct limit between it and the sound structure of the stomach, but most commonly the limit is very well marked. When scirrhus attacks a portion of the stomach only, it is generally towards the pylorus. The principal reason of this probably is, that there is more of glandular structure in that part of the stomach than in any other; and it would appear that glandular parts of the body are more liable to be affected with scirrhus than other parts.

"When the whole stomach, or a portion of it, is scirrhous, it is much thicker than usual, as well as much harder in its texture. When the diseased part is cut into, the original structure of the stomach is frequently marked with sufficient distinctness, but very much altered from the natural appearance. The peritoneal covering of the stomach is many times thicker than it ought to be, and has almost a gristly hardness. The muscular part is also very much thickened, and is intersected by numerous membranous septa. These membranous septa are, probably, nothing else than the cellular

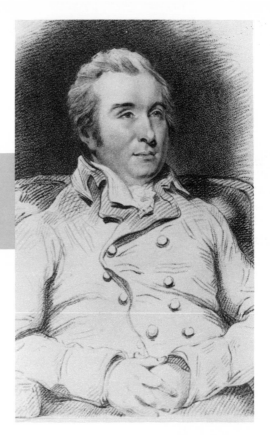

membrane intervening between the fasciculi of the muscular fibres, thickened from disease. The inner membrane is also extremely thick and hard, and not unfrequently somewhat tuberculated or irregularly elevated towards the cavity of the stomach.

"It frequently happens that this thickened mass is ulcerated upon its surface, and then a stomach is said to be cancerous. Sometimes the inner membrane of the stomach throws out a process which terminates in a great many smaller processes, and produces what has been commonly called a fungous appearance.

"It also happens that the stomach at some part loses entirely all vestige of its natural structure, and is changed into a very hard mass, of a whitish colour, with some appearance of membrane intersecting it: or it is converted into a gristly substance, like cartilage somewhat softened. The absorbent glands in the neighbourhood are at the same time commonly enlarged, and have a very hard white structure."

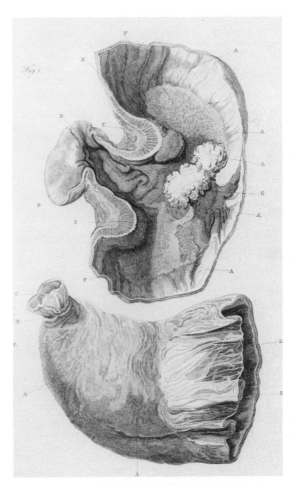

Cancer of the stomach, plate 7 of Baillie's engravings illustrating his *Morbid Anatomy,* 1799.

Matthew Baillie. **The Morbid Anatomy of Some of the Most Important Parts of the Human Body.** London: F. Johnson and G. Nicol, 1793.

A Series of Engravings, accompanied with Explanations which are intended to Illustrate the **Morbid Anatomy of Some of the Most Important Parts of the Human Body.** London: W. Bulmer and Co., 1799-1802.

Matthew Baillie. Classics in Oncology. **CA** 24: 47-56, Jan-Feb. 1974.

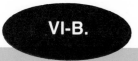

Medical Concepts

VI-B-1. Cancer a local disease: Gendron.

Claude Deshais Gendron (1663-1750) was a graduate of medicine at Montpellier, physician to the brother of the Sun King, Louis XIV, and later to the Duke of Orleans. His medical abilities and contributions were well recognized in his time. In 1700 he published his **Recherches sur la Nature et la Guerison des Cancer**, which was promptly translated into English.

After 8 years of observations and dissections, Gendron concluded that the 17th Century theory of cancer being due to acid ferments was not an improvement on the Galenical humors. He stated that cancer arises locally as a hard, growing mass, irreversible to drugs, that must be removed along with its "filaments." Successful treatment is possible only when "the very bottom of the callus and newly formed tumor can be removed from the flesh," which extends often more deeply than it is clinically suspected.

Gendron proposed no etiologic theory of cancer, but clearly indicated his belief that it was originally a localized, resectable entity. He illustrated his point by recounting the cure of a recurrent cancerous growth on the upper eyelid by a caustic substance while protecting the eye with gold leaf.

Gendron's words on one patient with advanced breast cancer retain currency, and, alas, only too much relevance:

"When the Queen Mother Ann of Astria developed a lump in her left breast, my Uncle, the late Abbott Gendron, was summoned to the Royal Palace. He examined her, and he informed the King that the lump was an adherent, incurable cancer moreover on the verge of ulcerating. . .

"But as members of the Royal Household could not tolerate the idea that incurable diseases should ever befall crowned heads, through intrigue and otherwise they managed to attract to the Palace workers of miracles. The latter promised the cure of the cancer with so much confidence that many thought it strange that the health of the Queen should be entrusted to someone who had declared her incurable and did nothing but endeavor to prolong her life, while there were others who promised a perfect cure.

Claude Deshais Gendron

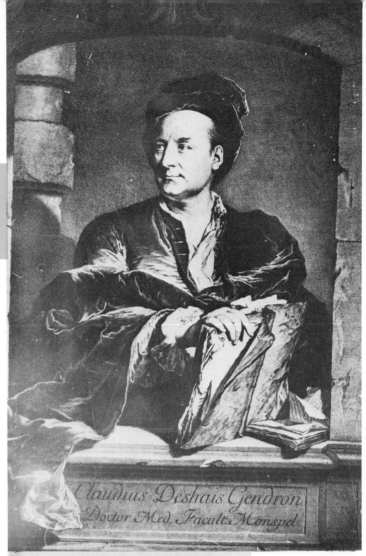

". . . The King discharged my Uncle. . .
and . . . my Uncle gave to the King a written account on what would be the effects
of this so-called secret drug, a remedy
well-known to him for a number of years.
And, without fail, the Queen did develop
every single complication my Uncle had
predicted, so that everyone could see,
though too late, there was a difference
between him who bookishly drew his
methods of treatment from the works of
Paracelsus and Van Helmont. . . my
Uncle who because of his long experience had relied mostly on his own better
understanding of the diseases. . .

"The cure of a disease, labeled incurable by those who master the Art of Healing, is not the privilege of those who
excel in the practice of deception."

Deshaies Gendron. **Enquiries Into the Nature,
Knowledge and Cure of Cancers.** London: J. Taylor, 1701.
P. Mustacchi and M. B. Shimkin. Gendron's Enquiries into
the Nature, Knowledge and Cure of Cancers. **Cancer** 9:
645-47, 1956.

RECHERCHES
SUR LA NATURE
ET
LA GUERISON
DES CANCERS.
Par Mr Deshaies GENDRON,
Docteur en Medecine de l'Uni-
versité de Montpellier.

A PARIS,
Chez ANDRE' CRAMOISY, ruë de
la Harpe, au Sacrifice d'Abraham.
M. DCC.

Gendron, *Recherches sur la Nature et la Guerison des Cancers,* 1700. Title page.

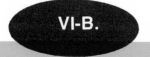

VI-B.

Medical Concepts

VI-B-2. Cancer and inflammation: Boerhaave

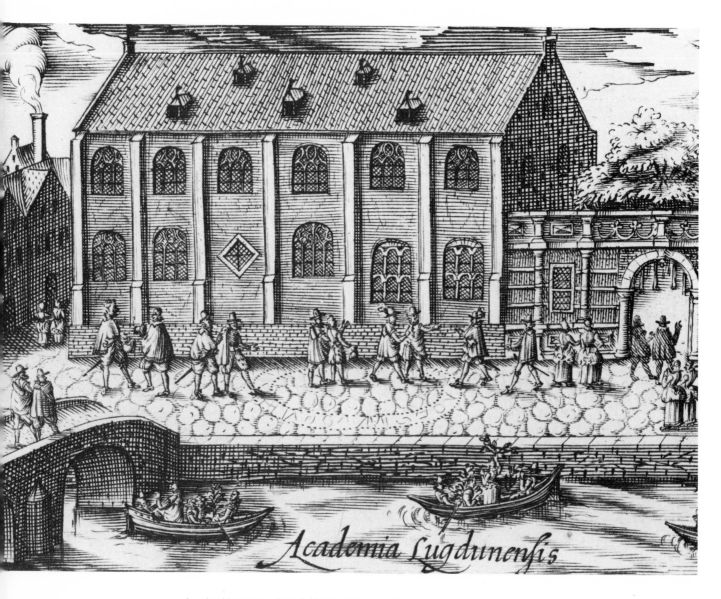

Leyden University, (from J. Meurs, Athenae batavae, Leyden, 1625).

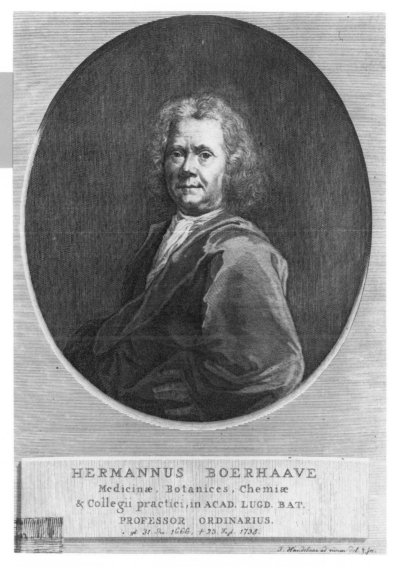

Hermann Boerhaave

Hermann Boerhaave (1668-1738) of Leyden was the most influential physician of his age, an intellectual descendant of Thomas Sydenham's return to Hippocratic medicine. He was an eclectic, without commitment to any medical theory. His teachings spread widely by his writings and by his pupils. Boerhaave's precepts were particularly influential in the schools in Vienna and Edinburgh, the latter attracting students from the American colonies.

Boerhaave's views on cancer linked it to inflammation, as summarized by Lindeboom:

"Inflammation might terminate in resolution, suppuration, gangrene, or scirrhus. A scirrhus is a hard, painless tumor ('tumor durus indolens'). It develops only in glands and may change to cancer under unfavorable circumstances. A scirrhus is caused by blocking of the excretory ducts, either by pressure from without or by shrivelling up, or coagulating the secretions. An example is the female breast, when, during lactation, the milk coagulates in the ducts. Any hard swelling which was not painful was considered to be a scirrhus."

Hermann Boerhaave. **Opera medica omnia.** Venice: 1742.
G. A. Lindeboom. **Hermann Boerhaave. The Man and His Work.** London: Methuen and Co., Ltd., 1968.

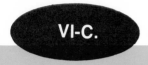

VI-C.

Surgery

VI-C-1. German cancer surgery: Heister.

Lorenz Heister (1683-1758) was among the leading German surgeons of the 18th Century, and professor of surgery at Altdorf and at Helmstedt. His **Chirurgie** of 1718 was one of the first systematic treatises on surgery, noted for its illustrations.

The operation for breast tumors he described was similar to that of Fabricius Hildanus and Scultetus. The instructions for the care of the patient begin with "Ordinary preoperative measures" of bleeding and purging. A special instrument could then be used to compress the breast at its base, or the breast was lifted by ligatures. The breast was then removed by a guillotine excision. Removal was recommended of the axillary lymph nodes and the underlying pectoral muscle. According to Cooper these methods must have resulted in some cures, but were largely abandoned for the less brutal and unfortunately less thorough operations of local excision with preservation of adequate amounts of skin for primary closure.

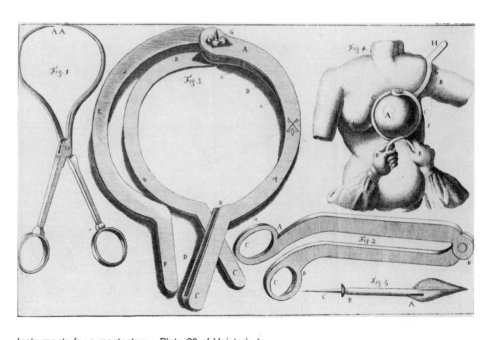

Instruments for a mastectomy. Plate 23 of Heister's *Institutiones Chirurgicae*, 1750.

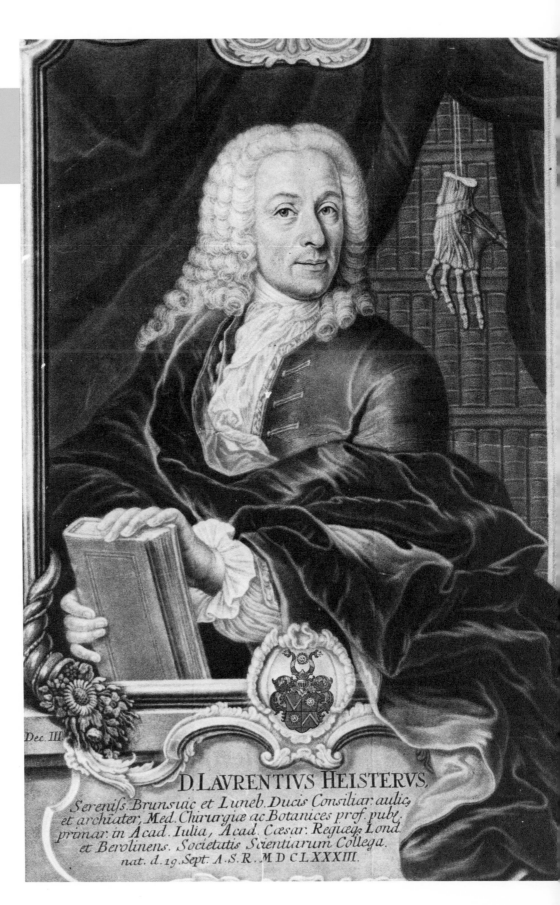

D. LAVRENTIVS HEISTERVS,

Sereniſſ. Brunſuac et Luneb. Ducis Conſiliar. aulic,
et archiater. Med. Chirurgiæ ac Botanices prof. publ,
pronar: in Acad. Iulia, Acad. Cæsar. Regiæ& Lond.
et Berolinens. Societatis Scientiarum Collega.
nat. d. 19. Sept. A. S. R. MDCLXXXIII.

Lorenz Heister. **Institutiones Chirurgicae.** Venice, 1750.
W. A. Cooper. The history of the radical mastectomy. **Ann.**
Med. Hist. 3: 36-54, 1941.

Lorenz Heister

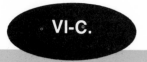

VI-C.

Surgery

VI-C-2. French cancer surgery: Petit and Le Dran.

Le Dran, *Memoire and Observations,* 1757.

Henri Francois Le Dran

Henri François Le Dran (1685-1770) is considered to be an important figure in the development of surgical concepts in the treatment of cancer. He divided cancer into 4 categories, cancer of the skin, cancer of the breast, cancer from reflux of menstrual products and cancer produced by abnormal lymph. He regarded cancer as a local disease in its early stage, which spread to regional lymph nodes and thence into the general circu-

lation, where it could involve the lungs. He dissected out enlarged axillary lymph nodes in breast cancer, but admitted that the outlook was bad when they were involved. Wide excision was recommended for cancer of the lip, or any other tumor, to clear up the area. The cancer indisposition was not only local, but could reside in the juices as an explanation for

Le Dran was a surgeon at the Hôpital Saint Côme, Paris, and his views were similar to those of Jean Louis Petit (1674-1750), first director of the French Academy and the commanding French surgeon of his age. For breast cancer, Petit recommended removal of not only the axillary nodes but some of pectoralis major muscle as well. Petit's observations were not published until 1774, twenty-four years after his death, but were well known to his contemporaries.

Petit, *Traité de Operations,* 1774. Title page.

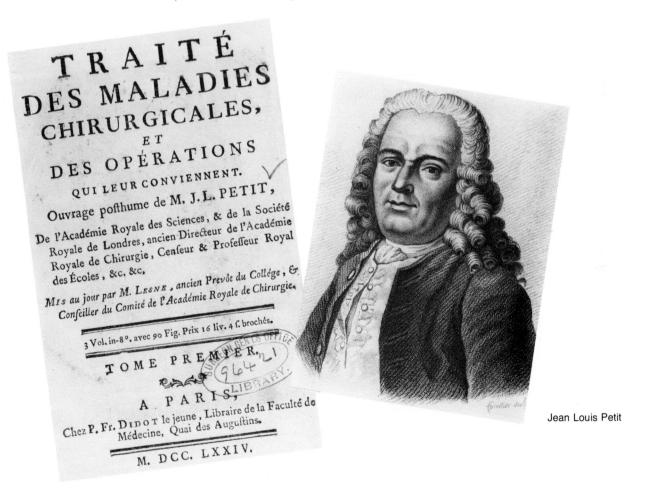

Jean Louis Petit

recurrence. Le Dran was an active opponent of all other forms of treatment for cancer instead of surgery, such as caustic pastes and internal remedies.

Le Dran's presentation is a slim memoir of 56 pages, prepared as a manual for students. It was translated into English and published within a year after the French original of 1757.

Henri F. Le Dran. Mémoire avec un précis de plusieurs observations sur le cancer. **Mem. acad. roy. de chir.** 3: 1-54, 1757.

Henri F. Le Dran. **Observations in Surgery**: Containing 115 different cases with particular remarks on each, for the improvement of young students. Transl. J. S., 3d ed. London: S. Crowder, 1758.

Jean Louis Petit. **Traité des malades chirurgicales**, et des **opérations qui leur conviennent** . . . Paris: Didot, 1774.

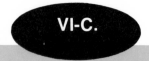

VI-C.

Surgery

VI-C-3. Rise of scientific surgery: John Hunter.

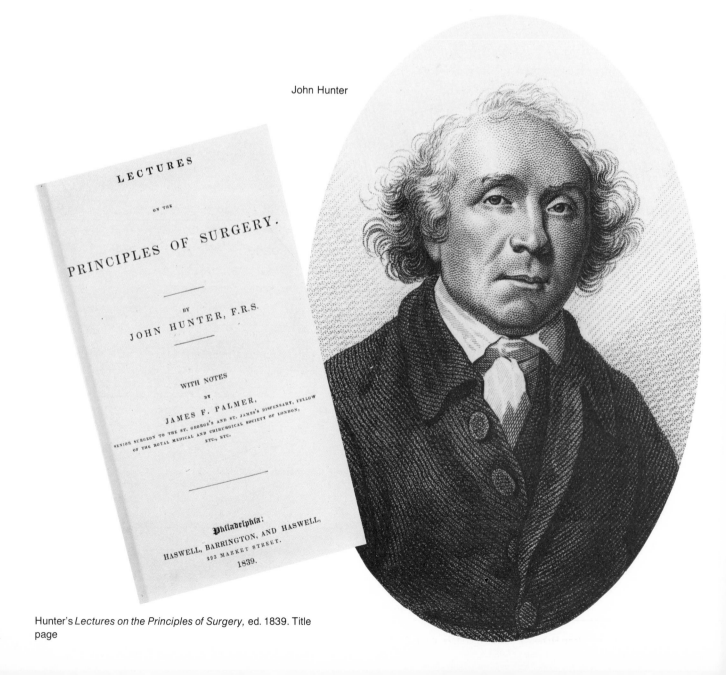

John Hunter

Hunter's *Lectures on the Principles of Surgery,* ed. 1839. Title page

John Hunter (1728-1793) was 5 foot 2 inches tall, but a giant in his contributions to anatomy and surgery. This Scotsman can be designated as the father of scientific surgery, but his influence permeated all of medicine.

Hunter's views on cancer reflect the shift from its interpretation as a manifestation of a generalized disease to one of more local origin, although in his lectures he retains both concepts. Following are excerpts on cancer from Hunter's **Lectures on the Principles of Surgery,** as summarized by Jessie Dobson.

"I would call that cancer which produces the following effects: viz, a circumscribed tumefaction with much hardness, and a drawing in of the skin covering it, as if the cellular membrane underneath it was destroyed; then a species of suppuration takes place in the centre and ulceration of the external surface . . . Cancer is one of the first class of our first division of poisons, viz, that which only produces local effects, though it has been supposed to contaminate the constitution; which would be terrible, indeed, as we have no specific nor even a palliative for it . . . .

"It most commonly attacks the conglomerate glands, the first the female breast; also the uterus, the lips, the external nose, the pancreas, and the pylorus; besides which the testicle is very subject to it, though that is not to be classed among the conglomerate glands . . ."

"It has been said that cancers are produced by ill health, as rheumatisms are; but this arises from the age of cancer being the age of such complaints and being thus the predisposing cause of both, but not particularly of the cancerous disposition. The predisposing causes are three in number, viz., age, parts of hereditary disposition; perhaps climate also has considerable effect, though not itself a predisposing cause. The cancerous age is from forty to sixty in both sexes, though it may occur sooner or later in certain cases. When cancer occurs in the breast of women under forty it is more rapid in its progress than when the patient is older and also more extensive; remote sympathy likewise takes place more readily in them than in the old, so that the operation succeeds better in the latter on this account. However, we seldom find it in the young or very old; though of the two it is most frequent in the latter . . .

"Some suppose cancers to be hereditary; but this I can only admit according to my principles of hereditary right; that is, supposing a person to possess a strong disposition or susceptibility for a particular disease, the children may also, but I have not yet ascertained the generality of this fact."

"Great attention should be paid to the tumour, whether it is moveable or not, for as the disease is further extended so the parts are more united to the tumour. If the tumour is not only moveable but the part naturally so, then there is no impropriety in removing it . . . if any consequent cancers easy of extirpation are found, they may safely be removed also. But it requires very great caution to know if any of these consequent tumours are within proper reach for we are apt to be deceived in regard to the lymphatic glands which often appear moveable when, on extirpation, a chain of them is found to run far beyond out of our reach which renders the operation unsuccessful. As this is not easily known, I would, in most cases, where the lymphatic glands are considerably enlarged, advise that the case should be let alone."

Jessie Dobson. John Hunter's views on cancer. **Ann. Roy. Coll. Surg. England** 25: 167-81, 1959.

John Hunter. **Lectures on the Principles of Surgery.** Philadelphia: Haswell, Barrington and Haswell, 1839.

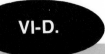

VI-D.

Cancer Hospitals

VI-D-1. French cancer charity: Rheims.

Jean Godinot, a canon of the Cathedran of Rheims, "a charitable and pious man who had devoted his whole life to caring for poor patients and relieving their misfortunes," in his will left a considerable sum of money to the city to be used for the erection and maintenance of a hospital exclusively for patients with cancer. The hospital, of 12 beds, was opened in 1740, and is recognized as among the earliest facilities for cancer.

The motivation for the special facility, other than charity, was the fear that cancer was contagious. This belief was not evident during the medieval period although cancer was classified as a tumor contrary to nature, which included carbuncles, tubercles, pustules, and other inflammatory conditions. During the 17th Century the contagiousness of cancer was expressed by Zacutus, Tulp and Sennert.

The inhabitants of Rheims, wanting to avoid patients with cancer, succeeded in having the hospital moved to outside the city in 1779. The next building, continuing under the direction of the personnel of the Hôtel Dieu, was named the Hôpital Saint Louis. It was used exclusively for patients with cancer until 1846.

R. Ledoux-Lebard. **La Lutte Contre Le Cancer.** Paris: Masson et Cie, 1906.

Les Centres Anti-Cancéreaux Français. **Vingt-Cinq ans d'Activité 1945-1970.** Rouen: Imp. Le Clerf.

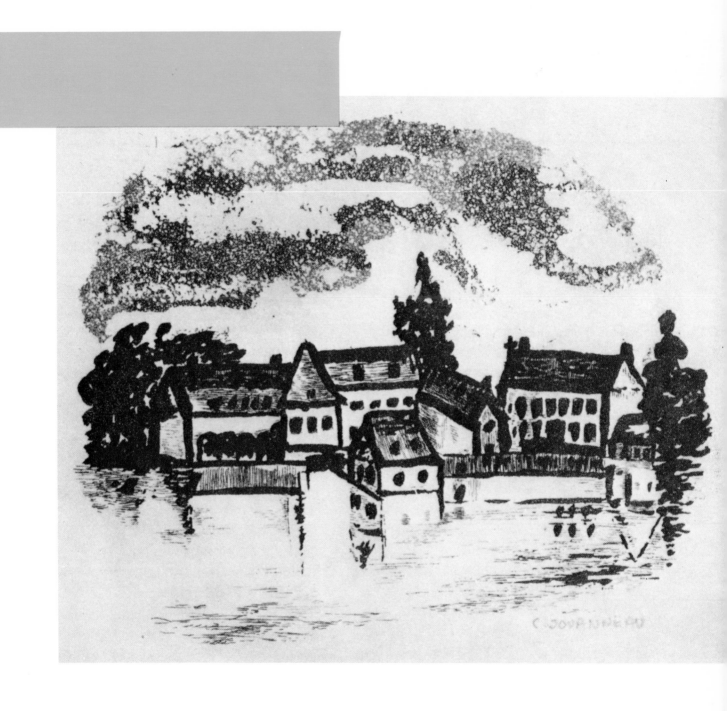

La Buerie, près de Reims (drawing by C. Jouanneau, from *Les Centres Anti-cancéreaux Français,* 1945-1970).

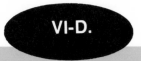

Cancer Hospitals

VI-D-2. First cancer institute: Middlesex.

In 1791, John Howard, a London surgeon and an ex-pupil of Percivall Pott, informed the Governors of the Middlesex Hospital that a friend of his, who wished to remain anonymous, desired to contribute a sum of money for the establishment of a cancer charity for the hospital. The principal objects of the bequest were "...the relief of persons afflicted with cancer, and the investigation of a complaint which, though extremely common, is, both with regard to its natural history and cure, but imperfectly known." Howard's generous friend was later known to be Samuel Whitbread (1720-96).

In June, 1792, a ward containing 12 beds was ready to receive cancer cases at the Middlesex Hospital. These included not only patients for whom there was a reasonable prospect of relief by operation or otherwise but also those whose disease was hopelessly advanced and who would be offered an asylum for life. The regulations stated that these patients "shall remain an unlimited time, until either relieved by art or released by death, unless it should be thought necessary to discharge them for ill-behaviour" (Wilson, 1845).

John Howard pointed out that such an institution would offer facilities for studying the natural history of cancer, and he emphasized the importance of keeping careful clinical records of all patients which should be made available for general inspection.

"This examination may be made by a medical gentleman of the hospital, with the patient before him, his notes to be corrected by himself, and kept as a record of the history and circumstances of each case, to be referred to as an authority by any intelligent or scientific person. A copy of these notes may be kept, fairly written for general instruction, and if anything extraordinary or worthy of more particular notice arises from these sources, let them be published to the world at large."

Howard stipulated that the nature of the disease should be investigated and trials made of new authentic methods of treatment. In 1853 the cancer wards contained 26 beds. By the beginning of the present century there was a wing with some 50 beds, and between 70 and 80 postmortem examinations were being carried out annually in the research laboratories (Coupland, 1902). The Middlesex Hospital Cancer Charity can be considered as the first cancer institute.

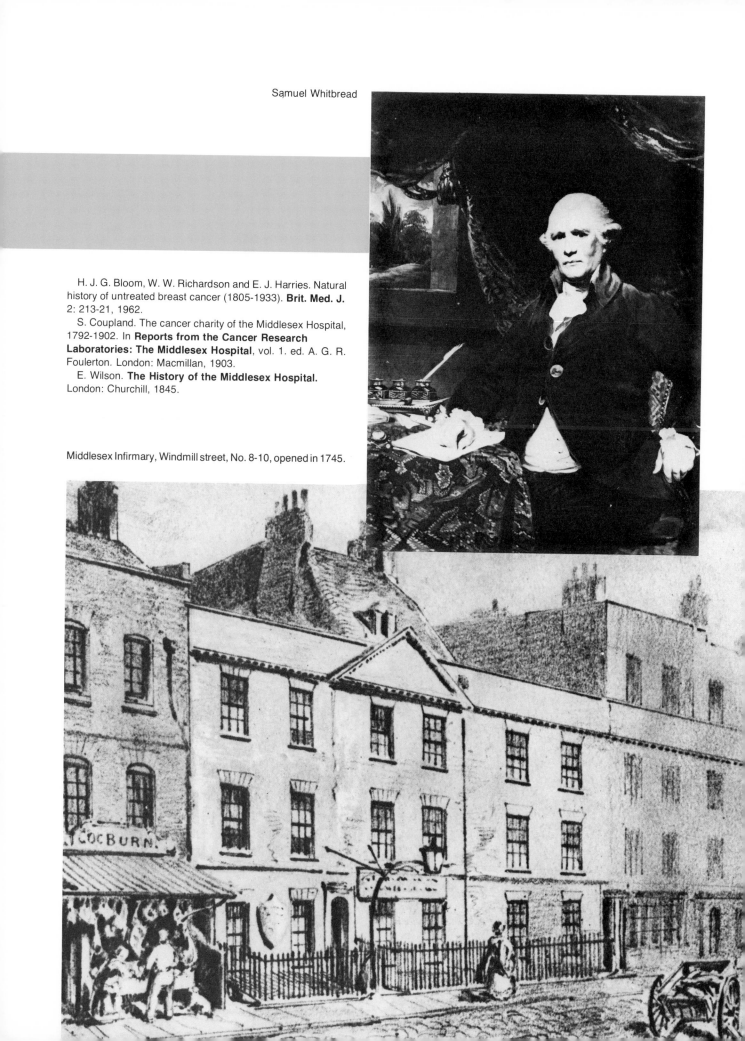

Samuel Whitbread

H. J. G. Bloom, W. W. Richardson and E. J. Harries. Natural history of untreated breast cancer (1805-1933). **Brit. Med. J.** 2: 213-21, 1962.

S. Coupland. The cancer charity of the Middlesex Hospital, 1792-1902. In **Reports from the Cancer Research Laboratories: The Middlesex Hospital**, vol. 1. ed. A. G. R. Foulerton. London: Macmillan, 1903.

E. Wilson. **The History of the Middlesex Hospital.** London: Churchill, 1845.

Middlesex Infirmary, Windmill street, No. 8-10, opened in 1745.

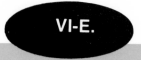

VI-E.

Carcinogenic Environments

VI-E-1. Breast cancer in nuns: Ramazzini.

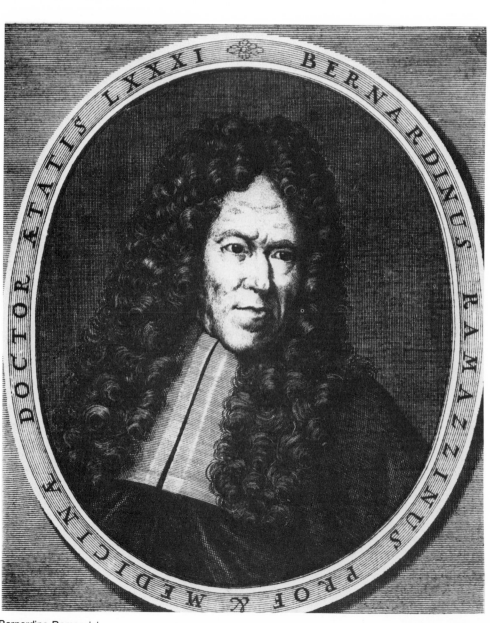

Bernardino Ramazzini

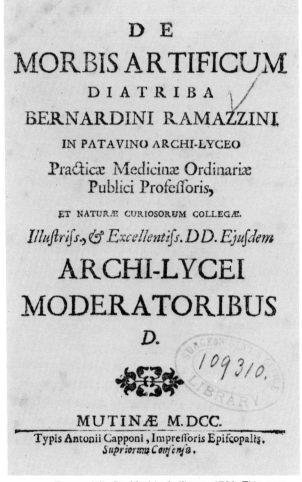

Ramazzini's *De Morbis Artificum,* 1700. Title page

Wilmer Cave Wright. **De Morbis Artificum by Bernardino Ramazzini. The Latin Text of 1713.** Revised with translations and notes. Chicago: University of Chicago Press, 1940. (p. 191).

Bernardino Ramazzini (1633-1714), introduced occupational medicine as a systematic study in his **De Morbis artificium** of 1700, although Paracelsus had called attention to stone-mason's and miner's phthisis and other diseases among industrial workers some 150 years earlier.

In Chapter XX, on diseases of wet-nurses, Ramazzini records the high occurrence of breast cancer among nuns: ". . . experience proves that as a consequence of disturbances in the uterus, cancerous tumors are very often generated in the woman's breast, and tumors of this sort are found in nuns more often than in any other women. Now these are not caused by suppression of the menses but rather, in my opinion, by their celibate life. For I have known several cases of nuns who came to a pitiable end from terrible cancers of the breast. . . . Every city in Italy has several religious communities of nuns, and you seldom can find a convent that does not harbor this accursed pest, cancer, within its walls."

This is perhaps the first record of associating an occupation, of being a nun, and a celibate way of life, with cancer of the breast.

Carcinogenic Environments

VI-E-2. Tobacco cancers: Hill and Soemmering.

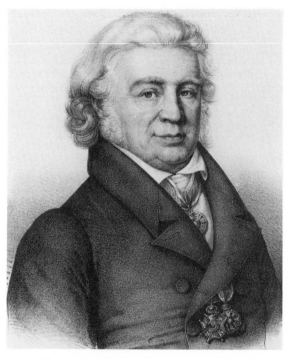

Samuel Thomas von Soemmering

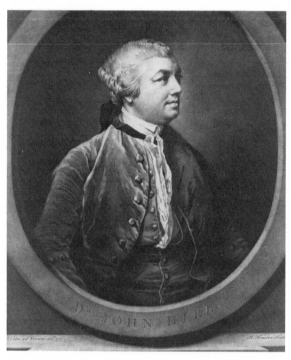

John Hill

John Hill (1716-1775) of London, in 1761 published his **Cautions Against the Immoderate Use of Snuff,** in which he reported six cases of "polypusses" related to indulgence in tobacco in the form of snuff. One polypus was described as a swelling in one nostril that was hard, black and adherent on a broad base. Painless at first, it later developed "all the frightful symptoms of an open cancer." The discussion included these wise and still current remarks: "Whether or not polypusses, which attend Snuff-takers, are absolutely caused by that custom: or whether the principles of the disorder were there before, and Snuff only irritated the parts, and hastened the mischief, I shall not pretend to determine: but

D. Eugene Redmond, Jr. Tobacco and cancer: the first clinical report, 1761. **New England J. Med.** 282: 18-23, 1970.

S. Th. Sommering. **De Morbis Vasorum Absorventium Corporis Humani.** Frankfurt/Main, 1795. (p. 109).

E. L. Wynder and D. Hoffman. Experimental tobacco carcinogenesis. **Adv. Cancer Res.** 8: 249-453, 1964.

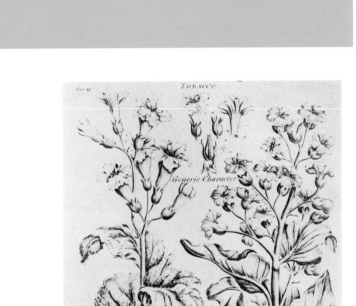

Tobacco plant (from D.E. Redmond, Jr., *New Engl. J. Med,* 1970)

CAUTIONS

Againſt the immoderate Uſe of

SNUFF.

Founded on the known Qualities of the

TOBACCO PLANT;

And the Effects it muſt produce when this Way taken into the Body:

AND

Enforced by Inſtances of Perſons who have periſhed miſerably of Diſeaſes, occaſioned, or rendered incurable by its Uſe.

By Dr. J. HILL.

THE SECOND EDITION.

LONDON:

Printed for R. BALDWIN in Pater-noſter Row, and J. JACKSON in St. James's-ſtreet.

MDCCLXI.

[PRICE ONE SHILLING.]

Hill's *Cautions against Snuff,* 1761. (from D.E. Redmond, Jr., *New Engl. J. Med,* 1970)

even supposing the latter only to be the case, the damage is certainly more than the indulgence is worth . . . . no man should venture upon Snuff, who is not sure that he is not so far liable to cancer: and no man can be sure of that."

Hill's report preceded by over a decade the description of chimney sweeps' scrotal cancer by Percivall Pott.

Samuel Thomas von Soemmering (1755-1830), Polish-born professor of anatomy at Mainz in 1795 added pipe smoking to identified environmental carcinogens. "Carcinoma of the lips occurs most frequently where men indulge in pipe smoking; the lower lips is particularly affected by cancer when it is compressed between the tobacco pipe and the teeth."

VI-E.

Carcinogenic Environments

VI-E-3. Chimney sweeps' cancer: Pott.

Percivall Pott (1714-1788), the eminent 18th Century surgeon of London's prestigious St. Bartholomew's Hospital, is the acknowledged first source of our knowledge about chemical carcinogenesis. His description in 1775 of cancer of the scrotum in chimney sweeps leaves no doubt that this was recognized as an occupational cancer caused by chronic exposure to an environmental agent, soot, in youngsters whose fate was "singularly hard" even for those days.

William Blake in his Songs of Innocence of 1789, wrote:

When my mother died I was very
    young
And my father sold me while my
    tongue
Could scarcely cry "weep, weep,
    weep, weep"
So your chimney I sweep and in soot
    I sleep.

There is no indication in Pott's essay of some 800 words that a new finding was being described, although it was not "publickly noted". The impression is that the condition was not unknown to surgeons of his time. Certainly the association of scrotal cancer to soot was recognized by the chimney sweepers, since "the trade call is the soot-wart".

Pott makes no mention of possible preventive measures such as avoidance of soot or better hygienic conditions. Scrotal cancer as a clinical entity continued to be described during the subsequent century. Its public health resolution was achieved through social conscience against child labor and appropriate legislative and regulatory actions.

Pott's description is devoid of numbers. Numerical expressions had to await the 19th Century, as in the lectures of Henry Butlin, and experimental replication in animals came during the 20th Century.

Percivall Pott. **Chirurgical Observations Relative to the Cataract, the Polypus of the Nose, the Cancer of the Scrotum, the Different Kinds of Ruptures, and the Mortification of the Toes and Feet.** London: Hawes, Clarke and Collins, 1775.

M. B. Shimkin and V. A. Triolo. History of chemical carcinogenesis: some prospective remarks. **Progr. Exp. Tumor Res.** 11: 1-20, 1969.

Michael Potter. Percivall Pott's contribution to cancer research. **NCI Monograph** No. 10, p. 1-13, 1963.

H. T. Butlin. Three lectures on cancer of the scrotum in chimney-sweeps and others. **Brit. Med. J.** 1: 1341-46, 2: 1-6, 66-71, 1892.

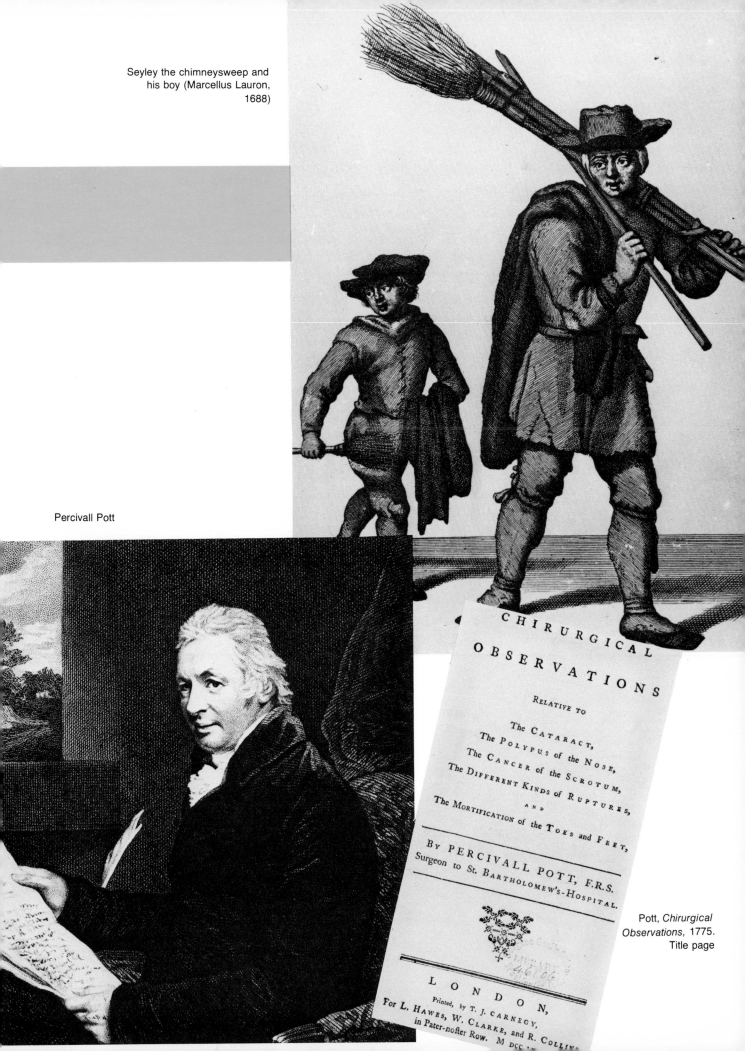

Seyley the chimneysweep and his boy (Marcellus Lauron, 1688)

Percivall Pott

Pott, *Chirurgical Observations*, 1775. Title page

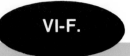

Experimental Oncology

VI-F-1. Cancer biochemistry: Astruc.

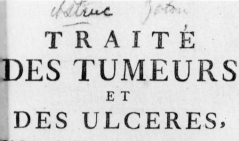

TRAITÉ
DES TUMEURS
ET
DES ULCERES,

Où l'on a tâché de joindre à une *Théorie solide*;
la Pratique la plus sûre & la mieux éprouvée:

AVEC DEUX LETTRES,

I. Sur la *Composition de quelques Remedes*, dont on
vante l'utilité, & dont on cache la préparation.

II. Sur la nature & le succès des nouveaux Remedes, qu'on
propose pour la guérison des *Maladies Vénériennes*.

TOME PREMIER.

*Ego fateor me ex eorum numero esse conari, qui proficiendo
scribunt, & scribendo proficiunt.* D. August. Epist. 143. n. 2.

A PARIS,

Chez P. GUILLAUME CAVELIER, Libraire,
rue S. Jacques, au Lys d'Or.

M. DCC. LIX.
Avec Approbation & Privilége du Roi.

DES TUMEURS. 69

arrive aux pommes de *momordica*, ne
puisse arriver à la masse chancreuse;
ou pour mieux dire, on ne peut pas
douter que cela n'y arrive, puisqu'on
le voit arriver sous ses yeux. Voilà qui
suffit, comme on l'a vû, pour rendre
raison de tous les symptomes du cancer, sans avoir besoin de supposer une
humeur âcre, rongeante, corrosive,
dont l'existence n'a nulle vraisemblan-
ce: car enfin d'où viendroit tout-à-
coup dans la masse qui commence à
dégénérer en cancer, une pareille humeur, dont il n'y avoit pas le moin-
dre vestige quelques jours auparavant,
tant que la masse n'étoit que squir-
rheuse?

.V. Autrefois, lorsque j'étois encore
prévenu pour l'opinion commune, sur
laquelle je ne laissois pas d'avoir beau-
coup de doutes, je fis une expérience
qui contribua à m'éclairer. Je pris une
mammelle chancreuse que j'avois fait
abattre, pesant environ sept livres,
& après l'avoir coupée en morceaux,
je l'exposai à la distillation dans une
cornue au bain de sable. Je ramassai
avec soin tous les principes que la

---

70   *TRAITÉ*

distillation me donna, de même que le
sel fixe que je retirai du *caput mortuum*
par la voie ordinaire. Je pris ensuite
le même poids de tranche de bœuf,
que j'exposai à une distillation sembla-
ble, en ramassant de même tous les
principes que la distillation fournit. Je
comparai exactement ces différens principes, sur-tout les sels, tant volatiles
que fixes. La quantité en étoit à-peu-
près égale, & la qualité me parut ab-
solument la même dans toutes les
épreuves que je fis, soit en les em-
ployant pour précipiter les métaux
dissous par des menstrues acides; soit
en les faisant fermenter avec les acides que j'y mêlai; soit en m'en ser-
vant pour tirer la teinture des résines;
soit en les mêlant avec le syrop vio-
lat, pour juger du changement de cou-
leur; soit enfin en le goutant avec attention. D'où je conclus que tout ce
qu'on dit de l'humeur âcre, rongeante, corrosive des cancers, étoit une
supposition fausse, & qu'il falloit par
conséquent chercher à expliquer par
quelque autre voie la génération de
ces tumeurs.

Astruc, *Traité des Tumeurs et des Ulceres,*
2 vols, 1759. Title page

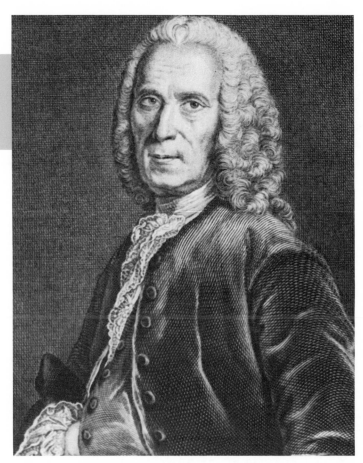

Jean Astruc

Jean Astruc (1684-1766), graduate of Montpellier, professor of anatomy in Paris, and physician to kings in France and in Poland, was a prolific writer. He is best known for his treatises on dermatology and venereal disease, but he also wrote on tumors.

His views were that lymphatic abnormality led to the formation of scirrhus, from which cancer developed. The initial thickening of lymph could be due to psychic depression as well as to trauma, scabies and obstipation! He separated true tumors from cysts, which he considered to be dilated lymphatics.

Astruc performed what Wolff called a naive experiment, recorded on pages 69 and 70 in the second volume of his treatise on tumors and ulcers. Astruc took a piece of cancerous breast, and a piece of beefsteak, incinerated these in retorts and found no difference in taste between the two. He thus disproved that cancer had bitter or salty materials in excess of those in normal meat. This wrote off both the black bile and the excess acid theories of cancer as far as he was concerned. Astruc can well be designated as the first biochemist to compare cancerous with normal tissue.

Jean Astruc. **Traité des Tumeurs et des Ulcères.** 2 vols. Paris: P. Guillaume Cavelier, 1759.

R. Süss, V. Kinzel and J. D. Scribner. **Cancer. Experiments and Concepts.** New York: Springer-Verlag, 1973. (p. 4).

Jacob Wolff. **Die Lehre von der Krebskrankheit.** Jena: Gustav Fischer, 1907. Vol. 1, p. 63-4.

VI-F.

Experimental Oncology

VI-F-2. Attempt to transfer cancer: Peyrilhe.

DISSERTATION
ACADÉMIQUE
SUR
LE CANCER,

QUI a remporté le prix double de l'A-
cadémie des Sciences, Arts & Belles-
Lettres de Lyon, le 8 Décembre 1773.

Par BER. PEYRILHE,

*Professeur - Royal au Collége de Chirurgie de
Paris, Conseiller du Comité de l'Académie
Royale de Chirurgie, Docteur en Médécine
de la Faculté de Toulouse, de l'Académie
des Sciences, Inscriptions & Belles-Lettres
de la même Ville, & de celle des Sciences
de Montpellier.*

Prolem fine matre creatam.

A P A R I S,

Chez RUAULT, Libraire, rue de la Harpe.

M. DCC LXXVI.

Peyrilhe, *Dissertation Academique sur le Cancer,* 1776. Title page

A

DISSERTATION

ON

CANCEROUS DISEASES.

BY

BER. PEYRILHE, M.D.

REGIUS PROFESSOR OF SURGERY, AND MEM-
BER OF THE ROYAL ACADEMY OF SUR-
GERY, AT PARIS; AND OF THE
ACADEMIES OF MONTPELLIER,
TOULOUSE, &c.

TRANSLATED FROM THE LATIN, WITH NOTES.

L O N D O N:

PRINTED FOR J. WILKIE, No. 71, St. PAUL'S CHURCH-YARD.

M.DCC.LXXVII.

Peyrilhe, *Dissertation* in English translation, 1777. Title page

In 1773 the Academy of Lyon in France offered a prize for the best thesis on the subject of What is Cancer? The winner was Bernard Peyrilhe (1735-1804), who identified himself as Professor of Chemistry at the Ecole de Sante and Professor-Royal at the College of Surgery in Paris, and who also wrote a text on the history of surgery.

Peyrilhe considered cancer to be a local process that invaded and generalized through the lymphatics. He recognized that there was no difference between scirrhus and cancer, other than scirrhus being an earlier manifestation before ulceration. He advocated surgical treatment for cancer. In breast cancer, removal of the axillary lymph nodes and even the underlying muscle were considered desirable.

To elucidate the nature of cancer, Peyrilhe recorded what was perhaps the first experimental approach to the problem. He took fluid from a mammary cancer of a woman and introduced the material under the skin of a dog. The wound opened after three days, and the dog began to howl enough to disturb Peyrilhe's housekeeper, who destroyed the animal.

Peyrilhe's thesis looms rather large by retrospective evaluation of his views and his minimal experiment. However, he seems to have been quite obscure during his time. For example, no portrait of him can be located in an age when likenesses of prominent academic clinicians were the rule.

Bernard Peyrilhe. **Dissertation Académique sur le Cancer.** Paris: Ruault, 1776.

VII. 19th Century: Invention And Industry

During the 19th Century biomedical sciences and medicine reached new heights of progress and achievement.

This was the century of Darwin, who redefined man in the world of living creatures, as Newton had defined man's place in the material universe. This was the century of Pasteur, who invented bacteriology and with Koch began man's conquest over infectious diseases. Virchow oriented pathology to the cellular level, and led German science to preeminence.

The greatest invention of the 19th Century, according to Whitehead, was the invention of the method of invention. Technology sparked the industrial revolution. Every pattern of life was permanently modified by railways, steamboats, telegraphs, telephones, spinning machines, and synthetic chemicals.

In medicine, quantitative methods began to be introduced, by Louis in his numerical method of evaluating treatment (1835), and by Wunderlich in his application of the thermometer to clinical practice (1868). Liebig and Wöhler demonstrated the unity of organic and inorganic chemistry (1828). Virchow and his associates developed cellular pathology as the basis for scientific medicine. Specificity of observations and experimentation gradually replaced simplistic, theoretical systems of medicine, iatrochemical, Brunonian or homeopathic. The latter did have influence against meddlesome, excessive drugging and bleeding of orthodox medicine.

Oncology was ushered into its histologic stage by Johannes Müller and the achromatic microscope. Surgery was made painless by the great American discovery of anesthesia, which preceded by 20 years the introduction in 1867 of antisepsis and asepsis by Joseph Lister. Now the great surgeons, led by Theodor Billroth of Vienna, could attempt to remove cancers of internal organs.

And at the very close of the Century, three discoveries were made that would guide oncology as well as all other biomedical sciences: Roentgen described X-rays in 1895, and the Curies isolated radium in 1898; filterable viruses entered the scene of infectious agents in 1892, with Ivanowski's work on tobacco mosaic; genetics became a new field of inquiry with the rediscovery by de Vries in 1900 of Mendel's publication of 1865.

J. D. Bernal. **Science in History.** 4 vols. Cambridge, Mass.: The MIT Press, 1971. Vol. 2, p. 634ff.

Edward McNall Burns. **Western Civilizations. Their History and Their Culture.** Ed. 8. New York: W. W. Norton, 1973. (p. 696ff).

Alfred North Whitehead. **Science and the Modern World.** New York: Macmillan, 1925. (p. 96ff).

THE ORIGIN OF SPECIES

BY MEANS OF NATURAL SELECTION,

OR THE

PRESERVATION OF FAVOURED RACES IN THE STRUGGLE FOR LIFE.

By CHARLES DARWIN, M.A.,

FELLOW OF THE ROYAL, GEOLOGICAL, LINNÆAN, ETC., SOCIETIES;
AUTHOR OF 'JOURNAL OF RESEARCHES DURING H. M. S. BEAGLE'S VOYAGE
ROUND THE WORLD.'

LONDON:
JOHN MURRAY, ALBEMARLE STREET.
1859.

DIE

CELLULARPATHOLOGIE

in ihrer Begründung auf

physiologische und pathologische Gewebelehre.

Zwanzig Vorlesungen,

gehalten

während der Monate Februar, März und April 1858 im pathologischen
Institute zu Berlin

von

RUDOLF VIRCHOW,

o. ö. Prof. der pathologischen Anatomie, der allgemeinen Pathologie u. Therapie an der
Universität, Direktor des patholog. Instituts u. dirigirendem Arzte a. d. Charité.

Mit 144 Holzschnitten.

BERLIN, 1858.
Verlag von August Hirschwald.
69 Unter den Linden (Ecke der Schadowstr.).

VII-A.

The London Group: New Questions of Cancer

English medicine at the end of the 18th Century was oriented around the giant figures of John and William Hunter. They laid the foundations for scientific surgery, anatomy, obstetrics and dentistry. Cancer was among the many interests of the Hunters and their associates.

In 1801, there was formed an "Institution for Investigating the Nature and Cure of Cancer," under the Society for Bettering the Condition and Increasing the Comforts of the Poor. Its medical committee published a report in 1802, in which it proposed 13 questions, as follows:

1. What are the diagnostic signs of cancer?

2. Does any alteration take place in the structure of a part, preceding that more obvious change which is called cancer? If there does, what is the nature of that alteration?

3. Is cancer always an original and primary disease, or may other diseases degenerate into cancer?

4. Are there any proofs of cancer being an hereditary disease?

5. Are there any proofs of cancer being a contagious disease?

6. Is there any well-marked relation between cancer and other diseases? If there be, what are those diseases to which it bears the nearest resemblance, in its origin, progress, and termination?

7. May cancer be regarded at any period, or under any circumstances, merely as a local disease? or, does the existence of cancer in one part, afford a presumption, that there is a tendency to a similar morbid alteration, in other parts of the animal system?

8. Has climate, or local situation, any influence in rendering the human constitution more or less liable to cancer, under any form, or in any part?

9. Is there a particular temperament of body more liable to be affected with cancer than others? and if there be, what is that temperament?

10. Are brute-creatures subject to any disease, resembling cancer in the human subject?

THE

EDINBURGH

MEDICAL AND SURGICAL

JOURNAL:

EXHIBITING

A CONCISE VIEW

OF THE LATEST AND MOST IMPORTANT

*DISCOVERIES IN MEDICINE, SURGERY,
AND PHARMACY.*

1806.

VOLUME SECOND

EDINBURGH:

PRINTED FOR ARCHIBALD CONSTABLE & COMPANY, EDINBURGH;
AND JOHN MURRAY, LONDON; AND GILBERT
& HODGES, DUBLIN.

1806.

Thomas Denman

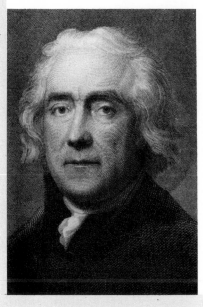

382   *Inſtitution for Inveſtigating the Nature of Cancer.*   July

The MEDICAL COMMITTEE of the SOCIETY for INVESTIGATING the
NATURE and CURE of CANCER, conſiſting of Drs Baillie, Sims, and
Willan; Meſſ. Sharpe, Home, Pearſon, and Abernethy, and Dr Denman,
Secretary, circulated in 1802 a ſet of Queries for obtaining information regarding theſe. Since that time they have been republiſhed, with Obſerva-
tions explanatory of their object. In reprinting a *Brochure* of ſo much
intrinſic value, we hope both to preſerve it, and to forward the views
of ſo laudable an Inſtitution.

EVERY perſon muſt be ſenſible of the various difficulties attending
the eſtabliſhment of a new inſtitution, and of the much greater and
more numerous difficulties which beſet our firſt ſteps in the acquiſition
of knowledge on a ſubject of which, it may be ſaid, we are even at
this time totally ignorant *. But, in order to form a baſis of inquiry, in which the nature and cure of cancer, it is preſumed, may be
purſued with all the advantages of reaſon and experience, the Medical Committee very early drew out and diſtributed the following
queries, for the conſideration not only of the correſponding members,
but of all medical men, to whom opportunities of anſwering them
might, by ſtudy or by accident, occur. A ſatisfactory anſwer to any
one of theſe queries would, in itſelf, be of great importance, and
might probably lead to an explanation of others. It is therefore ear-
neſtly requeſted, if any new obſervation or diſcovery reſpecting cancer ſhould be made, that it may be communicated to the ſecretary of
this inſtitution; and, if any progreſs in the inveſtigation of the nature and cure of cancer be made by or imparted to them, it will,
without delay, be laid before the public by the Medical Committee.
It may be neceſſary to obſerve that the promoters of this inſtitution
have never entertained the idea of creating the jealouſy, or of inter-
fering with the intereſts, of thoſe who are engaged in inſtitutions of
a ſimilar kind; their intention being ſolely that of co-operating in
the laudable endeavour to leſſen the maſs of human miſery, by calling
for the aſſiſtance of others, and by exerting themſelves to obtain a
remedy for a moſt painful and dreadful diſeaſe, againſt which all the
medicines and methods of treatment hitherto propoſed and tried
have been unavailing.

11. Is there any period of life absolutely exempt from the attack of
this disease?

12. Are the lymphatic glands ever affected primarily in cancer?

13. Is cancer under any circumstances susceptible of a natural
cure?

The committee was organized by
Thomas Denman (1733-1815), and consisted of Matthew Baillie (1761-1823),
James Sims (1741-1820), Robert Willan
(1757-1812), Everard Home (1756-
1832), John Pearson (1758-1826) and
John Abernathy (1764-1831), and a Mr.
Sharpe, who remains unidentified. An attempt by the group to set up a clinical
facility for cancer floundered in 1805.

Institution for Investigating the Nature and Cure of Cancer.
Edin. Med. Surg. J. 2: 382-89, 1802.

Thomas Denman. **Observations on the Cure of Cancer.**
London: J. Johnson, 1810.

M. B. Shimkin. Thirteen questions: some historical outlines
for cancer research. **J. Natl. Cancer Inst.** 19: 295-328, 1957.

V. A. Triolo. The Institution for Investigating the Nature and
Cure of Cancer. A study of four excerpts. **Med. Hist.** 13:
11-28, 1969.

105

VII-B.

The Paris School: Bichat and Laënnec.

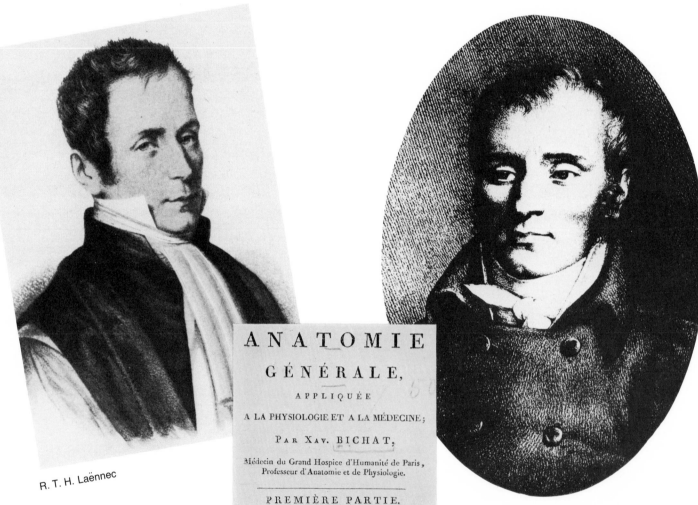

R. T. H. Laënnec

ANATOMIE
GÉNÉRALE,
APPLIQUÉE
A LA PHYSIOLOGIE ET A LA MÉDECINE;
PAR Xav. BICHAT,
Médecin du Grand Hospice d'Humanité de Paris,
Professeur d'Anatomie et de Physiologie.

PREMIÈRE PARTIE.

TOME PREMIER.

A PARIS,
Chez Brosson, Gabon et Cie, Libraires, rue Pierre-
Sarrazin, no. 6, et place de l'Ecole-de-Médecine.

AN X. (1801.)

Xavier Bichat

Bichat, *Anatomie Generale,* 1801. Title page.

The French revolution saw the rise of a group of medical leaders who rejected the theories of their predecessors for their own observations. Among these were Bichat and Laënnec.

Marie-François-Xavier Bichat (1771-1802) was the most important pathologist between Morgagni and Virchow, in founding a system of normal and pathologic anatomy based on tissues rather than on organs. Had he not died at the age of 31, the next step, of cellular pathology, might have been made in France rather than in Germany. He discarded the division of scirrhus and ulcerated cancer. He considered that tumors arose from connective tissue and had a common tissue structure.

René-Théophile-Hyacinthe Laënnec (1781-1826) will retain immortality as the discoverer of the stethoscope. He was a pathologist as well as a clinician, and carried forward Bichat's ideas on tissues. His descriptions of cancer were accurate, and his experience with it was wide. Tumors were classified into scirrhous, encephaloid and melanotic. He recognized that scirrhous tumors were not specific but had large amounts of connective tissue, whereas the soft encephaloid tumors, so called because of the resemblance to the brain, lacked scar tissue. Melanoma was considered to be a distinct form of cancer.

Neither Bichat nor Laënnec lived long enough to publish their contributions in full. The Paris school of the Revolutionary-Napoleonic period, initially auspiciously led by Pinel and by Corvisart, later was represented by Broussais, a notorious bleeder, and Dupuytren, an able but crude surgeon. The work of Pierre-Charles-Alexandre Louis (1787-1872), who began to use medical statistics as a guide to therapy, was more influential with American students than with his French colleagues.

Xavier Bichat. **Anatomie Générale Appliquée à la Physiologie et à la Médecine.** 2 vol. Paris: Brosson, Gabon et Cie, 1801.

Laënnec. Encephaloides. In **Dictionnaire des Sciences Medicales, par une soc. med. et chir.** 60 vol. Paris: Crapart and Panckoucke, 1812-22. 12: 165, 1815.

P-C-A Louis. **Recherches sur les Effets de la Saignée.** Paris: J. B. Bailliere, 1835.

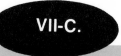

Pre-Listerian Surgery

VII-C-1. In the shadow of John Hunter: Home.

Everard Home (1756-1832), brother-in-law of the Hunters, is better known for injudiciously destroying some of John Hunter's manuscripts than for his own considerable accomplishments. Jane Oppenheimer has written astutely about this episode.

In many of his writings, Home freely and humbly acknowledged his debt to John Hunter. In his **Observations on Cancer,** published in 1805, he said "Much, certainly, originated with Mr. Hunter; perhaps the greatest part . . ." The book was a collection of cases, and represented the status of knowledge regarding cancer that existed among post-Hunterian surgeons. The clinical descriptions were accurate, treatment was limited to surgical excision when possible, and a number of autopsy reports were included.

Home's **Observations** were one of many monographs of surgical case reports of the period. Others of the time include the 1793 book by John Pearson, and the 1811 prize essay of Johnson.

In 1830 Home published another book on cancer, which contained the first

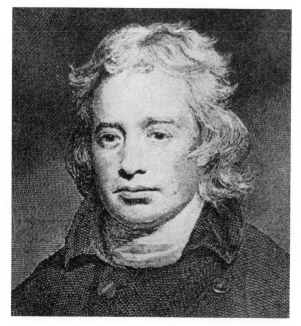

Everard Home

illustrations of the appearance of cancer under the microscope. Although the magnification was stated to be four hundred, no cellular details were recorded, and the round bodies of Figures 4 and 5 were interpreted as lymph globules, of the same size as the "blood globules deprived of their colouring matter" of his Figure 7. Home looked but did not see, as Müller did eight years later.

Everard Home. **Observations on Cancer, Connected with Histories of the Disease.** London: W. Bulmer and Co., 1805.

Everard Home. **A Short Tract on the Formation of Tumors.** London: Longman, Rees, Orme, Brown and Green, 1830.

Christopher Turner Johnson. **A Practical Essay on Cancer.** Philadelphia: Edward Parker, 1811.

John Pearson. **Practical Observations on Cancerous Complaints.** London: J. Johnson, 1793.

Jane M. Oppenheimer. **New Aspects of John and William Hunter.** New York: Henry Schuman, 1946.

Home, *Formation of Tumours,* 1830. Title page.

A SHORT TRACT

ON THE

FORMATION OF TUMOURS,

AND

THE PECULIARITIES

THAT ARE MET WITH IN THE STRUCTURE OF THOSE THAT
HAVE BECOME CANCEROUS;

WITH

THEIR MODE OF TREATMENT.

BY SIR EVERARD HOME, BART.

V.P.R.S. F.S.A. F.L.S.

SERGEANT SURGEON TO THE KING; SURGEON TO THE ROYAL HOSPITAL,
CHELSEA; CONSULTING SURGEON TO ST. GEORGE'S HOSPITAL; HONORARY
PROFESSOR TO THE ROYAL COLLEGE OF SURGEONS; TRUSTEE TO THE
HUNTERIAN COLLECTION; PROPRIETOR TO THE ROYAL INSTITUTION;
CORRESPONDING MEMBER OF THE ROYAL INSTITUTION OF FRANCE;
MEMBER OF THE ROYAL SOCIETY OF GOTTINGEN; MEMBER OF THE
PHYSICO-MEDICAL SOCIETY OF ERLANG; HONORARY MEMBER OF THE
MEDICAL SOCIETY, PHILADELPHIA; HONORARY MEMBER OF THE ROYAL
MEDICAL SOCIETY OF EDINBURGH; CORRESPONDING MEMBER OF THE
MEDICAL SOCIETY, DUBLIN; HONORARY MEMBER OF THE MEDICO-
CHIRURGICAL SOCIETY OF INVERNESS.

LONDON:

PRINTED FOR

LONGMAN, REES, ORME, BROWN, AND GREEN,

PATERNOSTER-ROW.

1830.

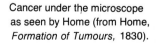

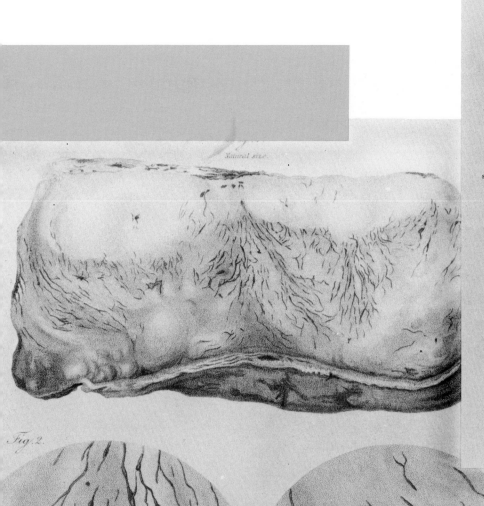

Cancer under the microscope
as seen by Home (from Home,
Formation of Tumours, 1830).

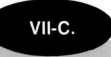

Pre-Listerian Surgery

VII-C-2. Soft cancers: Hey and Wardrop.

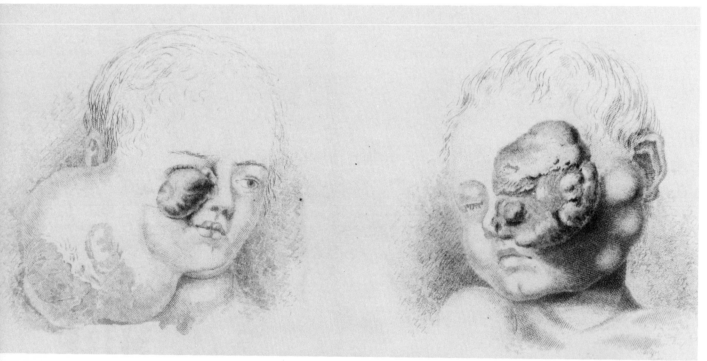

Fungous hematodes of eyeball, from Wardrop, *Observations on Fungous Hematodes*, 1809.

During the 18th Century, gross pathologic observations clearly differentiated cancers from inflammatory lesions, and assigned to scirrhus the role of an early stage of cancer before ulceration.

Gross pathology also revealed that some internal cancers were neither scirrhous nor ulcerated, but soft and of a mushroom or brain-like consistency. Thus the names of fungus hematodes of Hey, and encephaloides of Laënnec.

William Hey (1736-1819) was among the first to describe and name the soft,

vascular tumors. James Wardrop (1782-1869) extended this concept, using gliomas of the retina and testicular tumors as chief examples. Wardrop concluded that fungus hematodes was a disease separate from cancer because it occurred "in the liver, spleen, kidneys, and lungs, organs where the scirrhus structure has never been described." Some of the visceral tumors apparently were metastases, a concept unrecognized by Wardrop.

Classifications of tumors by gross structure were used in the anatomic-pathologic descriptions until replaced by histologic criteria. Abernethy categorized 8 types of "sarcoma," a word used to

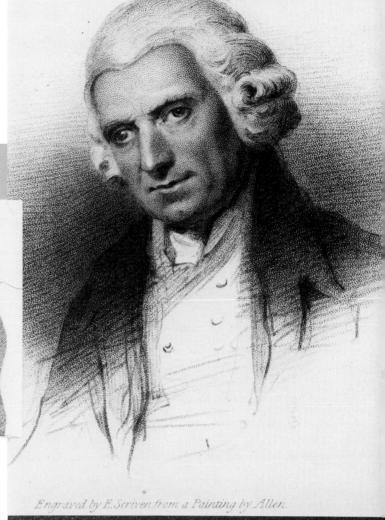

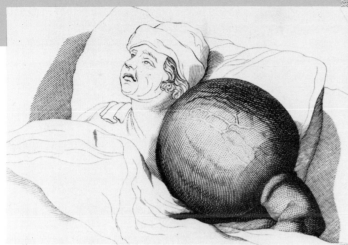

Fungous haematodi, from Hey, *Practical Observations in Surgery,* 1805.

William Hey

Engraved by E. Scriven from a Painting by Allen.

James Wardrop

connote the fleshy, soft nature of growth rather than its present malignancy.

The French school, typified by Laën-nec and his pupil at Strasbourg, Johann Georg Christian Fredrich Lobstein (1777-1835) divided tumors into the scir-rhus-cancerous, fungus-medullary, and melanomas.

Triolo has presented an excellent evaluation of this period of oncology.

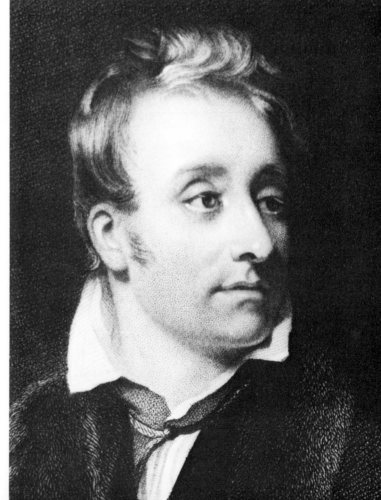

John Abernethy. **Surgical Observations Containing a Classification of Tumours, with Cases to Illustrate the History of Each Species.** London: Longman and Rees, 1804.

William Hey. **Practical Observations in Surgery**, illustrated by cases. London: Cadell and Davies, 1803.

J.-G.-C.-F. Lobstein. **Traité d'Anatomie Pathologique.** 2 vols. Paris: Levrault, 1829-33.

V. A. Triolo. Nineteenth century foundation of cancer research. Advances in tumor pathology, nomenclature, and theories of oncogenesis. **Cancer Res.** 25: 75-106, 1965.

James Wardrop. **Observations on Fungus Haematodes or Soft Cancer in Several of the Most Important Organs of the Human Body: Containing Also a Comparative View of the Structure of Fungus Haematodes and Cancer.** Edinburgh: Constable, 1809.

VII-C.

Pre-Listerian Surgery

VII-C-3. Recognition of metastases: Récamier.

RECHERCHES

SUR

LE TRAITEMENT

DU CANCER,

PAR LA COMPRESSION MÉTHODIQUE SIMPLE OU COMBINÉE,

ET

SUR L'HISTOIRE GÉNÉRALE DE LA MÊME MALADIE;

SUIVIES DE NOTES

1°. SUR LES FORCES ET LA DYNAMÉTRIE VITALES;
2°. SUR L'INFLAMMATION ET L'ÉTAT FÉBRILE.

PAR J. C. A. RÉCAMIER,

MÉDECIN DE L'HÔTEL-DIEU DE PARIS.

Chevalier de l'Ordre royal de la Légion-d'Honneur, Professeur de
Médecine au Collège royal de France, Professeur de Clinique
médicale à la Faculté de Médecine, Membre de l'Académie royale
de Médecine, etc., etc.

(Carcinoma,) Quidam ferro adusserunt, quidam scalpelo exsiderunt,
neque ulli unquàm medicina profuit. Adusta protinus concitata sunt
et increverunt donec occiderent. Excisa, etiam post inductam cicatri-
cem, tamen reverterunt et causam mortis attulerunt. (CELSE, edit.
Lugd. Bat., 1592, p. 594.)
Tota Chirurgia et Medicina desiderant medicamentum ad Cancrum,
ut suppuretur, vel in ambitu, ut aliquandò in ambracibus fit vel ut
substantia ejus vertatur in pus, et tamen continuum non salvatur:
Sed, proh dolor! Nullum datur.... (BOERHAAVIUS, Prax. Med.,
t. II, p. 558.)

TOME PREMIER.
—

PARIS,

CHEZ GABON, LIBRAIRE-ÉDITEUR,

Rue de l'École-de-Médecine, n° 10;

MONTPELLIER, MÊME MAISON;

BRUXELLES, au Dépôt de Librairie médicale française.

1829.

Récamier, *Recherches du Cancer,* 1829. Title page

110

recouvré en grande partie dans cet endroit son organisation primitive. »

Le fait de M. Parent, en montrant la réso-lution spontanée d'un engorgement carcinoma-teux, suivie d'un autre engorgement de même nature, peut conduire à admettre *des métastases cancéreuses.*

Le fait suivant conduit à penser que dans cer-tains cas la diathèse cancéreuse peut s'user sans métastase : madame G...., alors âgée de qua-rante-quatre ans, grêle, mal réglée et très-san-guine, portait, il y a douze ans, dans la région du colon droit, une tumeur fixe, qui était le siége d'élancemens spontanés très-vifs, avec des irradiations très-douloureuses, dont les exacer-bations, malgré le régime le plus sévère, rame-naient souvent la nécessité de la saignée, seul moyen de soulagement véritable pour elle. Je crus à l'existence d'une tumeur de nature can-céreuse dans cette région du canal intestinal, et MM. Fouquier et Marjolin, qui ont vu la malade avec moi, ont partagé la même opinion. On a con-tinué à saigner cette personne, très-affaiblie et très-maigre, lorsque l'intensité des accidens le de-mandait. L'époque de la cessation des règles est arrivée; les douleurs de la région cœcale ou coli-que ont diminué. Madame G.... a cessé d'être sai-

Joseph Claude Anselme Récamier (1774-1852), physician and gynecol-ogist, following service in the Napoleonic wars, was on the staff of Hôtel Dieu in Paris for 40 years, and professor of medicine at the College de France. He will retain a permanent place in oncology for recognizing clearly how cancer spreads and naming metastases.

Previous surgeons and anatomists de-scribed the extensions of cancer to sur-

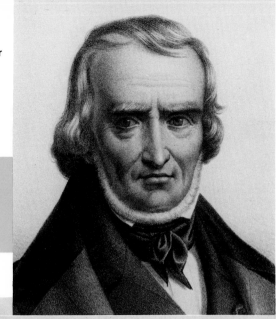

J. C. A. Récamier

Cancer of the uterus (from Récamier, *Recherches du Cancer,* 1829).

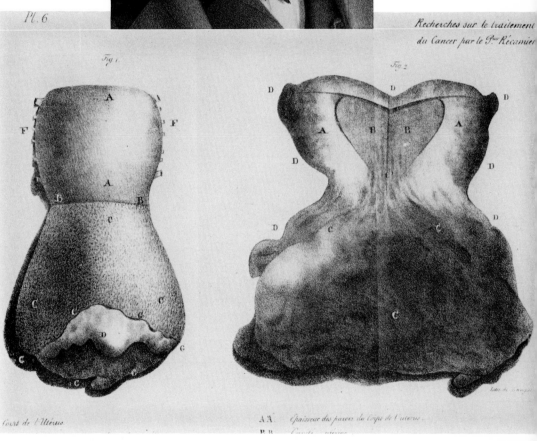

rounding tissues and lymph nodes, but distant deposits were not recognized as colonies of the primary tumors. Récamier described local infiltration, invasion of veins, and secondary growths in the brain in patients with mammary carcinoma. The specific introduction of the term "metastases" occurs in volume 2, page 110,, lines 3 to 7, of his **Recherches du Cancer** of 1829. A secondary deposit in the brain from a primary carcinoma of the breast is described as follows: "The case of M. Parent leads to the admission of cancer metastases: here a spontaneous eruption of carcinoma is succeeded by an identical eruption at another site."

In his extensive and exhaustive volumes, one of the main themes is the treatment of cancer of the breast by compression. This technique, almost guaranteed to promote metastases, did not become popular.

J. C. A. Récamier. **Recherches sur le Traitement du Cancer, par la Compression Méthodique Simple ou Combinée, et sur l'Histoire Générale de la Même Maladie.** 2 vols. Paris: Gabon, 1829.

R. J. Wilder. The historical development of the concept of metastasis. **J. Mt. Sinai Hosp. N.Y.** 23: 728-34, 1956.

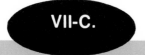

Pre-Listerian Surgery

VII-C-4. Cancer of breast and testis: Astley Cooper.

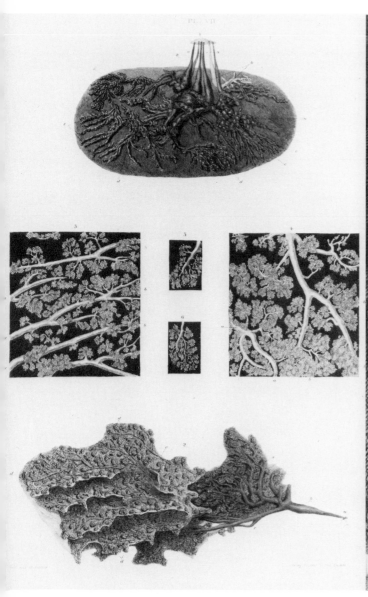

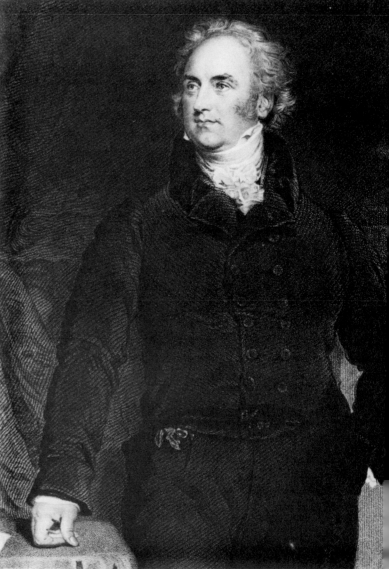

Anatomy of the breast (from Astley Cooper, 1840).

Astley Cooper

Astley Paston Cooper (1768-1841), a pupil of John Hunter, was the most popular surgeon in London during the first quarter of the 19th Century. He was a prodigious worker, teacher and writer, recognized and honored by his contemporaries. He was a pioneer in surgery on the vascular system and of the ear, and conducted experimental dissections and surgery.

Cooper's books on breast and on the testis were examples of continuing specialization, dealing with single organs, in which cancer was but one of the diseases. He clearly differentiated fibroadenoma of the breast, and chronic cystic mastitis, which he called "hydatid disease." He presented for the first time a clear and detailed description of the structure of the breast, including preparations of the lymphatic channels. Thus he recognized the need for a thorough knowledge of the anatomy of the normal organ as a basis for the study of its neoplasms.

Cooper's work on the testis was the best presentation of testicular tumors before histology. Hardness of the testicle was recognized as an important diagnostic sign. He described the natural history of the disease, including the path of metastases. Ten cases in which orchidectomy was performed were reported in detail. Beautiful lithographs in color added to the value of the book. Included was an illustration of a scrotal cancer in a chimney sweep.

Astley Cooper. **Illustrations of the Diseases of the Breast.** London: Longman, Rees, 1829.

Astley Cooper. **On the Anatomy of the Breast.** London: Longman, Orme, Green, Brown and Longman, 1840.

Astley Cooper. **Observations on the Structure and Diseases of the Testis.** London: J. Churchill, 1841.

G. Keynes. The life and works of Sir Astley Cooper. **St. Bartholomew's Hospital Reports**, 15: 9-36, 1922.

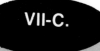

Pre-Listerian Surgery

VII-C-5. Oncology in the United States: Warren.

The first book of tumors published in the United States of America, in 1837, was **Surgical Observations on Tumours with Cases and Operations**, by John C. Warren.

John Collins Warren (1778-1856) of the illustrious medical family of Boston, was the second professor of anatomy and surgery at Harvard University. His education included study under Astley Cooper in London and Dupuytren in Paris. He was a founder of the Massachusetts General Hospital, and of the **Boston Medical and Surgical Journal**, now the **New England Journal of Medicine**. Warren was a principal in an incident that took place at the Massachusetts General Hospital on October 16, 1846. There he removed a vascular tumor from the left neck of a patient put to sleep with ether by William Thomas Green Morton. "Gentlemen, this is no humbug," exclaimed Warren, as he ushered anesthesia into history.

Warren's **Observations** were a collection of case reports, carefully presented in 607 pages with 16 color plates. This was before the histologic era of tumors. As such, it included entities that would not be considered under neoplastic diseases by presently-accepted criteria. The book eschewed theorization, and was a good example of phenomenologic compilations of cases that issued from post-Hunterian surgeons. It was reprinted in England and translated into German in 1839. It received good reviews and was well known to contemporary surgeons.

Rhoda Truax. **The Doctors Warren of Boston.** Boston: Houghton, Mifflin Co., 1968.

E. Warren **The Life of John Collins Warren, M.D.** 2 vols. Boston: Ticknor and Fields, 1860.

John C. Warren. **Surgical Observations on Tumours with Cases and Operations.** Boston: Crocker and Brewster, 1837.

URGICAL OBSERVATIONS

ON

TUMOURS,

WITH

CASES AND OPERATIONS.

BY

JOHN C. WARREN, M. D.

PROFESSOR OF ANATOMY AND SURGERY IN HARVARD UNIVERSITY,

AND SURGEON OF THE MASSACHUSETTS GENERAL HOSPITAL.

BOSTON:

CROCKER AND BREWSTER.

1837.

Warren, *Surgical Observations on Tumours*, 1837. Title page.

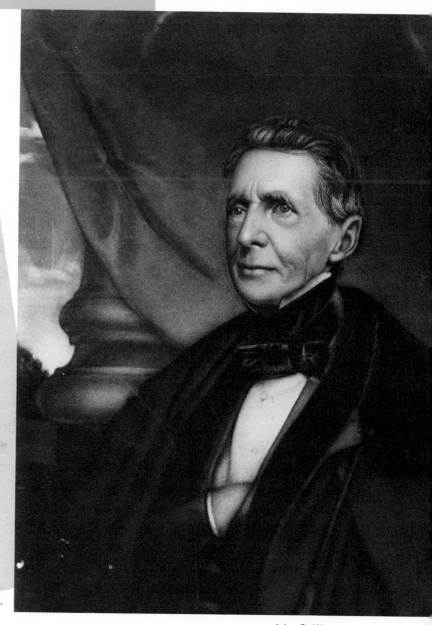

John C. Warren

VII-C.

Pre-Listerian Surgery

VII-C-6. Cancer of the uterus: Siebold and Wagner.

Cancer of the breast is the classical type of neoplastic disease in the surgical annals of history. Yet there is good indication that cancer of the uterus was the most common type of cancer among the women of Europe since the days of Paul of Aegina.

Cancer of the uterus was unapproachable surgically until the days of asepsis. Distinction was not made between cancer of the cervix and of the endometrium until the 20th Century; it is probable that some 90% of uterine cancer originated in the cervix.

Two German texts on uterine cancer during the mid-1800s straddle the gross and microscopic observations on the subject.

Adam Elias von Siebold (1775-1826) in 1824 summarized knowledge about the disease at his time. He thought that cancer of the uterus was more frequent in women who had frequent pregnancies, difficult labor and leukorrhea. He also regarded venery and the reading of romances as harmful, and was against pessaries. Although he considered the disease to be hopeless, and advised no treatment other than douches, he lamented that patients came to physicians only when the disease was advanced.

Ernst Leberecht Wagner (1829-1888) in 1858 published a book on uterine cancer based on autopsy material collected from Leipzig and Berlin. He described the path of metastases of cancer of the cervix. He traced the origin of the disease microscopically to the epithelium as well as to the connective tissue.

Adam Elias von Siebold. **Ueber den Gebärmutterkrebs, dessen Entstenhung und Verhütung.** Berlin: Ferdinand Dummler, 1824.

Ernst Wagner. **Der Gebärmutterkrebs.** Leipzig: B. G. Teubner, 1858.

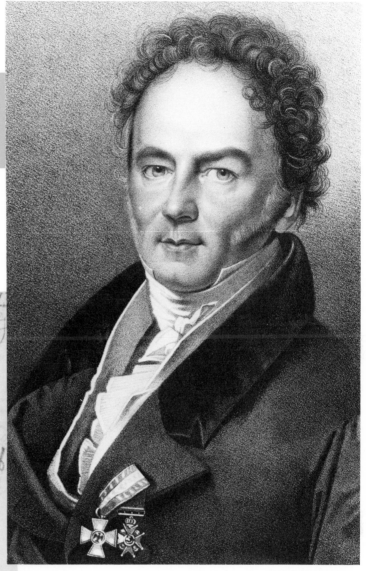

A. E. von Siebold

Ueber den

Gebärmutterkrebs,

dessen

Entstehung und Verhütung.

———

Ein Beitrag

zur

Diätetik des weiblichen Geschlechts

und zur

Beherzigung für Frauen und Gatten,
Mütter und Erzieherinnen;

von

Dr. Ad. Elias von Siebold,

Königl. Preuß. Geheim. Medicinal-Rathe, Ritter des rothen Adler-
Ordens und des Königl. Hannöverschen Guelphen-Ordens dritter
Klasse, öffentl. ord. Professor der Medicin und Geburtshülfe auf der
Universität zu Berlin, Director der Königl. Entbindungsanstalt, der
wissenschaftl. Medicinal-Deputation im Ministerium der geistlichen,
Unterrichts- und Medicinal-Angelegenheiten, und mehrerer
gelehrten Gesellschaften Mitglicde.

———

BERLIN,

bei Ferdinand Dümmler.

1824.

Siebold, *Ueber den Gebärmutterkrebs,* 1824. Title page.

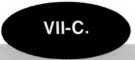

VII-C.

Pre-Listerian Surgery

VII-C-7. Cancer of the prostate: Adams and Thompson.

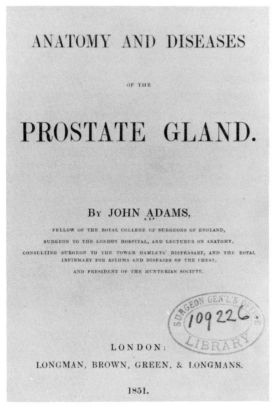

ANATOMY AND DISEASES

OF THE

PROSTATE GLAND.

By JOHN ADAMS,

FELLOW OF THE ROYAL COLLEGE OF SURGEONS OF ENGLAND,

SURGEON TO THE LONDON HOSPITAL, AND LECTURER ON ANATOMY,

CONSULTING SURGEON TO THE TOWER HAMLETS' DISPENSARY, AND THE ROYAL
INFIRMARY FOR ASTHMA AND DISEASES OF THE CHEST,

AND PRESIDENT OF THE HUNTERIAN SOCIETY.

LONDON:

LONGMAN, BROWN, GREEN, & LONGMANS.

1851.

Adams, *Anatomy and Diseases of the Prostate Gland,* 1851.
Title page.

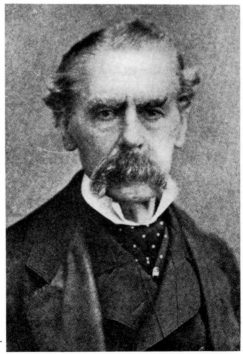

Henry Thompson

John Adams (1806-1877) in 1851 wrote a book on the prostate gland, which included a 13-page chapter on prostatic cancer. He stated that the disease was comparatively rare, and quoted Tanchou's 5 cases among 8289 deaths from cancer collected in Paris. He did not indicate the number seen by him, but included "two cases of cancerous prostate occurring in children at the early age of three years," which probably were embryonal rhabdomyosarcomas.

Adams presented a thorough clinical description of prostatic cancer, starting with the symptoms, which "are of the most distressing character."

"A schirrhous prostate conveys to the finger, passed per anum, a sense of gristly hardness, and is usually irregularly nodulated, one lobe being especially affected. As the disease progresses, the symptoms become exacerbated, the pulse increases in frequency, the bladder becomes more intolerant of its contents, or retention of urine arises, blood frequently escapes with the urine, pain and restlessness become more constant, and even opium ceases to exert its benignant influence; the disease makes its appearance either in the inguinal glands or in other parts of the body, and the patient is gradually worn out by the constant pain and irritation, or, ulceration having occurred, a more rapid termination of the case may be anticipated." "Of the treatment, unfortunately, little of a satisfactory nature can be said." Elastic catheters and opiates may procure "relief from such horribly distressing symptoms as always attend this most intractable disease."

Henry Thompson (1820-1904) in 1873 also considered cancer of the prostate a rare disease, recording only 2 cases in his book on diseases of the prostate. Thompson was an English surgeon, who obtained his medical degree from the University of London in 1851 and rose to professor of pathology and surgery of the Royal College of Surgeons. He was knighted in recognition of his services.

The frequency of cancer of the prostate was not truly appreciated until the report in 1935, by Arnold R. Rich (1893-1968) of Baltimore, which recorded occult carcinoma in 14% of all autopsies, and in 28% of autopsies on men over 70 years old.

John Adams. **The Anatomy and Diseases of the Prostate Gland.** London: Longman, Brown, Green and Longman, 1851.

A. R. Rich. On the frequency of occurrence of occult carcinoma of the prostate. **J. Urol.** 33: 215-223, 1935.

Henry Thompson. **Diseases of the Prostate.** ed. 4. London: J & A. Churchill, 1873.

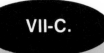

VII-C.

Pre-Listerian Surgery

VII-C-8. Wider mastectomy again: Velpeau and Moore.

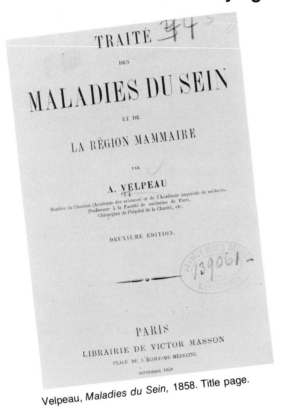

Velpeau, *Maladies du Sein*, 1858. Title page.

Charles Moore on inadequate operations for breast cancer, 1867.

Alfred-Armand-Louis-Marie Velpeau (1795-1867) was a leading French surgeon, with a large experience in breast cancer. He advocated the removal of the pectoral muscle along with the breast. In his treatise on the subject, he clearly distinguished fibroadenoma of the breast, which he called adenoid tumors, from carcinoma. In 1854 he summarized his own and contemporary results, which were less than 5% successful. Yet to Velpeau these poor results were challenges to improvement.

Charles Hewitt Moore (1821-1870) insisted upon the complete, en-block removal of the breast for cancer, along with the axillary contents, pectoral muscle and adequate skin, without cutting into the tumor itself. "It was mistaken kindness which led to a change in this mode

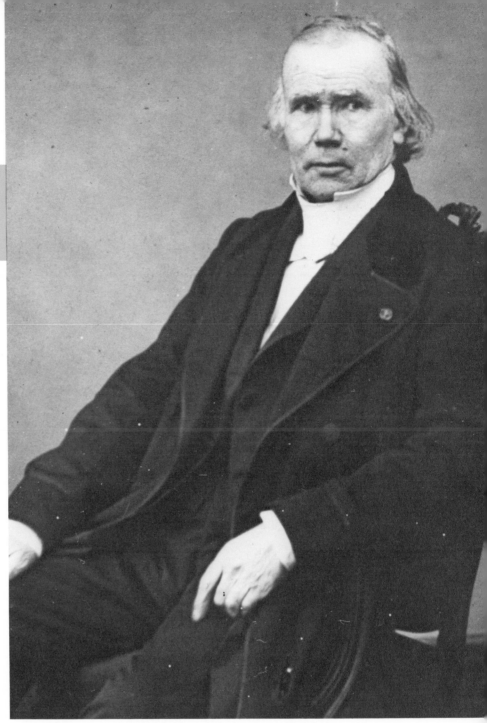

A. Velpeau

of operating," he wrote. Moore was in charge of the Middlesex Hospital cancer facility, probably the first cancer institute in the world.

The recommendations of Velpeau and of Moore came during the period when microscopic diagnosis of cancer was still developing. Hermann Lebert (1813-1878) applied the microscope to Velpeau's material, but he was so often in error that Velpeau relied primarily on gross appearance of his surgical specimens.

Anesthesia became available during the latter part of Velpeau's experience, but both he and Moore preceded aseptic surgery that allowed acceptable post-operative risk for the patients. Even in 1879, in Billroth's clinic, the postoperative mortality in cancer of the breast was 24 percent, primarily from erysipelas.

Charles H. Moore. On the influence of inadequate operations on the theory of cancer. **Med.-Chir. Trans.** 50: 245-280, 1867.

A. Velpeau. **Traité des Maladies du Sein et de la Région Mammaire.** Paris: Victor Masson, 1854.

VII-C.

Pre-Listerian Surgery

VII-C-9. Cancer at mid-century: Walshe.

Walter Hayle Walshe (1812-1892) was an Irishman who obtained his medical degree in Edinburgh, and who studied under Louis in Paris. He settled in London and was on the staff of the Brompton Hospital, became professor of pathological anatomy, and was dean of the University of London Medical School from 1846 to 1847.

In 1841 Walshe contributed the section on cancer to Costello's **Cyclopedia of Practical Surgery.** The material was expanded, with additions by J. Mason Warren of Boston, for an American audience as **The Anatomy, Physiology, Pathology and Treatment of Cancer.** It was again expanded in 1846 for English readers to **The Nature and Treatment of Cancer.**

Walshe's books were in sharp contrast with the post-Hunterian collections of surgical and pathological cases, offering a systematic treatment of the whole subject of oncology. He developed a classification of the diseases, in keeping with the early period of histology, summarized theories of causation, included microscopic observations and even some biochemical data, and dealt with statistical considerations. It was a complete reflection and one view of the subject for that time.

Concerning treatment of cancer, Walshe wrote in the American version:

"1. There is no existing evidence to show that carcinoma of an internal organ has ever been cured. 2. Cancer has never been removed by medicinal agents alone. 3. Morbid productions possessing the anatomical and pathological character of scirrhus have been removed with the knife, and no return of the disease has been observed. . . ." As to prophylaxis, "In the present state of the science this cannot be done."

Walshe reproduced a plate of microscopic observations on tumor cells taken from Johannes Müller's classic of 1838. His cancer statistics came primarily from the data collected by Tanchou around Paris.

Walter Hayle Walshe

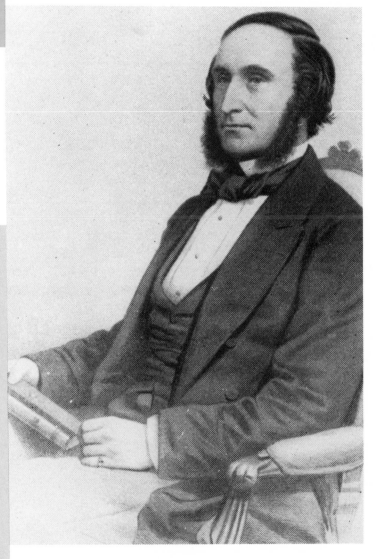

THE

NATURE AND TREATMENT

OF

CANCER.

BY

WALTER HAYLE WALSHE, M.D.

PROFESSOR OF PATHOLOGICAL ANATOMY IN UNIVERSITY COLLEGE,
PHYSICIAN TO UNIVERSITY COLLEGE HOSPITAL,
AND TO THE HOSPITAL FOR CONSUMPTION AND DISEASES OF THE CHEST.

LONDON:
PRINTED FOR TAYLOR AND WALTON,
BOOKSELLERS AND PUBLISHERS TO UNIVERSITY COLLEGE,
UPPER GOWER STREET.

1846.

Walshe, *Nature and Treatment of Cancer,* 1846. Title page.

William B. Costello, ed. **The Cyclopedia of Practical Surgery**, vol. 1, p. 590-692. London: Sherwood, Gilbert and Piper, 1841.

J. R. Reynolds. Walter Hayle Walshe (obituary). **Lancet**, 2: 1535-38, Dec. 31, 1892.

Walter Hayle Walshe. **The Anatomy, Physiology, Pathology and Treatment of Cancer.** Boston: William D. Ticknor & Co., 1844.

Walter Hayle Walshe. **The Nature and Treatment of Cancer.** London: Taylor and Walton, 1846.

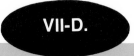

VII-D.

Microscopic Pathology

VII-D-1. The achromatic microscope.

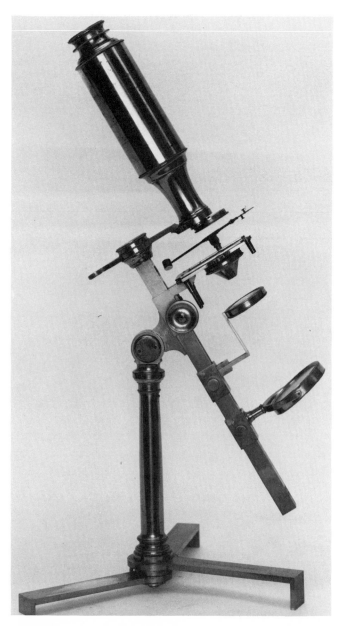

Compound microscope, Dollond, London, circa 1825 (from Blumberg, 1967).

The history of magnification by lenses stretches back to ancient times. In 1590, Zaccharias Janssen of Middleburg, Holland, while experimenting with a telescope, found that elongating the tube of the instrument also enlarged near objects. Galileo in 1610 mounted the tube so it could be focused, and a member of the Accademia dei Lincei named it "microscope."

Antoni van Leeuwenhoek (1632-1723), was among the first to use his simple microscopes for systematic, serious studies. Marcello Malpighi (1628-1694) was among the first biological scientists to use the microscope. The development of an achromatic microscope on a practical scale, however, occurred during the first quarter of the 19th Century. The developments were stimulated by the Royal Microscopical Society, which offered prizes for better optical designs.

Among the first men to start manufacture of microscopes was C. L. Chevalier, of France, who in 1825 constructed and presented his instrument to the Royal Society in London, of which he was an honorary member. The firm of Chevalier and Son was established in Paris, and the R. & J. Beck Company in England.

The cell concept in normal and pathologic anatomy arose from the use of the microscope by Johannes Müller and his students. Virchow in his eulogy of his teacher recounts that the first microscope used by Müller was presented to him by Rudolphi. Karl Asmund Rudolphi (1771-1832) was a Swede, and professor of anatomy and physiology at the University of Berlin from 1810. The gift of the microscope can be dated at 1823, when Müller completed his medical education at the age of 22. And the microscope was stated to be of English make, although in his 1838 publication Müller specifically and patriotically mentions the Shieck instrument of Berlin. Perhaps his first microscope could have been a Dollond model from London, similar to one pictured here as the emblem of the period.

The role of the microscope in biological sciences grew increasingly larger as the instrument improved. The introduction of improved methods of preserving, cutting and staining tissue preparations were equally important contributions to the development of histology.

J. M. Blumberg. The Billings Microscope Collection of the Medical Museum, Armed Forces Inst. Path., Washington, D. C. **Am. Registry Path.**, 1967, Fig. 56, p. 30.

Frank J. Muñoz and H. A. Charipper. **The Microscope and Its Use.** Brooklyn, N.Y.: Chemical Publ. Co., Inc., 1943.

Rudolph Virchow. Johann Müller, the Physiologist: an éloge pronounced in the hall of the University of Berlin. Transl. A. Mercer Adam. **Edinburgh Med. J.** 4: 458-63 and 527-44, 1858.

VII-D.

Microscopic Pathology

VII-D-2. Rise of science in Germany: Johannes Müller.

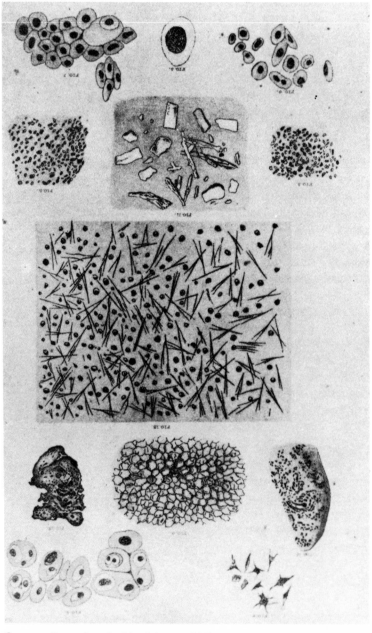

Cancer cells, as described by Johannes Müller, 1838.

Johannes Müller

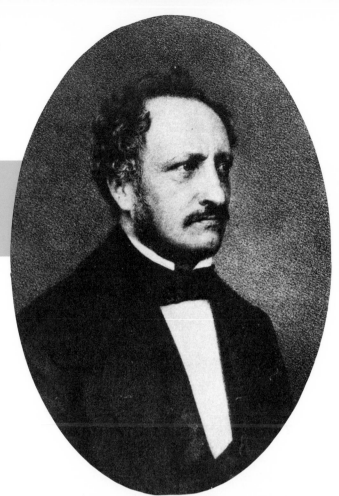

Johannes Müller (1801-1858) was one of the fountainheads of modern medicine, and one of the greatest teachers of the 19th Century. Born in Coblenz, he received his medical education at the University of Bonn, and after a short, unhappy attempt at practicing medicine entered an academic career. He was professor of pathology, physiology and comparative anatomy, and eventually dean of the faculty at the University of Berlin. According to Garrison, Müller was strongly built with broad shoulders and a large head, a striking, magnetic, impressive teacher of rare personal charm. From the circumstances of his death, it is possible that he terminated his own life.

Müller was a philosopher as well as a prolific investigator, writer and teacher. His pupils are a roll-call of scholars that elevated biological science in Germany to a pinnacle: Schwann, Henle, Kölliker, Virchow, DuBois-Reymond, Helmholtz and Brücke.

Among the more important contributions were his explanation of color sensation on the retina (1826), the law of eccentric projection of sensation from the peripheral sense organs (1833), his experiments on phonation and the vocal cords (1835) and the law of specific nerve energy (1840), which states that every sensory organ responds to the stimulus with its particular sensation.

In 1836, Müller began observing through the microscope the large collec-tions of tumors in the museums of Berlin, Halle, Brunswick and London. In 1838 he published his findings, the same year as Schleiden's work on plant cells appeared in **Müller's Archiv** and a year before his student, Schwann, described cells in all animal tissues, including those of embryos. Müller clearly recognized that tumors were composed of disorganized, abnormal cells. The stage was set for Virchow.

Müller's slight book, of which only the first volume was published, ushered in the histologic period of oncology and, indeed, of all pathology. It is strange that this genius could so wrongly evaluate his work, in stating that "microscopical and chemical analyses can never become the means of surgical diagnosis. . ."

Howard W. Haggard and G. M. Smith. Johannes Müller and the modern conception of cancer. **Yale J. Biol. & Med.**, 10: 419-36, 1938.

Johannes Müller. **Ueber den feinern Bau und die Formen der krankhaften Geschwülste.** Berlin: G. Reimer, 1838.

J. Müller. **On the Nature and Structural Characteristics of Cancer.** Transl. Charles West. London: Sherwood, Gilbert, and Piper, 1840.

Hans G. Schlumberger. Origins of the cell concept in pathology. **Arch. Path.** 37: 396-407, 1944.

VII-D.

Microscopic Pathology

VII-D-3. Dean of pathology: Virchow.

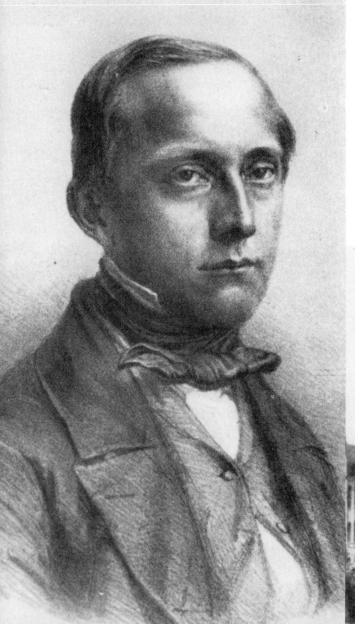

Rudolf Virchow (1821-1902) of Berlin was the founder of cellular pathology, and one of the great medical figures of all time. **Die Cellularpathologie in ihren Begründung auf physiologische und pathologische Gewebelehre** (1858) set in motion a new way of looking at the body as a cell-state in which every cell is a citizen, diseases being merely a conflict of citizens in this state brought about

Rudolf Virchow as a young professor, 1850 (from Lubarsch).

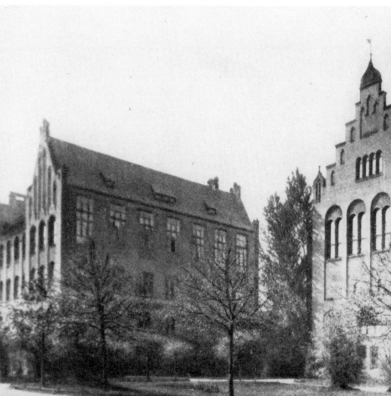

by the action of external forces. Virchow's aphorism, **Omnis cellula e cellula**, means that cell development is not discontinuous and there are no specific cells in disease, but only modifications of physiologic types. This view is the basis of Virchow's work on tumors, **Die krankhaften Geschwülste**, which treats of these formations as physiologically independent new growths of homologous or heterologous structure. Homologous tumors were proliferations of cells already present, and were in general benign. Heterologous tumors arose as a result of a change in character to cells of a

different type, and were malignant. However, Virchow believed that these malignant tumors arose from connective tissue elements. It took the work of many pathologists to establish that carcinomas were derived from epithelial elements. Virchow also believed that dissemination of cancer was due to the transportation of a non-cellular infection from the primary tumor to distant sites, rather than seeding of tumor cells. Oncogenic viruses, unknown to Virchow, may yet show that this mechanism may be involved in some neoplastic diseases.

Virchow's writing include contributions to pathology, parasitology, anthropology, as well as to public health and politics. At the age of 26 he founded the **Archiv für pathologische Anatomie**, known as **Virchow's Archiv.**

Garrison describes Virchow as a small, elastic, professional figure, with snappy, black eyes, quick in mind and body, something of a martinet in the morgue or lecture-room, often transfixing inattention or incompetence with a flash of sarcasm. Yet he was generous, whole-souled, and broad-minded withal and none who made good was ever lost from sight or memory. All his long life he was keen and ardent in controversy. In extreme old age Virchow, always liberal in politics, became reactionary in science; but love of truth, generosity in word and deed, were the essence of his youth and mature manhood. His lifelong championship of the rights of industrial humanity, valiantly upheld in the very stronghold of the Prussian military government, shows the kind of fiber he was made of.

Pathology Institute and Museum, Berlin (from Lubarsch).

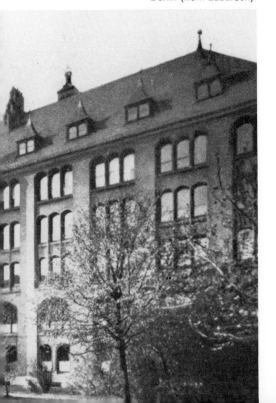

O. Lubarsch. Biographische Einleitung. **Virchows Arch.** 235: 1-30, 1921.

V. A. Triolo. Nineteenth century foundations of cancer research. Advances in tumor pathology, nomenclature, and theories of oncogenesis. **Cancer Res.** 25: 75-106, 1965.

Rudolph Virchow. **Die Krankhaften Geschwülste**. Berlin: August Hirschwald, 1863.

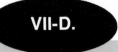

Microscopic Pathology

VII-D-4. Epithelial origin of carcinoma: Remak, Thiersch and Waldeyer.

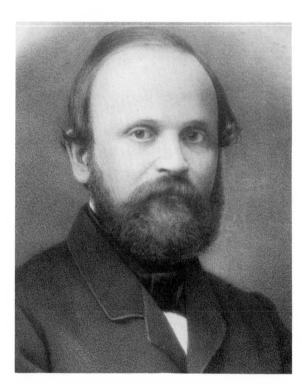

Robert Remak

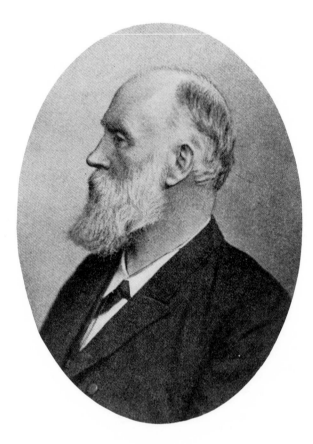

Karl Thiersch

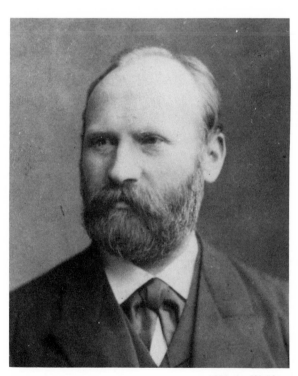

Wilhelm Waldeyer

The derivation of carcinomas from epithelial tissues, rather than from connective tissue as postulated by Virchow, was established by meticulous reconstructions and observations by other contemporary pathologists.

Robert Remak (1815-1865) provided demonstrations of three primary germ layers from his studies in embryology, and proposed that epitheliomas arose from the epithelial germ layer.

Karl Thiersch (1822-1895), a surgeon of Erlangen, made serial sections of tumors with razors and showed in stained reconstructions that epithelial tumors were continuous with and had origin in epithelium.

Wilhelm Waldeyer (1837-1921), a great anatomist, a pupil of Henle and eventually professor at Berlin, confirmed the epithelial origin of epithelial tumors of internal organs. He also added observations establishing that metastases of cancers were by embolization of tumor cells via lymphatic and blood vessel channels.

R. Remak. Ein Beitrag zur Entwickelungsgeschichte der krebshaften Geschwülste. **Deut. Klin.** 6: 70-174, 1854.

C. Thiersch. **Der Epitheliakrebs, namentlich der Haut.** Leipzig: Engelmann, 1865.

W. Waldeyer. Die Entwicklung der Carcinoma. **Virchows Arch.** 41: 470-523, 1867 and 55: 67-159, 1872.

VII-D.

Microscopic Pathology

VII-D-5. The embryonal theory: Cohnheim.

Julius Cohnheim (1839-1884) of Pomerania, studied medicine at Berlin and in 1861 fell under the spell of Rudolf Virchow. After service as surgeon in the Prussian-Danish war of 1864, he returned to the Pathological Institute of the Charité. Subsequently, after accepting the Christian faith, he was professor of pathology at Kiel (1868-1872), Breslau (1872-1878) and Leipzig (1878-1884). He was a pioneer in experimental pathology, especially on inflammation and suppuration. In 1877 he successfully inoculated tuberculosis in the anterior chamber of the eye of the rabbit.

Cohnheim is noted in oncology for his hypothesis that tumors arose from "cell rests" or superfluous groups of embryonic cells that failed to mature and persisted in the tissues. In Cohnheim's words, "the real cause of the subsequent tumor is to be sought in a fault or irregularity of the embryonic rudiment." This theory is no longer accepted except as it may apply to teratomatous neoplasms.

The last years of Cohnheim's life were clouded by severe complications of gout, and his brilliant career was cut short at the age of forty-five. He is described as a man of robust, cheerful, energetic disposition, swift and sure of speech, with great powers of wit and sarcasm.

Julius Cohnheim. **Lectures on General Pathology.** 3 vols. London: New Sydenham Society, 1889.

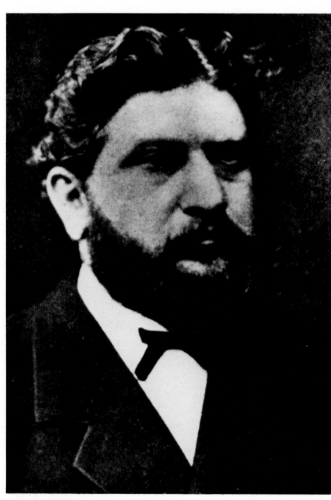

Julius Cohnheim

Cohnheim, *Allgemeine Pathologie,* 1877. Title page.

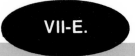

VII-E.

Special Neoplasms

VII-E-1. Mycosis fungoides: Alibert.

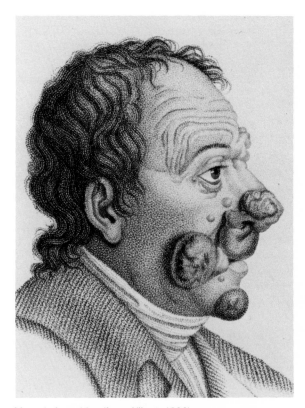

Mycosis fungoides (from Alibert, 1806).

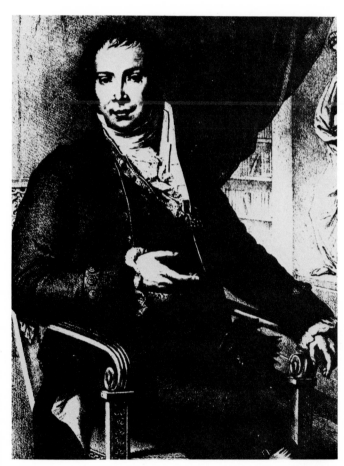

J. L. M. Alibert

In 1806, Alibert described a 56-year-old man with "une eruption furfuracee," followed by the appearance of small, smooth, painless nodules on various parts of the body. The first appeared on the face, and successively involved the axillae, groins, popliteal fossae, scrotum and inner aspects of the thighs. The masses were sessile and "secreted a green ichorous humor," and some sloughed and involuted. Others progressed to non-healing, painful ulcers. The patient had a progressively deteriorating course, with emaciation, diarrhea and fever, and died five years after the onset of the disease.

Alibert considered this a form of yaws and named it "pian fungoide." In 1832 he renamed the disease "mycosis fungoides," from the mushroom-like appearance and its fungating proclivity.

Jean-Louis Alibert (1768-1837) was a leading French dermatologist who became physician to Louis XVIII and was made a Baron by Charles X. He classified dermatologic diseases, and published an excellent atlas of patients with dermatologic afflictions.

Mycosis fungoides is regarded as a cutaneous manifestation of malignant lymphoma. The name is, of course, a misnomer, since it has no mycotic etiology and with radiation and chemotherapeutic treatment, the lesions seldom fungate. However, long usage will probably retain the term.

J. L. M. Alibert. **Descriptions des Maladies de la Peau Observées. à l'Hôpital Saint-Louis.** Paris: Barrois, 1806-14, pl. 36, p. 157.

J. L. M. Alibert. **Monographie des Dermatoses.** Ed. 2. Paris: G. Bailliere, 1835, p. 413.

S. M. Bluefarb. **Cutaneous Manifestations of the Malignant Lymphomas.** Springfield, Ill.: C. C. Thomas, 1959.

VII-E.

Special Neoplasms

VII-E-2. Hodgkin's disease: Hodgkin.

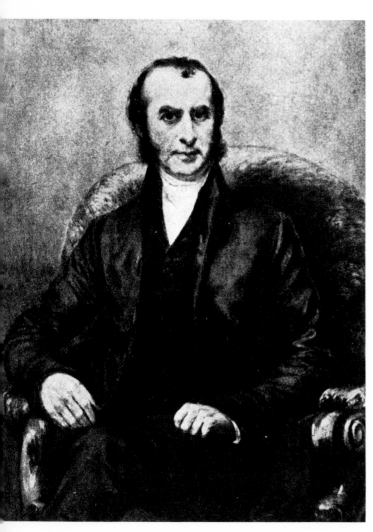

Thomas Hodgkin

Thomas Hodgkin (1798-1866), a member of the Society of Friends and pathologist at Guy's Hospital, in 1832 reported 7 cases with enlargement of the spleen and lymph nodes. Hodgkin was calling attention to a set of changes, and did not consider that he was describing a new disease. He left Guy's after failing to receive a promotion in 1837.

Samuel Wilks (1824-1911), a devoted historian of Guy's, rediscovered Hodgkin's manuscript in 1856, and in his kind manner, designated the syndrome as Hodgkin's disease (he also linked the names of Bright and Addison eponymically to diseases).

Among the 7 cases were tuberculosis and leukemia, but at least 2 met the histologic criteria for Hodgkin's disease. Tissues had been preserved for a hundred years, first in alcohol and then in formalin, and have been reexamined on many occasions.

Case II was of Ellenborough King, a boy of 10, and a patient of Dr. Bright. He had been ill for 13 months, when he began to fail. A tumor was observed in the left hypochondrium, in the area of the spleen, and the glands of the neck were

Histologic appearance of Hodgkin's
Case II (Guy's Hospital
No. 1523, 1828).

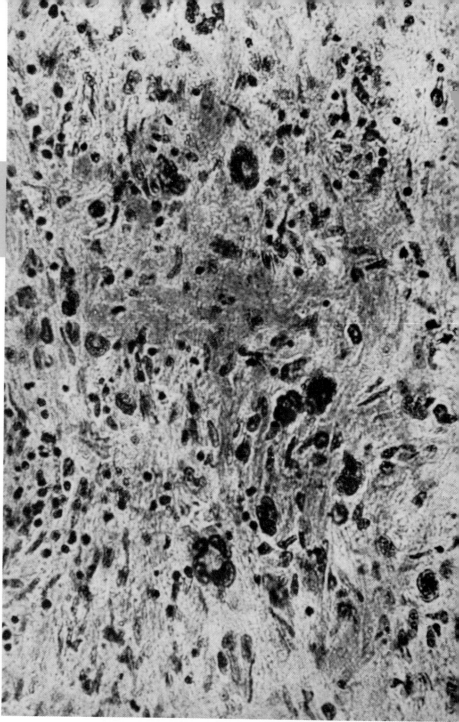

swollen.

"The glands in the neck had assumed the form of large smooth ovoid masses, connected together merely by loose cellular membrane and minute vessels; when cut into they exhibited a firm cartilaginous structure. . . with no softening or suppuration." Glands in the chest and abdomen "were in the same state and greatly enlarged. . . The spleen was enlarged to at least four times its natural size. . ."

Despite resistance to eponyms, the dozen or so other names, such as lymphomatosis granulomatosa, have never been successfully substituted for what appears to be a definite entity. Intensive radiotherapy and chemotherapy have changed dramatically the outlook of this previously fatal affliction.

Thomas Hodgkin. On some morbid appearances of the absorbent glands and spleen. **Med.-Chir. Trans.** 17: 68-114, 1832.

H. Jackson, Jr. and F. Parker. **Hodgkin's Disease and Allied Disorders.** New York: Oxford Univ. Press, 1947.

Henry S. Kaplan. **Hodgkin's Disease.** Cambridge, Mass.: Harvard Univ. Press, 1972.

E. R. Long. **Selected Readings in Pathology**, ed. 2. Springfield, Ill.: C. C. Thomas, 1961.

Samuel Wilks. Cases of enlargment of the lymphatic glands and spleen (or Hodgkin's disease). **Guy's Hospital Rept.**, 3d ser. 11: 56-67, 1865.

VII-E.

Special Neoplasms

VII-E-3. Leukemia: Virchow and Bennett.

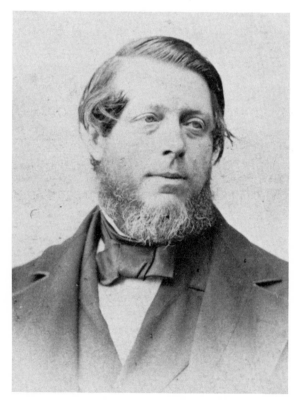

John Hughes Bennett

Leukemia "was first described almost simultaneously by two brilliant young men who, after applying their great gifts to a meticulous exploration of its features in the living and the dead, engaged at once in an almost venomous wrangle over the honor of having been the first to identify this fatal disease." Thus is the event described by Dameshek and Gunz.

The two men who described leukemia were John Hughes Bennett (1812-1875) of Scotland and Rudolf Virchow (1821-1902) of Germany. Their simultaneous publications in 1845 were case reports, and in both the unusual feature was the post-mortem appearance of the blood, with a preponderance of colorless corpuscles rather than red corpuscles. In both cases the spleen was greatly enlarged.

Bennett interpreted his case, and an older case reported by Craigie after seeing Bennett's autopsy, as "suppuration of the blood." Virchow rejected the pyemic explanation and called the condition by its descriptive characteristic as "white blood."

Further cases were rapidly gathered including older reports recognized retrospectively. By 1852, Bennett published a monograph "Leucocythemia," on 37 cases. Virchow in 1856 introduced the term "Leukemia" in a review. He also recognized that there were two kinds of leukemia, one associated with splenomegaly and the other with enlargement of lymph nodes. Thus the myelocytic and lymphocytic varieties were identified before the white blood cells were characterized microscopically.

Acute leukemia was recognized by N. Friedreich (1826-1882) in 1857, and the aleukemic form of lymphocytic disease, lymphosarcoma, was described by H. Kundrat (1845-1893) in 1893.

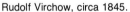

Rudolf Virchow, circa 1845.

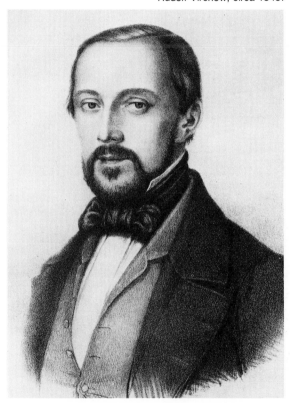

J. H. Bennett. Case of hypertrophy of the spleen and liver, in which death took place from suppuration of the blood. **Edinburgh Med. & Surg. J.** 64: 413-23, 1845.

J. H. Bennett. **Leucocythaemia or White Cell Blood.** Edinburgh: Sutherland and Knox, 1852.

D. Craigie. Case of disease of the spleen, in which death took place in consequence of the presence of purulent matter in the blood. **Edinburgh Med. & Surg. J.** 64: 400-13, 1845.

W. Dameshek and F. Gunz. **Leukemia.** . Ed. 2. New York: Grune & Stratton, 1964.

N. Friedreich. Ein neuer Fall von Leukämie. **Virchow's Arch. Path. Anat.** 12: 37-58, 1857.

Kundrat. Ueber Lympho-Sarkomatosis. **Wien Klin. Wchnschr.** 6: 211-3, 234-9, 1893.

R. Virchow. Weisses Blut. **Froriep's Notizen** 36: 151-56, 1845.

R. Virchow. Die Lukämie. In **Gesammelte Abhandlungen zur wissenschaftlichen Medicin.** Frankfurt: Meidlinger, 1856.

VII-E.

Special Neoplasms

VII-E-4. Multiple myeloma: Bence-Jones.

Multiple myeloma was the first neoplastic entity in which a specific biochemical characteristic was identified.

The events were as follows:

Mr. Thomas Alexander McBean, 43 years of age, in 1844 developed severe chest pain following a minor trauma, relieved by a plaster cast. Severe pain recurred a month later, and then became intractable until his death in 1846. He was cared for by Dr. Thomas Watson, who took him to Dr. William MacIntyre for a consultation. The examination included a urinalysis, with unexpected findings of opacity on boiling. The opacity disappeared upon addition of nitric acid, but reappeared on cooling. A urine specimen was sent by Dr. Watson to a young physician-pathologist, Henry Bence-Jones (1814-1873), with a note asking, "What is it?" Bence-Jones identified the protein as the "hydrated deutoxide of albumen." An autopsy on the patient showed softening of the cancellous bones, which were studied by John Dalrymple and recorded in the literature.

The story, including the name of the patient, was reconstructed by Clamp in 1967, and is well presented by Snapper and Kahn. It seems that every participant except the family physician published his observations. In retrospect, the biochemical analysis by Bence-Jones was the signal contribution.

The disease was characterized in greater detail during the subsequent century, including the recognition of more localized plasmacytomas. The next step was taken by Waldenström, in 1944, who described macroglobinemia and led multiple myeloma into immunology and molecular biology.

H. Bence-Jones. On a new substance occurring in the urine of a patient with "mollities ossium." **Phil. Tr. Royal Soc. London**, 138: 55-62, 1848.

J. R. Clamp. Some aspects of the first recorded case of multiple myeloma. **Lancet** ii: 1354-56, 1967.

J. Dalrymple. On the microscopical character of mollities ossium. **Dublin J. Med. Sci.** 2 (no. 3 NS): 85-95, 1846.

W. MacIntyre. Case of mollities and fragilitas ossium accompanied with urine strongly charged with animal matter. **Med. Chir. Soc. Tr.** 33: 211-32, 1850.

I. Snapper and A. Kahn. **Myelomatosis.** Baltimore: Univ. Park Press, 1971.

J. Waldenström. Incipient myelomatosis or 'essential' hyperglobulinemia with fibrinogenopenia—a new syndrome? **Acta Med. Scand.** 117: 216-47, 1944.

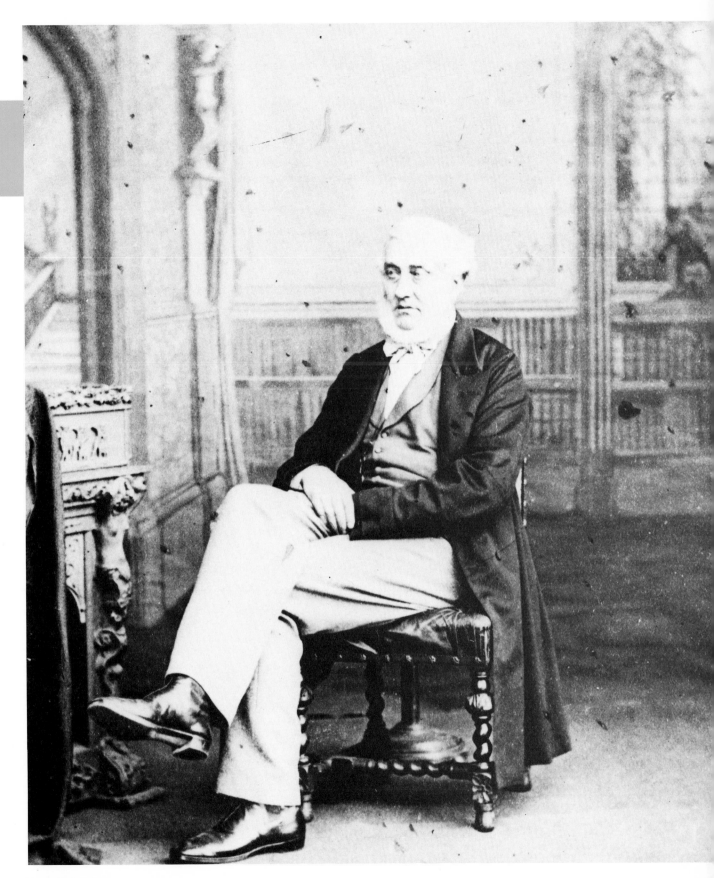

Henry Bence-Jones

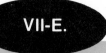

Special Neoplasms

VII-E-5. Kaposi's sarcoma: Kaposi.

Moriz Kaposi (1837-1902), born Moriz Kohn in Hungary, graduated in medicine from the University of Vienna in 1861. He became assistant to Ferdinand von Hebra (1816-1880), professor and founder of the histologic school of dermatology, married Hebra's daughter, completed Hebra's textbook, and inherited Hebra's chair of dermatology in 1881, a post he retained until his death.

Kaposi was the undisputed master of Viennese dermatology, and a superb teacher. His minute clinical descriptions include many to which his name was eponymically attached, or to which he added the Latin suffix "mihi," meaning "belonging to me."

In 1872 Kaposi described and named "Idiopathic Multiple Pigment Sarcoma of the Skin," for which there are over 30 synonyms. The eponymic name has prevailed for the entity, in view of its obscure nature and unknown etiology.

Kaposi's sarcoma presents clinically as multiple soft bluish nodules of the skin with hemorrhages, symmetrically involving the extremities. The photograph of a 43-year old barber is taken from a monograph of 12 cases published by Tomasso De Amicis (1838-1924) in 1882, and rediscovered by F. Ronchese.

Kaposi's sarcoma predominates in adult males. It occurs sporadically in many countries. A. Quenum and R. Camain pointed out its high frequency among the Bantu, and further studies confirmed its concentration in equatorial and south Africa.

The histopathology of Kaposi's sarcoma has been studied extensively, and there is a general consensus that the entity is a cutaneous neoplasm of connective tissue origin, which may involve internal organs. The spindle cell is an integral part of the lesion, but the exact nature of the cell of origin is unestablished; it may be the pericyte, the Schwann cell or the reticuloendothelial cell.

L. V. Ackerman and J. F. Murray (eds). **Symposium on Kaposi's Sarcoma.** Basel: S. Karger A.G., 1963.

S. M. Bluefarb. **Kaposi's Sarcoma.** Springfield, Ill.: C. C. Thomas, 1957.

M. Kaposi. Idiopathisches, multiples Pigmentsarkom der Haut. **Arch. Dermat. Syph.** 4: 265-73, 1872.

A. Quenum and R. Camain. Les aspects africains de la maladie de Kaposi, réticulopathie maligne systématisée. **Ann. d'anat. path.** 3: 337-68, 1958.

F. Ronchese. Kaposi's Sarcoma. An overlooked essay of 1882. **Arch. Dermat.** 77: 542-45, 1958.

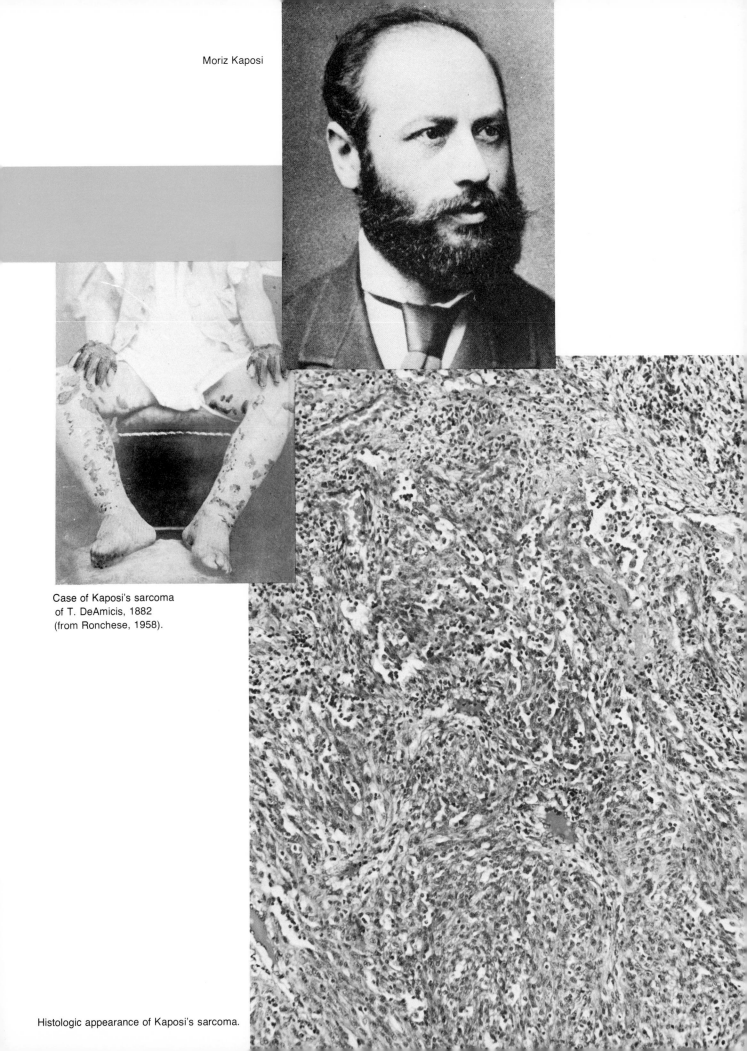

Moriz Kaposi

Case of Kaposi's sarcoma
of T. DeAmicis, 1882
(from Ronchese, 1958).

Histologic appearance of Kaposi's sarcoma.

VII-E.

Special Neoplasms

VII-E-6. Neurofibromatosis: Recklinghausen.

Friedrich Daniel von Recklinghausen (1833-1910), was one of the foremost among the German pathologists who were students of Rudolph Virchow. He obtained his medical degree in 1855, and became an assistant at the pathological institute in Berlin from 1858 to 1864. He was then chosen professor of pathological anatomy successively at Konigsberg, Wurzburg, and Strassburg, where he remained from 1872 until retirement in 1906.

Recklinghausen's influence was on all pathology, and his name is eponymically associated with two unrelated entities. Neurofibromatosis, the first Recklinghausen's disease, was described in 1882. In 1891 osteitis fibrosa became the second Recklinghausen's disease.

General neurofibromatosis was described clinically long before Recklinghausen's monograph, which reviews the literature starting with the 1793 case of Tilesius. It includes the 2 cases reported in 1849 by Robert William Smith of Dublin, which John Fulton discovered.

Recklinghausen showed that neurofibromas arose from nerves, which had been suggested by previous writers. He traced degenerating nerve fibers by histological techniques and stated that all these tumors arose from nerve trunks or filaments. His conclusion has been fully verified by many later studies, and is the basis for the eponymic association. Multiple neurofibromatosis is one of the early neoplastic entities that were shown to have an important genetic component. Some of the lesions eventually become biologically and morphologically malignant.

F. D. von Recklinghausen. **Ueber die multiplen Fibrome der Haut und ihre Beziehung zu den multiplen Neuromen.** Berlin: A. Hirschwald, 1882.

F. W. Crowe, J. W. Schull and J. V. Neel. **A Clinical, Pathological, and Genetic Study of Multiple Neurofibromatosis.** Springfield, Ill.: C. C. Thomas, 1956.

J. F. Fulton. Robert W. Smith's description of generalized neurofibromatosis (1849). **New Engl. J. Med.** 200: 1315-17, 1929.

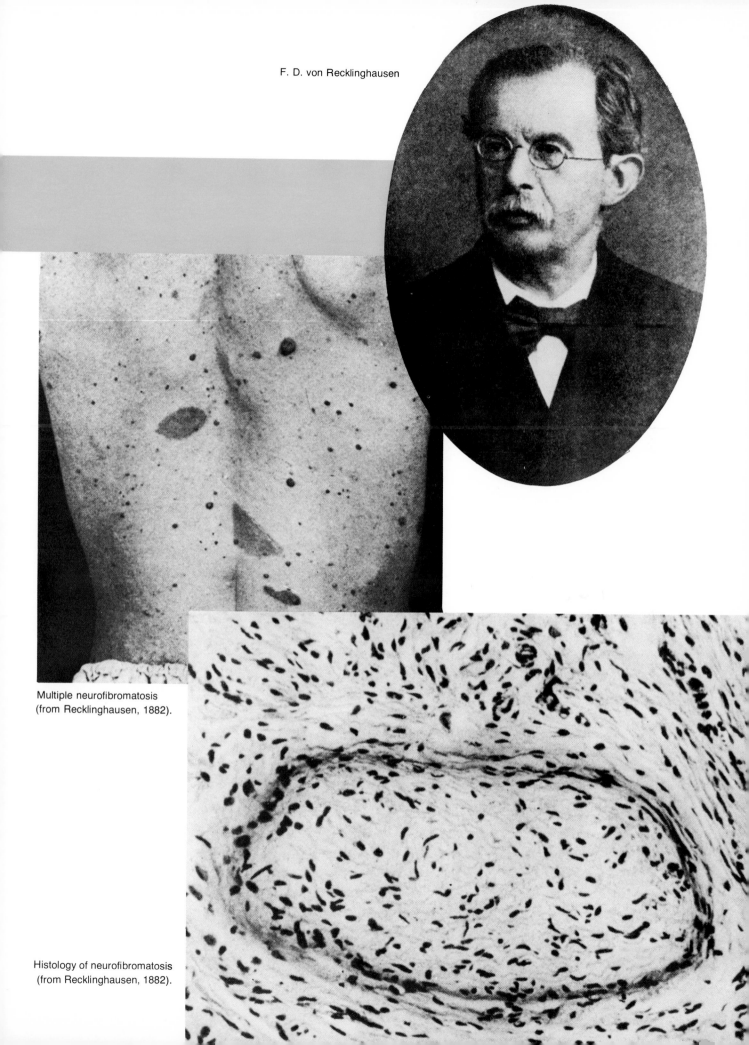

F. D. von Recklinghausen

Multiple neurofibromatosis
(from Recklinghausen, 1882).

Histology of neurofibromatosis
(from Recklinghausen, 1882).

Max Wilms

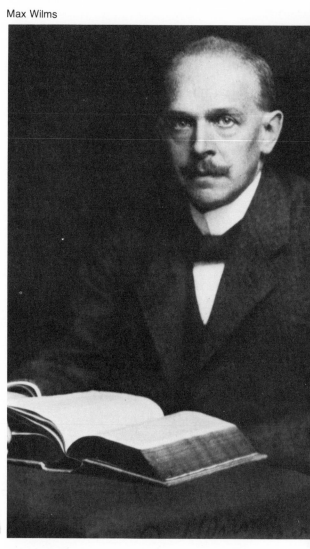

VII-E-7. Wilms' tumor: Wilms.

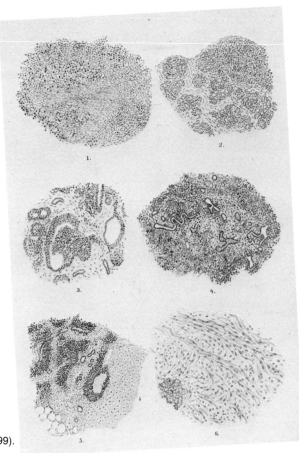

Cell types in Wilms'
tumor (from Wilms, 1899).

"The patient was a 3-year old girl with a kidney tumor which had grown to immense proportions in a short time. The child, anemic and emaciated, was admitted with an enormous mass in the right abdomen and with definite ascites. After nephrectomy, the little child recovered uneventfully. A few months later, however, a recurring abdominal mass was again palpable and shortly afterward the child died. The removed tumor had nearly the size of a man's head and was surrounded by an external capsule which was invading the renal capsule. The kidney lay compressed at the hilus of the neoplasm, the tumor situated like a shell around the kidney. The boundaries to the renal parenchyma were sharp, but the neoplasm had grown into the renal vein,

Lars Röhl. Max Wilms, (1867-1918). **Invest. Urol.** 4: 194-96, 1966.

M. Wilms. **Die Mischgeschwülste.** Heft. 1: Die Mischgeschwülste der Niere. Leipzig: A. Georgi, 1899.

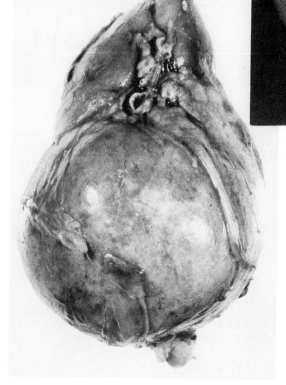

Child with Wilms' tumor.

Gross specimen of tumor.

partially obstructing its lumen. The renal pelvis was free of tumor.''

This typical description of the first of seven cases of nephroblastoma was published by Max Wilms in 1899, in his monograph on mixed tumors.

Wilms was not the first to describe the embryonic renal tumor that became known as Wilms' tumor. T.F. Rance recorded one in 1814 and Wilms reviewed published cases starting with Eberth in 1872, Cohnheim in 1875, and others. The nomenclature of these tumors was based upon the dominant histologic structures, and included chondroma, rhabdomyoma and similar terms. The complex structures were attributed to metaplasia according to Virchow's views,

and to displaced germinative tissue according to Cohnheim. Wilms pointed out that the tumors were derived from embryonic mesoderm. It is this clarification of their origin that related his name eponymically to the tumor.

Max Wilms (1867-1918) was born near Aachen, and obtained his medical degree at Bonn in 1890. He worked in pathology at Giessen and at Cologne, and in 1899 published his monograph on mixed tumors. He subsequently trained in surgery at Leipzig, being appointed professor of surgery in Basel in 1907 and at the University of Heidelberg in 1910. He died at age 51 from an infection contracted during an operation on a French prisoner of war.

Post-Listerian Surgery

Anesthesia, introduced in 1846, and antisepsis, introduced in 1867, revolutionized surgery, including surgery for cancer.

The troubled history of anesthesia has been oft told. It is one of the great contributions to humanity made in the United States. The history of antisepsis and asepsis is linked with Joseph Lister (1827-1912). In amputations of the lower extremity, mortality dropped from 16 to 35 cases before antisepsis, to 6 of 40 after the adoption of the antiseptic method. The proposals encountered opposition, until tested during an epidemic of trauma, the Franco-Prussian War. Yet even then, one wonders whether Lister may have eventuated with Semmelweis as an eccentric had his discoveries not occurred during the bacteriologic explanations of Pasteur and of Koch. For, indeed, Lister's interpretation of his principle was that "all the local inflammatory mischief and general febrile disturbance which follow severe injuries are due to the irritating and poisoning influence of decomposing blood or sloughs."

Many of the great advances in cancer surgery straddle the 19th and the 20th Centuries.

J. Lister. On the antiseptic principles in the practice of surgery. **Lancet** 2: 353-56, 1867.

Joseph Lister. **Collected papers**, 2 vols. London: Oxford Univ. Press, 1909.

ON THE ANTISEPTIC PRINCIPLE IN THE PRACTICE OF SURGERY.*

By JOSEPH LISTER, Esq., F.R.S.,
PROFESSOR OF SURGERY IN THE UNIVERSITY OF GLASGOW.

In the course of an extended investigation into the nature of inflammation, and the healthy and morbid conditions of the blood in relation to it, I arrived, several years ago, at the conclusion that the essential cause of suppuration in wounds is decomposition, brought about by the influence of the atmosphere upon blood or serum retained within them, and, in the case of contused wounds, upon portions of tissue destroyed by the violence of the injury.

To prevent the occurrence of suppuration, with all its attendant risks, was an object manifestly desirable; but till lately apparently unattainable, since it seemed hopeless to attempt to exclude the oxygen, which was universally regarded as the agent by which putrefaction was effected. But when it had been shown by the researches of Pasteur that the septic property of the atmosphere depended, not on the oxygen or any gaseous constituent, but on minute organisms suspended in it, which owed their energy to their vitality, it occurred to me that decomposition in the injured part might be avoided without excluding the air, by applying as a dressing some material capable of destroying the life of the floating particles. Upon this principle I have based a practice of which I will now attempt to give a short account.

The material which I have employed is carbolic or phenic acid, a volatile organic compound which appears to exercise a peculiarly destructive influence upon low forms of life, and hence is the most powerful antiseptic with which we are at present acquainted.

The first class of cases to which I applied it was that of compound fractures, in which the effects of decomposition in the injured part were especially striking and pernicious. The results have been such as to establish conclusively the great principle, that *all the local inflammatory mischief and general febrile disturbance which follow severe injuries are due to the irritating and poisoning influence of decomposing blood or sloughs.* For these evils are entirely avoided by the antiseptic treatment, so that limbs which otherwise would be unhesitatingly condemned to amputation may be retained with confidence of the best results.

Lister, *On the antiseptic principle,* 1867.

Radical mastectomy at Grace-New Haven Hospital, Connecticut, 1894.

VII-F.

Post-Listerian Surgery

VII-F-1. A giant of surgery: Billroth.

Christian Albert Theodor Billroth (1829-1894) occupies an unchallenged place among the greatest of surgeons, and a pioneer in treatment of cancer of internal organs that aseptic surgery made possible.

Billroth, born on the island of Rügen, graduated in medicine from Berlin in 1852, and became an assistant to Langenbeck at Göttingen. He was made professor of surgery at Zürich (1860-1867), and then at Vienna, where he spent the rest of his life and achieved his surgical triumphs. These included resection of the esophagus in 1871, complete excision of the larynx in 1873, partial gastrectomy in 1881, and gastrojejunostomy in 1885. He performed many intestinal resections and enterorrhaphies, pelvic operations and mastectomies.

Among his many pupils were Mikulicz, Czerny, Wölfler, Kocher, Hacker, Eiselberg and Narath. He was a prolific writer and a talented musician; his friendship with Johannes Brahms was one of his attachments to Vienna.

It was Billroth's practice to publish uncompromisingly his surgical results on an annual basis. Alexandre von Winiwarter (1848-1916) of Belgium, one of his assistants, compiled these data into one of the first statistical reviews of operative results in cancer, especially of patients with mammary and gastric cancer. The end-results on 548 patients with carcinoma treated in Billroth's clinic between 1867 and 1876 are presented. In cancer of the breast, 4.7% of 170 patients were alive and well three years or more later.

T. Billroth. Ein Beitrag zur den Operationen am Magen. Gasteroraphie. **Wien Med. Wchnschr.** 27: 913-16, 1877.

T. Billroth. Offenes Schreiben an Herrn Dr. L Wittelshöfer. **Wien Med. Wchnschr.** 31: 161-65, 1881.

T Billroth. Ueber die Resection des Oesophagus. **Arch. Klin. Chir.** 13: 65-69, 1871.

Ruth J. Mann. Theodor Billroth, 1829-1894. **Mayo Clin. Proc.** 49: 132-35, 1974.

A von Winiwarter. **Beiträge zur Statistik der Carcinome.** Stuttgart: Enke, 1878.

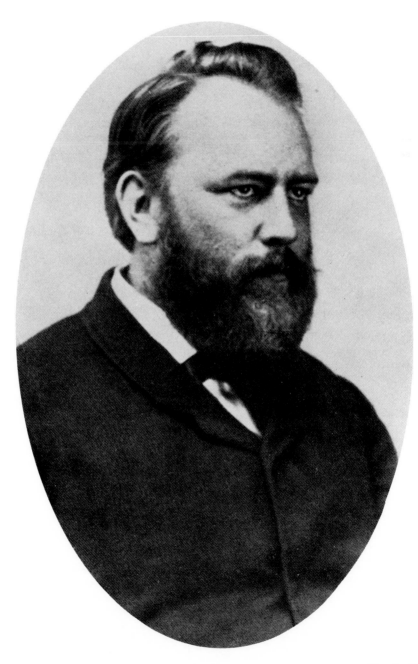

Theodor Billroth

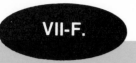

VII-F.

Post-Listerian Surgery

VII-F-2. Radical mastectomy: Halsted.

Cancer of the breast has been a prime example of malignant disease and its treatment since antiquity. The primitive and brutal amputations described in the older medical writings can be compared with the legend of the martyrdom of Saint Agatha.

As the information concerning breast cancer and its spread grew during the late 18th and early 19th Centuries, surgeons began to emphasize the need to remove the axillary lymph nodes in breast cancer. The results, however, remained poor.

It remained for William Stewart Halsted (1852-1922) to develop the radical mastectomy in which the breast is removed en-bloc with the axillary contents and the pectoral muscles. Halsted reported his operation in 1891 and more completely in 1894. At the latter time, Willy Meyer of New York published a similar approach.

With the introduction of the radical mastectomy, the end-results in breast cancer improved, from an average of under 20% to almost 40% 3-year survival. Halsted's procedure for breast cancer

remained unchallenged for half a century.

Halsted was born in New York, and was professor of surgery at Johns Hopkins University from 1889 on. He was a prodigious worker, quiet and unobtrusive, whose surgical "touch" was delicacy and meticulous technique. His contributions extended over a wide range of general and experimental surgery.

The history of breast cancer and its treatment is beautifully recorded by Cooper and by Lewison.

W. A. Cooper. The history of the radical mastectomy. **Ann. Med. Hist.** 3: 36-54, 1941.

W. S. Halsted. The treatment of wounds. IV. Operations for carcinoma of the breast. **Johns Hopkins Hosp. Repts.** 2: 277-280, 1890-91.

W. S. Halsted. The results of operations for the cure of cancer of the breast performed at the Johns Hopkins Hospital from June 1889 to January 1894. **Ann. Surg.** 20: 497-555, 1894.

E. F. Lewison. Saint Agatha, the patron saint of diseases of the breast in legend and art. **Bull. Hist. Med.** 24: 409-20, 1950.

E. F. Lewison. **Breast Cancer and Its Diagnosis and Treatment.** Baltimore: The Williams and Wilkins Co., 1955. Chapter 1, p. 1-27.

W. Meyer. An improved method of the radical operation for carcinoma of the breast. **Med. Rec.** 46: 746-49, 1894.

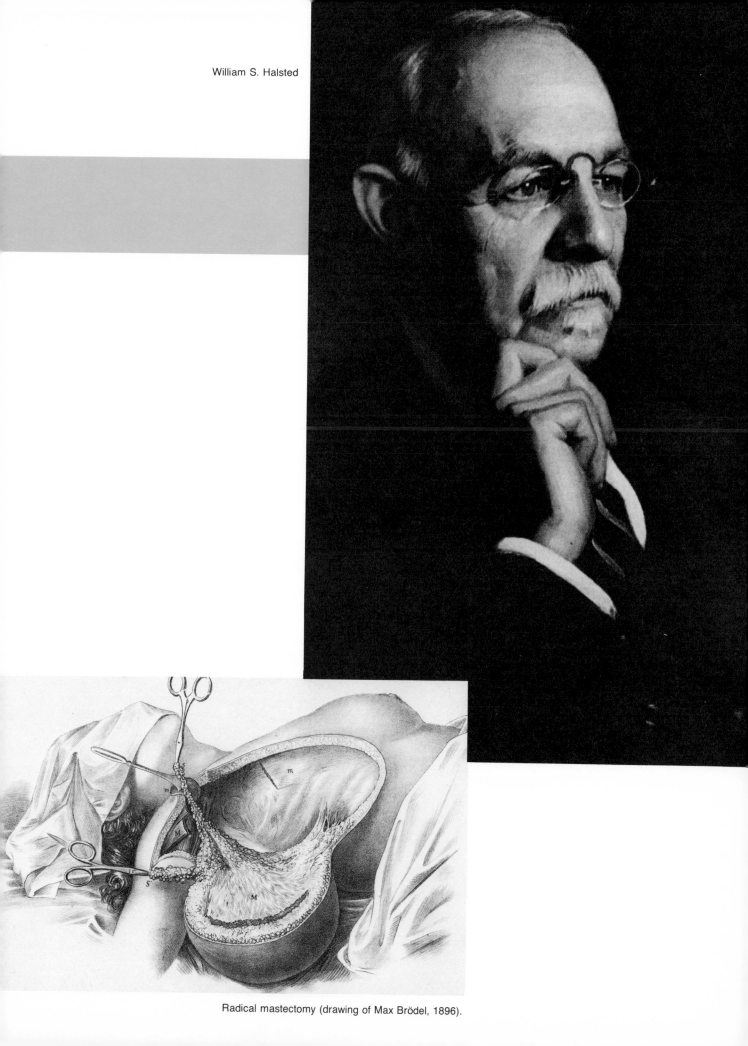

William S. Halsted

Radical mastectomy (drawing of Max Brödel, 1896).

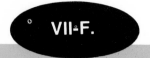

Post-Listerian Surgery

VII-F-3. Rectal cancer: Lisfranc to Quénu.

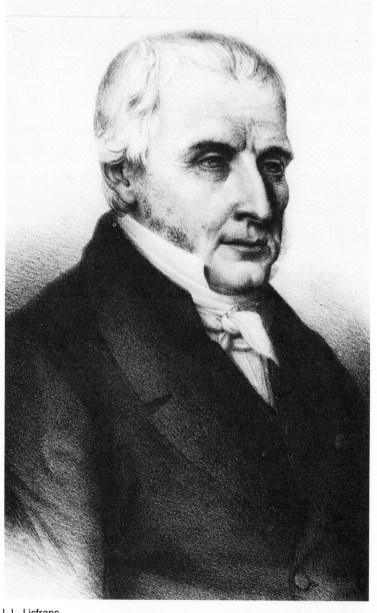

J. L. Lisfranc

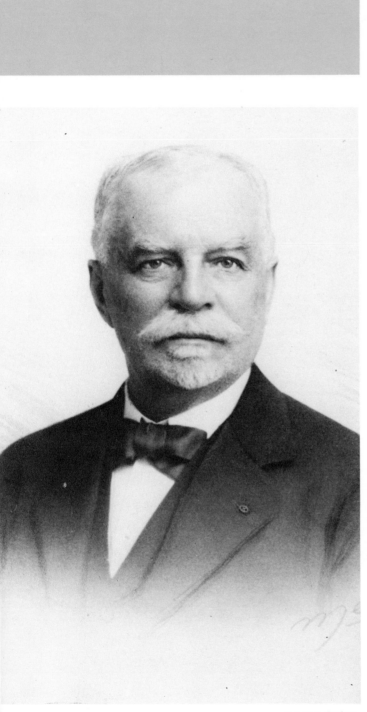

E-A-V-A Quénu

Cancer of the colon and rectum were approached surgically during the 19th Century, but definitive methods had to await the 20th Century.

Jacques L. Lisfranc (1790-1847) performed perineal removal of the rectum for cancer, by excision of the anus and lower rectum below the peritoneal reflection. He operated on 9 patients, with 3 operative deaths. It was obviously a palliative, last-ditch relief of complete obstruction, and his patients died of carcinomatosis within 2 years of operation.

Jean François Reybard (1790-1863) in 1833 resected a carcinoma of the sigmoid in a man of 28, performed an end-to-end anastomosis, and the patient recovered from the operation to live for six months until recurrence. The case was reviewed by the Royal Academy of Medicine and deemed authentic, but no attempts to repeat the procedure are on record.

Edouard-André-Victor-Alfred Quénu (1852-1933) elected to resect cancer of the rectum by the abdomino-perineal route in order to provide better access to the higher rectal cancers and the lymph nodes along the iliac vessels. He did not attempt systematic resection of the regional lymph nodes. Quénu did his first operation in 1896 and had 8 cases by 1899.

J. Lisfranc. Mémoire sur l'excision de la partie inferieure du rectum devenue carcinomateuse. **Mém. acad. roy. méd.** 3 :291-302, 1833.

J. F. Reybard. Mémoire sur une tumeur cancéreuse affectant l'S iliaque du côlon; ablation de la tumeur et de l'intestin; réunion directe et immédiate des deux bouts de cet organe, guérison. **Bull. acad. roy. méd.** 9: 1031-43, 1843-44.

E. Quénu et H. Hartmann. **Chirurgie du Rectum.** Paris: G. Steinheil, 2 vol., 1895 and 1899.

VII-G.

Statistics and Epidemiology

VII-G-1. Cancer death rates: Tanchou and Rigoni-Stern.

della periodicità delle stesse, ed in causa specialmente
della maggior facilità alle meccaniche offese?

Parlando in primo luogo dei cancri delle donne
non posso far utili confronti tra la quantità totale di
quelli dell' utero e di quelli delle mammelle. Giova
piuttosto osservare la differente frequenza degli uni e
degli altri circa l'età: quelli dell' utero sembrano rag-
giungere il maximum tra i 40 e 50 anni, quelli delle
mammelle fra i 60 e i 70.

I rapporti tra la popolazione femminina esistente
nei diversi periodi di età, e la frequenza delle ma-
lattie cancerose, sono, rappresentata la popolazione
stessa in ciascbedun periodo da diecimila, come segue:

Età.	Cancro d'utero.	Cancro delle mammelle.
		1,10
da 20 a 30 anni.	3,59	5,54
30 » 40	21,05	20,57
40 » 50	44,25	29,16
50 » 60	40,82	53,70
60 » 70	24,21	50,46
70 » 80	11,58	28,66
80 » 90	2,20	30,35
90 » 100	0,00	

Dalle quali proporzioni deducesi che la frequenza
dei cancri dell'utero è in ragione affatto diversa da
quella dei cancri delle mammelle: quelli sono già

Rigoni-Stern's report of 1842, showing age distribution of uterine and mammary cancer deaths.

512

sufficientemente numerosi dai 30 ai 40 anni, e lo di-
ventano poi il doppio più nei due successivi decennj,
mentre dopo i 60 anni vanno rapidamente diminuen-
do; questi poi sotto i 40 anni sono pochissimi, mentre in seguito vanno aumentando specialmente dopo i
60 anni e forse anche dopo i 70. Forse la diminu-
zione che osservasi dopo gli 80 anni non è che ap-
parente. Comunque la cosa sia, egli è certo che dopo
i 60 anni i cancri d'utero stanno a quelli delle mammelle come 1 a 4, o meglio come 3 a 13 circa.

Io considero queste deduzioni come importantis-
sime per la storia del cancro.

Seguitando a dire dei cancri dell'utero e delle
mammelle nelle femmine ebbi a notare della frequenza
relativa di questa malattia a seconda dello stato loro
diverso. Le quantità precise sono le seguenti:

Morirono di cancro.

Stato.	Dell'utero.	Delle mam.	Totale.
nubili comprese le monache	20	86	106
maritate	225	114	339
vedove	108	99	207
stato non indicato	12	10	22
Somme	365	309	674

confrontando la frequenza relativa dei cancri,
specialmente sott'occhio la proporzione di quelli
e della mammella nelle nubili e nelle ma-

Vital statistics have their roots in John Graunt (1620-1674) and in Johann Peter Süssmilch (1707-1777). But it was not until the 19th Century that cancer statistics in a modern sense emerged.

Cancer statistics were gathered around Paris between 1830 and 1840, by Stanislas Tanchou (1791-1850) and data for 1760 to 1839 around Verona were accumulated by Domenico Antonio

Rigoni-Stern (1810-?).

Tanchou recorded a total of 382,851 deaths, of which 194,735 were among males and 158,116 among females. Cancer was the cause of death in 9,118; 2,161 in males and 6,957 in females. The distribution of cancers by over 20 sites of origin showed the 5 most frequent ones as follows:

Uterus	2,996
Stomach	2,303
Breast	1,147
Liver	578
Rectum	251

The cancer death percentage had risen from 1.96 to 2.40 during the decade, leading Tanchou to conclude that cancer deaths were increasing.

Rigoni-Stern pointed out that such statistics had possible sources of error, including those of terminology. His data were on 150,673 deaths, of which 76,489 were males and 74,184 were females. There were 1,142 deaths from cancer, 142 in males and 994 in females, which he divided into four types: uterus (365 cases), breast (319 cases), face and "other." The preponderance of cancers of the uterus around Verona was not as marked as around Paris, but still uterus was the most frequent site. The analyses of his figures, by age, sex, occupation and other features, resemble modern demographic studies on cancer. Among his conclusions, as summarized by

Scotto and Bailar were:

1. The incidence of cancer generally increases with age.
2. This is mainly due to a very rapid increase observed for uterine cancers.
3. The frequency of breast cancer is inversely related to the incidence of uterine cancer for different age groups.
4. Breast cancer increases with age. A notable increase is also observed 10 to 15 years after the usual time of menopause.
5. Unmarried persons generally have a greater chance of contracting cancer, especially breast cancer in women.
6. Married women contract uterine cancer more often than unmarried women.
7. Cancer in general seems to be less frequent in the country and suburbs than in the cities.
8. The incidence of skin cancer is equal for both males and females.
9. Cancer of different anatomical sites probably has different etiologies.
10. Cancer is much more frequent in females than in males.

Tanchou's data on cancer were used by Walshe in England and by LeConte in the United States, but the contributions of Rigoni-Stern were forgotten, until resurrected by Clemmesen in 1951.

Johannes Clemmesen. **Statistical Studies in the Aetiology of Malignant Neoplasms.** 4 vols. København: Munksgaard, 1965, vol. 1, p. 2.

John LeConte. Statistical researches on cancer. **Southern Med. and Surg. J.** n.s. 2: 257-93, 1846.

P. Mustacchi. Ramazzini and Rigoni-Stern on parity and breast cancer. **Arch. Int. Med.** 108: 639-42, 1961.

D. Rigoni-Stern. Fatti statistici relativi alle mallattie cancerose che servirono di base alle poche cose. **G. Progr. Patol. Terap.** 2: 499-517, 1842.

Joseph Scotto and John C. Bailar III. Rigoni-Stern and medical statistics. A nineteenth-century approach to cancer research. **J. Hist. Med.** 24: 65-75, 1969.

S. Tanchou. Recherches sur la fréquence du cancer. **Gaz. des Hôpitaux** 16 (ser. 2,5): 313, July 6, 1843.

W. H. Walshe. **The Nature and Treatment of Cancer.** London: Taylor and Walton, 1846.

Statistics and Epidemiology

VII-G-2. Classification of cancer: Farr and Bertillon.

The development of vital registration systems, essential for the understanding of the rates of diseases in different communities, began in England, where in 1836 was established the General Register office. William Farr (1807-1883), who worked for over 40 years in the office, practically founded modern vital statistics.

In 1853, Farr and Jacob Marc d'Espine (1806-1860) of Geneva drew up a classification of diseases for international use, which went through a series of modifications. Adolphe Louise Jacques Bertillon (1851-1922) of France continued the task. In 1900 the Bertillon Classification of the Causes of Death was accepted in Paris for international use.

Cancer was included under II. Other General Diseases (I being Epidemic Diseases), as follows:

25A. **Cancer of the mouth**. This title includes: Cancer of the lips, tongue, roof of the mouth, or of the velum palati; cancer of the jaw; epithelioma, carcinoma, or cancroid of those parts; smokers' cancer.

25B. **Cancer of the stomach; of the liver.** This title includes: Cancer of the esophagus; cancer of the cardiac portion of the stomach; cancer of the pylorus; carcinoma; scirrhus, colloid or encephaloid tumor of those parts; gastrocarcinoma; tumor of the stomach.
This title does not include: Organic lesion of the stomach (81); hematemesis (81).

25C. **Cancer of the intestines; of the rectum**. This title includes: Cancer of the colon; cancer of the anus; carcinoma, scirrhus, encephaloid, cancroid or epithelioma of those parts.

25D. **Cancer of the female genital organs**. This title includes: Cancer of the womb; cancer of the ovary; cancer of the vagina; cancer of the vulva; carcinoma, scirrhus, encephaloid, colloid, heteromorphous or neoplastic tumor, sarcoma or epithelioma of those organs.

A. L. J. Bertillon

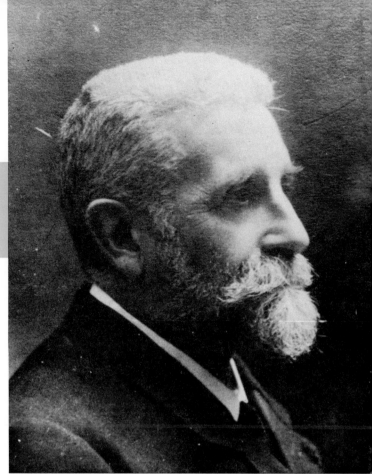

25E. **Cancer of the breast**. This title includes: Carcinoma, scirrhus, encephaloid, colloid, heteromorphous or neoplastic tumor, cancroid or epithelioma of the breast or mammary gland.

25F. **Cancer of the skin**. This title includes: Cancroid (without epithet); epithelioma or epithelial tumor (without epithet); cancer of the face or cervico-facial cancer; noli-me-tangere.

This title does not include: Lupus (22 D); estiomene (22D).

25G. **Cancer of other organs**. This title includes: Cancer of the peritoneum; cancerous peritonitis; pelvic cancer; cancer of the kidney, bladder or prostate; cancerous goitre; thyreo-sarcoma; sarco-hydrocele; cancer of bone; osteosarcoma; cancerous tumor or sarcoma of the neck; carcinoma, scirrhus, encephaloid, cancerous ulcer, malignant tumor, sarcoma, or malignant fungus of these parts or of unspecified part of the body.

This title does not include: Cancer of the esophagus (25 B); cancer of the anus (25 C); cancer of the ovary, vagina or vulva (25 D).

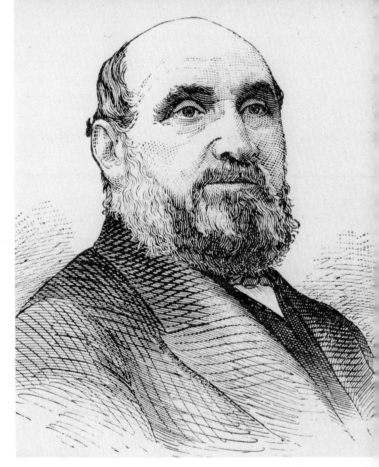

William Farr

The Bertillon Classification of Causes of Death.
Lansing: Robert Smith Printing Co., 1899.
C. Singer and E. A. Underwood. **A Short History of Medicine.** ed. 2. New York: Oxford, 1962. (p. 715-17).

VII-H.

Carcinogenic Environments

VII-H-1. Lung cancer among miners: Härting and Hesse.

The mines of the Black Forest regions of Schneeberg and Joachimsthal have been worked for their riches for at least 500 years. Silver for the coffers of princelings, and later cobalt and uranium, were paid for heavily in the health of the workers. The fatal Mala Metallorum was well known to Paracelsus in 1531 and to Agricola in 1556.

In 1879, F. H. Härting, physician to the Schneeberg miners, and W. Hesse, a district doctor, analyzed 150 deaths among 650 men during 1869-1877, and reported that 75 percent of all deaths were due to a malignant neoplasm of the lung. The original diagnosis was recorded as lymphosarcoma of the mediastinum with extension to the lungs. Reviews of pathology by subsequent investigators reclassified the great majority of the cases as bronchogenic carcinoma. The epidemiological conclusion, however, was unequivocal from the inordinate relative frequency of cancer.

The investigations of Härting and Hesse are the first clear record of an internal neoplasm being caused by environmental exposure to a complex carcinogen. The exact nature of the carcinogen was debated for many years. The most probable chief stimulus that is accepted currently is radioactivity from uranium. A similar situation of greatly increased risk to lung cancer is becoming evident among uranium miners on the Colorado plateaus.

Epidemiological investigations have added several other industrial situations that increase the risk to lung cancer, including inhalation of chromates, ferrous ore, and asbestos. Tobacco smoke, however, is the more widely distributed pulmonary carcinogen for man.

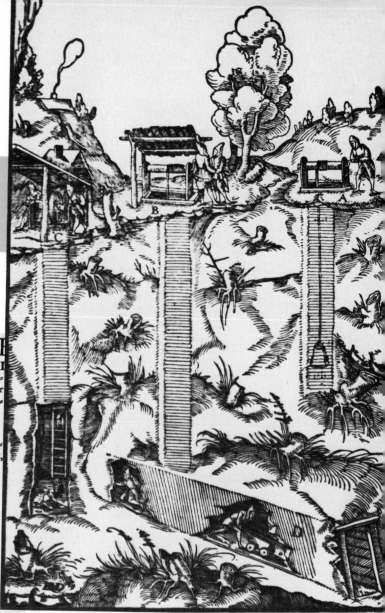

Mining in the Black Forest, from Agricola, 1556.

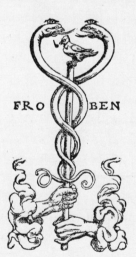

Agricola, *De Re Metallica,* 1556. Title page.

Gregorius Agricola. **De Re Metallica, 1556.** Transl. by
Herbert C. Hoover and Lou H. Hoover. London: Mining
Magazine, 1912.

M. G. Hanna, Jr., P. Nettesheim, and J. R. Gilbert, (eds).
Conference on Inhalation Carcinogenesis. AEC
Symposium Series #18, U. S. Atomic Energy Commission,
Div. Tech. Info., Oak Ridge, Tenn., 1970.

G. H. Härting and W. Hesse. Der Lungenkrebs, die
Bergkrankheit in den Schneeberger Gruben. **Vrtljschr.
gerlichtl. Med.** 30: 296-309 and 31: 102-32, 1879.

E. Lorenz. Radioactivity and lung cancer: a critical review of
lung cancer in the miners of Schneeberg and Joachimsthal. **J.
Natl. Cancer Inst.** 5: 1-15, 1944.

J. K. Wagoner, V. E. Archer, B. E. Carroll, D. A. Holaday,
and P. A. Lawrence. Cancer mortality patterns among U. S.
uranium miners and millers, 1950 through 1962. **J. Natl.
Cancer Inst.** 32: 787-801, 1964.

VII-H.

Carcinogenic Environments

VII-H-2. Arsenical cancer: Paris and Hutchinson.

Arsenical cancer, described in man as an occupational and an iatrogenic hazard, has not been reproduced in experimental animals.

John Ayrton Paris (1785-1856) in 1822 described the consequences of arsenical fumes around copper smelting works of Cornwall and Wales. "... horses and cows commonly lose their hoofs, and the latter are often seen in the neighboring pastures crawling on their knees and not infrequently suffering from a cancerous affection of their rumps.'. . . It deserves notice that the smelters are occasionally affected with a cancerous disease in the scrotum, similar to that which infests chimney sweepers. . . ."

Jonathan Hutchinson (1828-1913) of the London Hospital in 1888 reported 6 patients who had been treated for many years with potassium arsenite in the form of Fowler's solution. This was the universal tonic during Victorian times. Three patients with psoriasis developed skin cancer, and 3 patients with psoriasis, pemphigus and cancer of the tonsil developed keratosis.

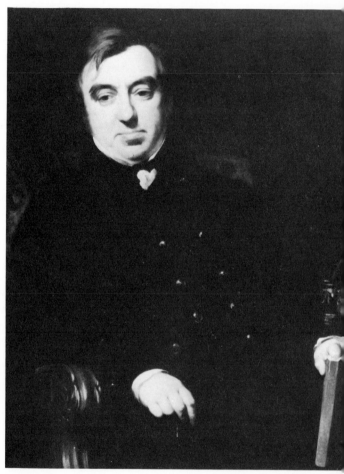

John Ayrton Paris

J. Hutchinson. On some examples of arsenic-keratosis of the skin and of arsenic-cancer. **Trans. Path. Soc. London** 39: 352-63, 1888.

John Ayrton Paris. **Pharmacologia; or the History of Medicinal Substances.** New York: F. and R. Lockwood, 1822.

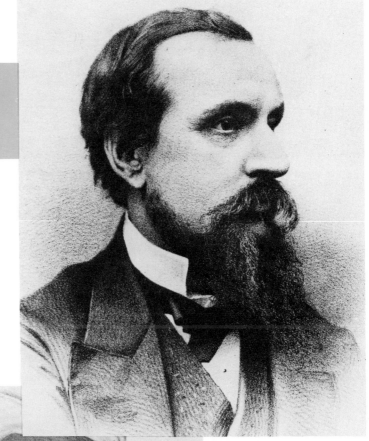

Hutchinson was especially known as a dermatologist and syphilologist, although he also was a surgeon. His name is eponymically associated with the triad of congenital syphilis: notched teeth, interstitial keratitis and sclerosis of the ear drum.

Jonathan Hutchinson

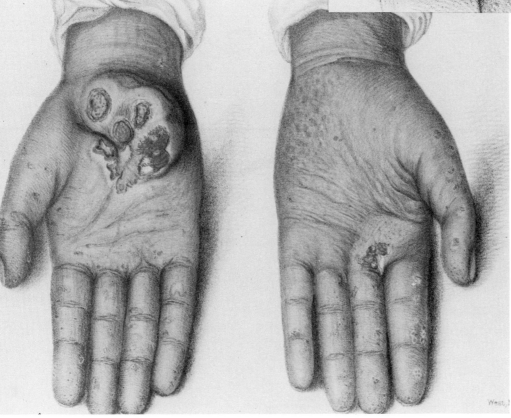

Arsenical cancers of the hand (from Hutchinson, 1888).

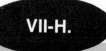

VII-H.

Carcinogenic Environments

VII-H-3. Aniline bladder cancer: Rehn.

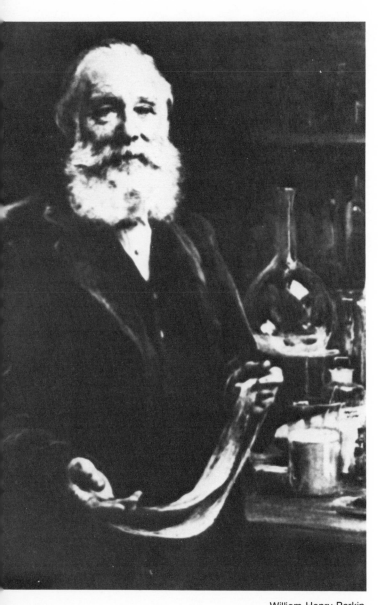

William Henry Perkin

The coal tar dye industry was founded by William Henry Perkin (1838-1907), in England in 1856, when he discovered pigments of the aniline group. The chemical industry of Germany up to World War I supplied more than 80% of the world's production of aniline, its derivatives and related aromatic amines.

A German surgeon of Frankfurt-am-Main, Ludwig Rehn (1849-1919), reported in 1895 the occurrence of bladder cancer in 3 of 45 workers in the aniline dye industry. The occupational cancer hazard was soon demonstrated in Switzerland, England and other industrial countries.

Epidemiologic studies incriminated several aromatic amines, especially napthylamines and benzidine, as carcinogens. Attempts to reproduce the human experience in animals were unsuccessful until 1938, when W. C. Hueper and his associates reported that dogs developed bladder cancer following repeated subcutaneous injections of 2-napthylamine.

The industrial epidemic of chemical bladder carcinogenesis has been reduced but not eliminated by appropriate legal prohibitions and improvements in industrial hygiene regulations.

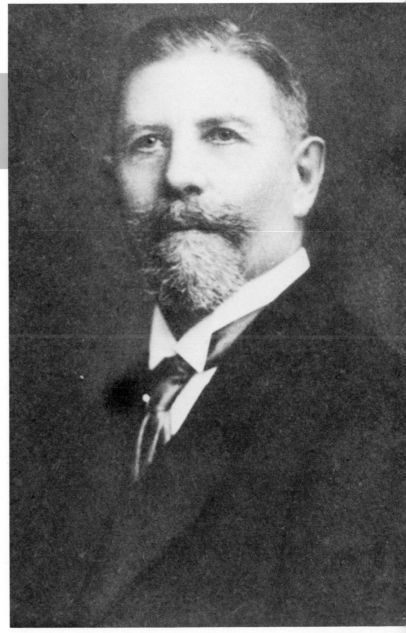

Ludwig Rehn

W. C. Hueper, F. H. Wiley, and H. D. Wolfe. Experimental production of bladder tumors in dogs by administration of beta-naphthylamine. **J. Indust. Hyg.** Toxicol. 20: 46-84, 1938.

O. Leichtenstern. Ueber Harnblasenentzündung und Harnblasen—geschwülste bei Arbetern in Farbfabriken. **Deut. Med. Wchnschr.** 24: 709-13, 1898.

James M. Price. Etiology of bladder cancer. p. 189-261. In E. Maltry, Jr. (ed). **Benign and Malignant Tumors of the Urinary Bladder.** Flushing, N. Y. Med. Examin. Publ. Co., Inc., 1971.

L. Rehn. Blasengeschwülste bei Fuchsin-Arbeitern. **Arch. Klin. Chir.** 50: 588-600, 1895.

Experimental Oncology

VII-I-1. Inoculations with cancer: Nooth and Alibert.

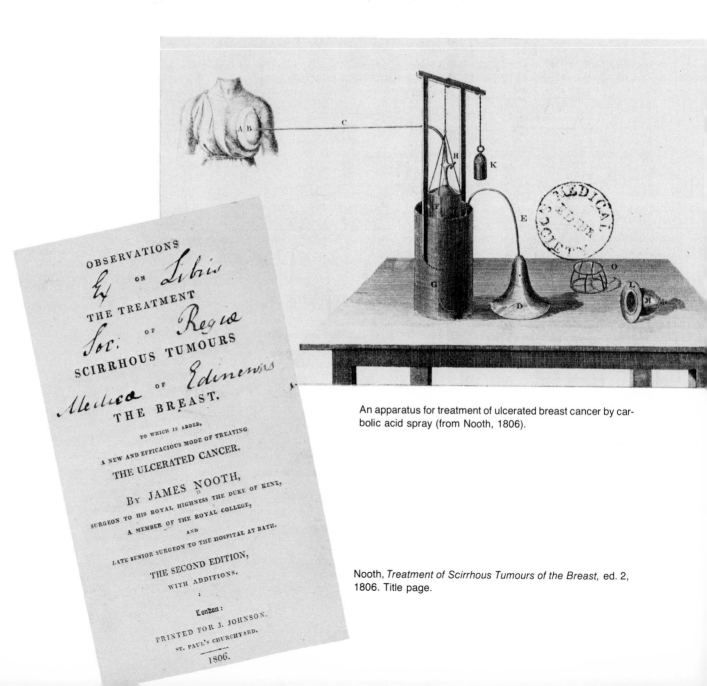

An apparatus for treatment of ulcerated breast cancer by carbolic acid spray (from Nooth, 1806).

Nooth, *Treatment of Scirrhous Tumours of the Breast*, ed. 2, 1806. Title page.

The first attempts to test by experiment whether cancer was transferable from man to man were recorded by Nooth and by Alibert.

James Nooth was a surgeon who practiced in Dorchester and at Bath, and was surgeon to the Duke of Kent. In the second edition of his **Observations on the Treatment of Scirrhous Tumours of the Breast** he wrote:

"The structure of scirrhous tumours, and the morbid state they are in when under examination, precludes a very nice or satisfactory investigation. Being anxious to know what effects this matter would produce, if inserted by inoculation into the arm of a healthy person, (but not being entitled to make that experiment on any human being except myself,) I conveyed a minute portion of it into a small incision on my arm; two hours afterwards I felt the part uneasy, with a strong pulsation. On the following day, it was more uneasy, and much more inflammation appeared than generally attends so small a wound inflicted by a sharp instrument; on the third, it remained nearly in the same state; on the fourth day the wound became easier, and the inflammation and pulsation began to subside. A few days afterwards a large dry scab was formed, which I removed, and found the sore perfectly healed. Not choosing to rely on a single experiment as a sufficient proof that a cancerous disposition could not be conveyed into the habit, I repeatedly inoculated myself from the year 1777, without ever producing any effects dissimilar to those in the first experiment. I am convinced, that those persons who give their attendance to cancerous subjects, are not so liable to get this cruel disease by absorption, as has been too generally supposed."

Jean Louis Alibert (1768-1837) records the following events, as described by Woglom:

"On October 17, 1808, at the Hôpital de St. Louis, and in the presence of several physicians and students, Alibert allowed himself to be injected with ichorous material from a cancer of the breast. The experiment was performed at the same time upon M. Fayet, a medical student, and the next morning upon MM. Lonoble and Durand. Except for an inflammatory reaction the experiment was without sequelae. A week later Alibert inoculated himself a second time, and his colleague, M. Biett. He himself escaped with a result similar to that which followed the first trial, but M. Biett developed a somewhat more severe infection, which involved the axillary and cervical lymph nodes."

J. L. Alibert. **Description des Maladies de la Peau observeés à l'Hôpital St.-Louis.** Paris: Chez Barrois l'âine et fils. 1806-1814, p. 118.

James Nooth. **Observations on the Treatment of Scirrhous Tumors of the Breast.** Ed. 2. London: J. Johnson, 1806, p. 13.

M. B. Shimkin. An historical note on tumor transplantation in man. **Cancer** 35: 540-1, 1975.

W. H. Woglom. **The Study of Experimental Cancer. A Review.** George Crocker Special Research Fund No. 1, New York: Columbia University Press, 1913, p. 43.

VII-I.

Experimental Oncology

VII-I-2. Inoculations between species: Dupuytren and Leidy.

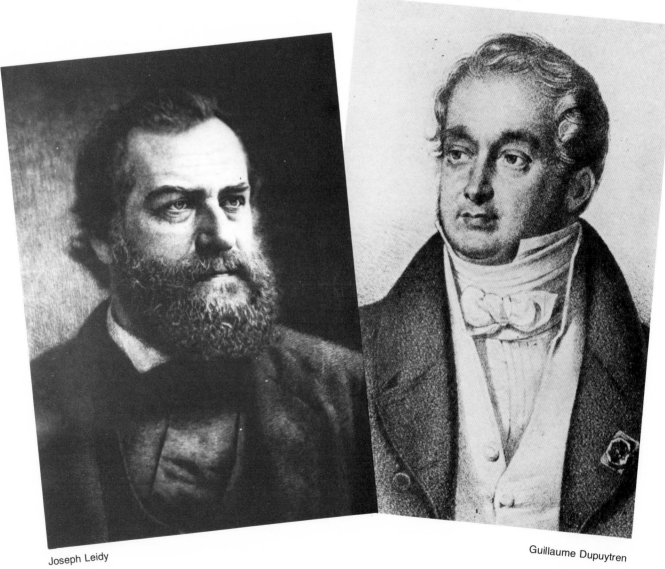

Joseph Leidy

Guillaume Dupuytren

Experimental medicine is dependent upon the use of animals. Living animals were first used for physiological experiments in antiquity. Galen used apes, pigs and dogs in his work, and Vesalius repeated many of the same experiments for comparison.

The first recorded use of an experimental animal in cancer was Peyrilhe's injection of human cancerous material into a dog, in 1775. Woglom cites attempts to transfer human cancer to animals in 1807 by Guillaume Dupuytren (1777-1835), the outstanding French surgeon of his day, and in 1840 by Conrad Langenbeck (1776-1851).

Joseph Leidy (1823-1891), of Philadelphia, in 1851 inoculated human breast cancer under the skin of a frog, and five months later found vascular attachments to the fragments, which had been transformed into fibrous tissue. Thus, attempts to transfer cancer between different species were uniformly unsuccessful.

According to Lombard, Gessner in 1553 described a skin tumor in a carp, and by the middle of the 18th Century there were detailed accounts of occurrences of cancer in animals. The fact that animals developed cancers was well known by the early 19th Century. Johannes Müller, in his microscopic examinations of tumors, included specimens from the veterinary anatomical museums in Germany. By the end of the century, Sticker assembled over a thousand carcinomas in larger domestic animals, primarily from veterinary and abattoir sources in Germany from 1858 to 1900.

Credit for the first description of a mammary tumor in the mouse is usually given to Edwards Crisp (1806-1882). His complete report of 1854 was "The animal caught in a trap was of the usual size, and upon the right pectoral muscle was a hard scirrhous like tumor, the size of a large nut. When microscopically examined it had many of the appearances supposed to be characteristic of scirrhus."

E. Crisp. Malignant tumour on the pectoral muscle of a mouse. **Tr. Path. Soc. London** 5: 384, 1854.

Joseph Leidy. Transplantation of malignant tumors. **Proc. Acad. Natural Sci. Philadelphia** 4: 212, 1850 and 5: 201, 1851.

Charles Lombard. **Cancérologie Comparée.** Paris: G. Doin and Cie, 1962.

A. Sticker. Ueber den Krebs der Thiere insbesondere ueber die Empfanglichkeit der verschiedenen Hausthierarten und ueber die Unterschiede des Thier- und Menschenkrebses. **Langenbecks Arch. Klin. Chir.** 65: 616-96, 1902.

Ellen B. Wells. **Animal Experimentation in Medicine Through the 18th Century.** Bethesda, Md.: National Library of Med., 1965.

W. H. Woglom. **The Study of Experimental Cancer.** New York: Columbia Univ. Press, 1913.

VII-I.

Experimental Oncology

VII-I-3. First transplantation of cancer: Novinsky.

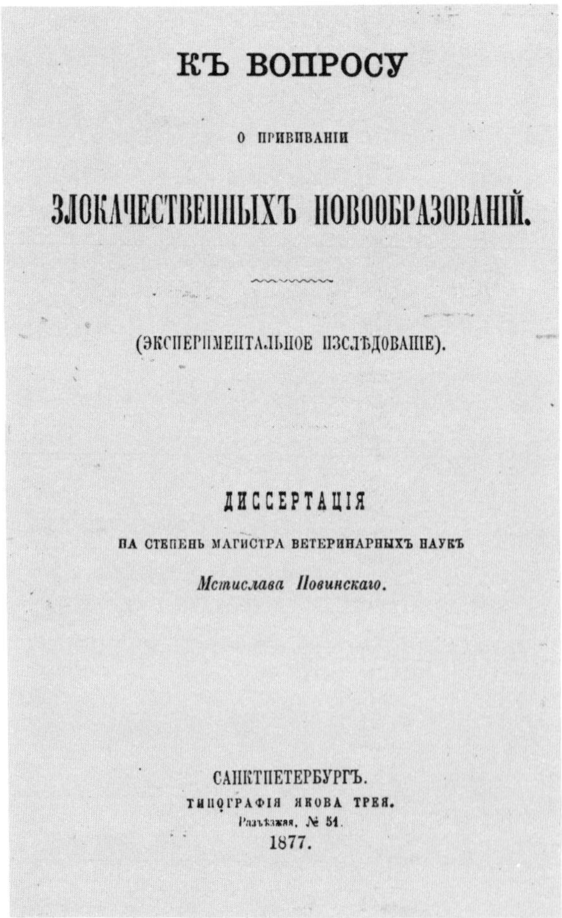

КЪ ВОПРОСУ

О ПРИВИВАНІИ

ЗЛОКАЧЕСТВЕННЫХЪ НОВООБРАЗОВАНІЙ.

(ЭКСПЕРИМЕНТАЛЬНОЕ ИЗСЛѢДОВАНІЕ).

ДИССЕРТАЦІЯ

НА СТЕПЕНЬ МАГИСТРА ВЕТЕРИНАРНЫХЪ НАУКЪ

Мстислава Новинскаго.

САНКТПЕТЕРБУРГЪ.
ТИПОГРАФІЯ ЯКОВА ТРЕЯ.
Разъѣзжая, № 51.
1877.

Novinsky, *On the Question of Inoculation of Malignant Neoplasms,* 1877. Title page.

M. Novinsky

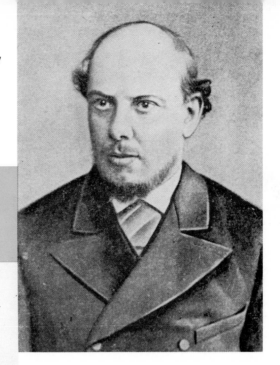

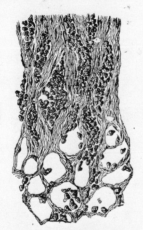

Рис. 1—изображает привитую
опухоль мозговидного рака.
Препарат взят из опухоли
собаки, см. опыт № 2-й

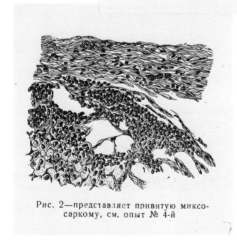

Рис. 2—представляет привитую миксо-
саркому, см. опыт № 4-й

Microscopic appearance of transplanted tumors
in dogs (from Novinsky, 1877).

M. Novinsky. **On the Question of Inoculation of
Malignant Neoplasms.** (thesis). St. Petersburg: Yakov Trey,
1877.

M. Nowinsky. Zur Frage über die Impfung der Krebsigen
Geschürdste. **Centralbl. f.d. med. Wissensch.** 14: 790-91,
1876.

L. M. Shabad. **M. A. Novinsky, Forefather of
Experimental Oncology.** Moscow: Acad. Med. Nauk USSR,
1950.

M. B. Shimkin. M. A. Novinsky: A note on the history of
transplantation of tumors. **Cancer** 8: 653-55, 1955.

In December of 1875, Novinsky in St.
Petersburg obtained a dog with an invasive carcinoma of the nose. Small fragments of the tumor were implanted subcutaneously into a puppy. The mass
grew and 2 months later fragments were
transplanted into 3 other puppies, where
it again grew. The histological appearance was the same as that of the original
tumor, and the first transplant showed
metastases to a lymph node.

A year later a tumor of the uterus and
vaginal vault in a dog was successfully
transplanted through 2 generations of
puppies. Thus, transplantation of tumors
in animals of the same species was
clearly demonstrated.

Mistislav Aleksandrovich Novinsky
(1841-1914) was a student in the veterinary department of the Medical-Surgical
Academy in St. Petersburg, and the work
was a thesis for the degree of Master of
Veterinary Science. Novinsky entered
government service and conducted no
further research. His work was recognized, but on the basis of his brief report
in German rather than his complete
thesis. Later authors extended the priority of tumor transplantation to Hanau,
and Novinsky's contribution was almost
forgotten.

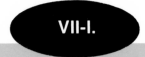

VII-I.

Experimental Oncology

VII-I-4. Tumor transplants in rodents: Hanau and Morau.

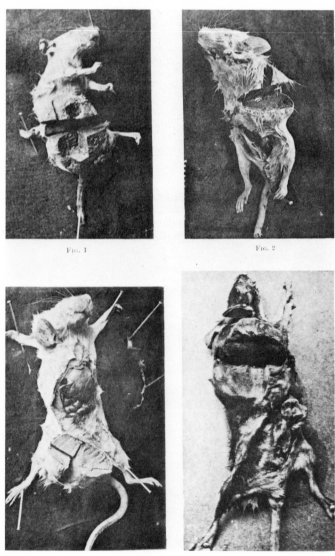

Transplanted tumors in mice (from Morau, 1894).

A decade after Novinsky's successful transplantation of tumors in dogs, Hanau reported transplantation of a tumor in a rat. The experiment consisted of inculcating two rats with a metastasis of a vulvar epidermoid carcinoma. Hanau recognized that Novinsky's work was "almost certainly positive."

Arthur Nathan Hanau (1858-1900) was a graduate at Bonn and worked with Cohnheim, Weigert and Kühne. He became an assistant in pathology in Zurich, where he did his tumor work. A romantic legend arose that Hanau committed suicide because his work was neglected. In fact, Hanau had two operations for rectal cancer, and on autopsy was found to have a large gastric carcinoma.

In 1896 Jenny reviewed Hanau's histologic material, and this review focused attention on the contribution.

Successful transplantation of mammary tumors in mice was reported in 1894 by Henry Morau of Paris. However, his interpretation of the results, as well as some of the results, were erroneous. Morau believed he was transferring some tumor-producing agent rather than the tumor itself. Since he used old mice, and since some of his tumors arose distant to the site of inoculation, the experiments were confounded by the appearance of spontaneous tumors as well as representing transplantation.

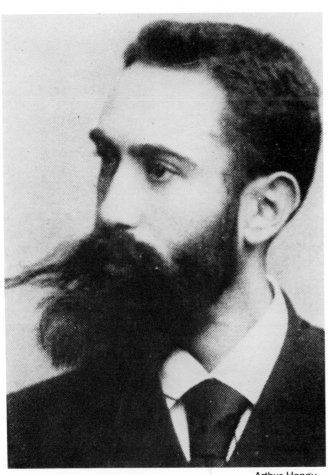

Arthur Hanau

Arthur Hanau. Erfolgreiche experimentalle Uebertragung von Carcinom. **Fortschr. Med.** 7: 321-39, 1889.

H. Jenny. Beiträge zur Lehre von Carcinom. **Arch. Klin. Chir.** 51: 269-315, 1896.

Henry Morau. Recherches expérimentales sur la transmissibilité de certains néoplasmes. **Arch. Med. Exper. et d'Anat. Path.** 6: 677-705, 1894.

M. B. Shimkin. Arthur Nathan Hanau: A further note on the history of transplantation of tumors. **Cancer** 13: 211, 1960.

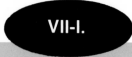

Experimental Oncology

VII-I-5. Bacteriology of cancer:

CANCER PARASITES.

BACTERIA: Bacillus of Rappin,[35] 1886; Scheurlen,[36] 1887; Francke,[37] 1888; Lampiasi,[38] 1888; Koubassof,[39] 1889.
Micrococcus neoformans, Doyen,[40] 1902.
COCCIDIA: Coccidium of Darier,[41] 1889; Albarran,[42] 1889; Thoma,[43] 1888; Sjobring,[44] 1890.
Coccidium sarcolytum, Adamkiewicz,[45] 1892; Soudakiewitsch-Metchnikoff,[46] 1892; Monsarrat,[47] 1905.
SPOROZOA (unclassified): Bird's-eye inclusion, Foa,[48] 1891; Plimmer's bodies, 1892.
Sporozoon, Ruffer,[49] 1892; Sawtschenko,[50] 1893.
Amœbasporidium, L. Pfeiffer,[51] 1893.
Rhopalocephalus carcinomatosus, Korotneff,[52] 1893.
Sporozoon, Kourloff,[53] 1894; Bosc,[54] 1897.
Hæmatozoon, Kahane,[55] 1894.
Cancriamœba macroglossia, Eisen,[56] 1900.
Leydenia gemmipara, Schaudinn,[57] 1896.
Intranuclear parasite, Schuller,[58] 1901–4.
BLASTOMYCETES: *Saccharomyces neoformans*, Sanfelice,[59] 1896; Plimmer,[60] Leopold,[61] Roncali,[62] Bra.[63]
Russell's fuchsin bodies.[64]
Mucor racemosus, Schmidt,[65] 1906.
MYCETOZOA: *Plasmodiophora brassicæ*, Behla,[66] Podwyssoski,[67] Feinberg,[68] Gaylord,[69] Robertson and Wade,[70]
SPIROCHÆTÆ: Gaylord,[71] Calkins,[72] 1907.
Cyanide-fast bodies, Robertson,[73] 1907.

Cancer Parasites, a partial listing according to Ewing, 1907.

James Ewing. Cancer problems. **Harvey Lectures** 3: 34-88, 1907-08.

Harvey R. Gaylord. On the presence of a characteristic organism in cancer. **First Ann. Rept. N.Y. State Path. Lab.**, 1899. (p. 13).

Harvey R. Gaylord. A spirochete in primary and transplanted carcinoma of the breast in mice. **J. Infect. Dis.** 4: 155-70, 1907.

The fourth quarter of the 19th Century belongs medically to Pasteur and to Koch, and the new science of bacteriology.

It was inevitable that the concepts and techniques of bacteriology were applied to neoplastic diseases. Between 1886 to 1907, the literature is replete with reports claiming or implying the identification and isolation of every variety of micro-organism as the cause of cancer. In the early nineties, it appeared to have been a question, not so much as to the infectious origin of cancer, but rather as to which of the many parasites was the real causative agent.

Ewing, in his review of 1907, listed 38 representative papers on cancer parasites, which included bacilli, molds, spirochetes and protozoa among the candidates. G. Rappin in France maintained the claims for his bacillus for three decades, as did F. Sanfelice of Italy for his blastomycete, against which he devised a vaccine.

In the United States, Harvey R. Gaylord (1872-1924), director of the major research program at the cancer laboratory founded in Buffalo in 1898, assumed that cancer was an infectious process caused by a protozoan. Some years later, after this hypothesis was no longer tenable, a new candidate appeared—a spirochete in mammary tumors in mice. This organism also disappeared from the scene on further examination.

Little of positive value remained from the search for infectious agents in cancer. By 1910 scientific consensus was for a non-infectious nature of cancer. This view seriously hampered the acceptance of the role of filterable viruses in neoplastic disease. At the same time, there still remain proponents for bacterial causation of cancer, the organisms usually being described as having complex life cycles.

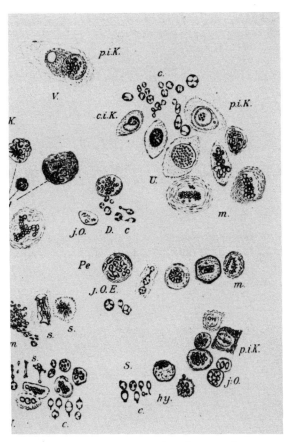

Schuller's intranuclear parasite of carcinoma and sarcoma (from Ewing)

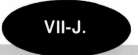

VII-J.

Clinical Investigations

VII-J-1. Oophorectomy for breast cancer: Beatson.

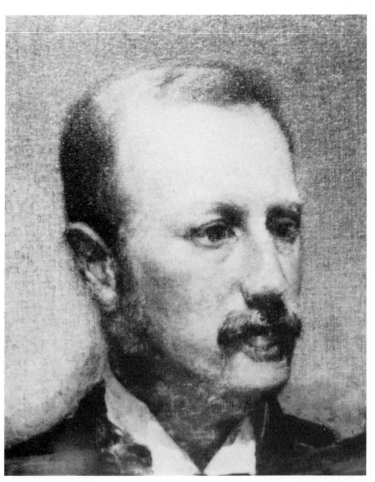

George T. Beatson

George Thomas Beatson (1848-1933) of Glasgow in 1896 described the regression of advanced mammary cancer in premenopausal women following ovariectomy. This was the first demonstration of partial hormonal dependence of a neoplasm in man, made long before the endocrine functions of the ovary were defined. Beatson was born in Scotland and received his doctorate in 1878 at Edinburgh. There he was house surgeon to Joseph Lister at the Royal Infirmary.

The reasons that led Beatson to perform oophorectomy in breast cancer remain moot, even after the meticulous review of the evidence by Simmer. It is evident that Albert S. Schinsinger (1827-1911) of Freiburg in 1889 suggested the procedure in order to make "the ladies prematurely old by removing their ovaries," since he thought that the prognosis was better among older women. Schinsinger did not perform oophorectomy, and it is not known whether his suggestion influenced Beatson.

By 1905, Lett gathered 99 cases of inoperable breast cancer treated by oophorectomy, substantiating real but temporary regressions in about one-third of premenopausal patients. The procedure fell into disuse until the advent of chemical sex hormones in the 1930s. Beatson's place in oncology, however, will remain firm. His work was honored in 1951, when the Glasgow Royal Cancer Hospital was renamed the Beatson Institute for Cancer Research.

It is worthy of note that at the same time, J. W. White (1850-1916) of Philadelphia showed that castration shrank the prostate gland in dogs and had a beneficial effect on prostatic hypertrophy in man. This procedure also was abandoned until the work of Huggins in 1940.

George T. Beatson. On the treatment of inoperable cases of carcinoma of the mamma: suggestions for a new method of treatment with illustrative cases. **Lancet** ii: 104-7, 162-5, 1896.

H. Lett et al. An analysis of 99 cases of inoperable carcinoma of the breast treated by oophorectomy. **Lancet** i: 227-8, 1905.

H. H. Simmer. Oophorectomy for breast cancer patients: its proposal, first performance, and first explanation as an endocrine ablation. **Clio Medica** 4: 227-247, 1969.

J. W. White. The present position of the surgery of the hypertrophied prostate. **Ann. Surg.** 40: 782-95, 1904.

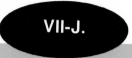

VII-J.

Clinical Investigations

VII-J-2. Systemic cancer therapy: Lissauer and Coley.

A wide variety of herbal and chemical concoctions were given to cancer patients since antiquity. Such agents can be divided into salves and other topically applied preparations, usually containing arsenic or other metals and having an escharotic effect on the cancer as well as surrounding tissue. The second class were preparations given systemically.

Perhaps the first chemical agent to be used with objective response in any form of neoplastic disease was arsenic, in the form of potassium arsenite (Fowler's solution) in leukemia. Two such cases were reported in 1865 by Lissauer of Bendorf. There is no further identification of Dr. Lissauer, but the treatment persisted since no other approaches emerged until

ionizing radiation and benzol were added during the first decade of the 20th Century.

William B. Coley (1862-1936), a prominent surgeon of New York, in 1893 observed regression of a lymphosarcoma in a patient under attack of erysipelas. Coley devised a mixture of streptococci and Bacillus prodigiosus (Coley's mixed toxins) which had objective effects in patients with sarcomas; the treatment was dangerous and the effects were unpredictable. A major research endeavor to characterize the active material was launched during the 1940s by M. J. Shear, and a polysaccharide eventually extracted, but its place in cancer therapy remains undefined.

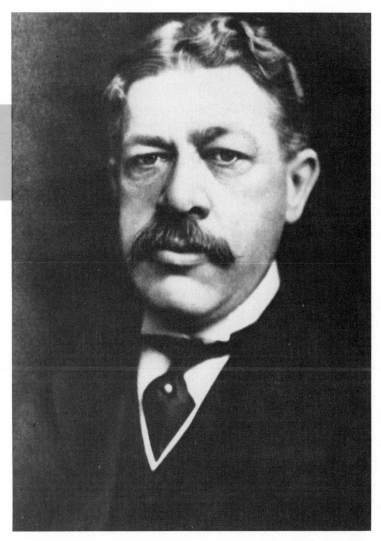

William B. Coley

BERLINER KLINISCHE WOCHENSCHRIFT. 2. October 1865.   403

II. Zwei Fälle von Leucaemie.

Mitgetheilt
von
Dr. **Lissauer** in Bendorf.

Der in Nr. 31. dieser Wochenschrift von Dr. Valentiner mitgetheilte Fall von Leucaemie, bei welcher zur Coupirung des Fiebers Liq. arsenic. Fowler. angewandt wurde, brachte mir zwei Fälle derselben Krankheit in Erinnerung, die ich kurz nach einander im Landkrankenkause in Cassel zu beobachten Gelegenheit hatte, von welchen bei einem Liq. arsen. Fowler. eine Zeit lang versuchsweise von gutem Erfolge war. Ich theile beide Eälle hier kurz mit, theils als einen kleinen Beitrag zur Kenntniss dieser im Ganzen immer noch selten diagnosticirten Krankheit, theils, um zur weiteren Anwendung obigen Mittels anzuregen.

N. N., 32 Jahre alt, weiblichen Geschlechts, wurde im October v. J. aufgenommen. Sie gab an, früher stets gesund, mit 17 Jahren regelmässig menstruirt gewesen zu sein, und vor ungefähr einem Jahre ein uneheliches Kind geboren zu haben, das bald nach der Geburt gestorben sei. Von ihrem Liebhaber, der ihr die Ehe versprochen, hintergangen, habe sie sich sehr gegrämt und viel Sorgen gemacht. Zugleich will sie seit dieser

Lissauer, on the treatment of leukemia with potassium arsenite (Fowler's solution), 1865.

W. B. Coley. The treatment of inoperable sarcoma with the mixed toxins of erysipelas and *Bacillus prodigiosus*: immediate and final results in 140 cases. **J. Am. Med. Assn.** 31: 389-95, 456-65, 1898.

Claude E. Forkner. **Leukemia and Allied Disorders.** New York: The Macmillan Co., 1938.

Lissauer. Zwei Fälle von Leucaemie. **Berl. Klin. Wchnschr.** 2: 403-4, 1865.

M. J. Shear *et al*. Some aspects of a joint institutional research program on chemotherapy of cancer: current laboratory and clinical experiments with bacterial polysaccharide and with synthetic organic compounds. In F. R. Moulton (ed). **Approaches to Tumor Chemotherapy.** Washington, D. C.: Am. Assn. Adv. Sci., 1947. (p. 236-84).

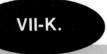

VII-K.

Preludes to the Next Century

VII-K-1. Filterable viruses: Ivanowski and Beijerinck.

During the bacteriological era, many obviously communicable diseases, such as smallpox and hydrophobia, could not be related to microorganisms visible under the microscope. Pasteur in 1884 suggested that an "infinitesimally small" microorganism was involved in hydrophobia.

The existence of such organisms was demonstrated by a Russian botanist, Dmitri Alexievich Ivanowski (1864-1920), working in St. Petersburg in 1892 and using the tobacco mosaic disease. He showed that the sap from diseased plants would transmit the disease after passage through a filter with pores too small to allow passage of bacteria. Ivanowsky's report was published 2 years after he read a paper at the Academy of Sciences in St. Petersburg.

In 1898, Martinus Willem Beijerinck (1851-1931), in Delft, the Netherlands, made similar observations on tobacco mosaic and called the filterable factor a "contagium vivum fluidum." Beijerinck, an irascible botanist, claimed that he had no knowledge of Ivanowsky's earlier discovery.

In 1898, G. Sanarelli, an Italian working in Uruguay, described multiple myxomatosis of rabbits as being due to a submicroscopic agent. This was the first tumor-like disease to be ascribed to a filterable virus. The term "virus," used in a general sense for a poison or a noxious influence since medieval times, became restricted to a specific group of pathogenic agents. It was not until the 1930s that viruses were visualized under the electron microscope, and were isolated.

The role of viruses in cancer research is well told by Ludwik Gross.

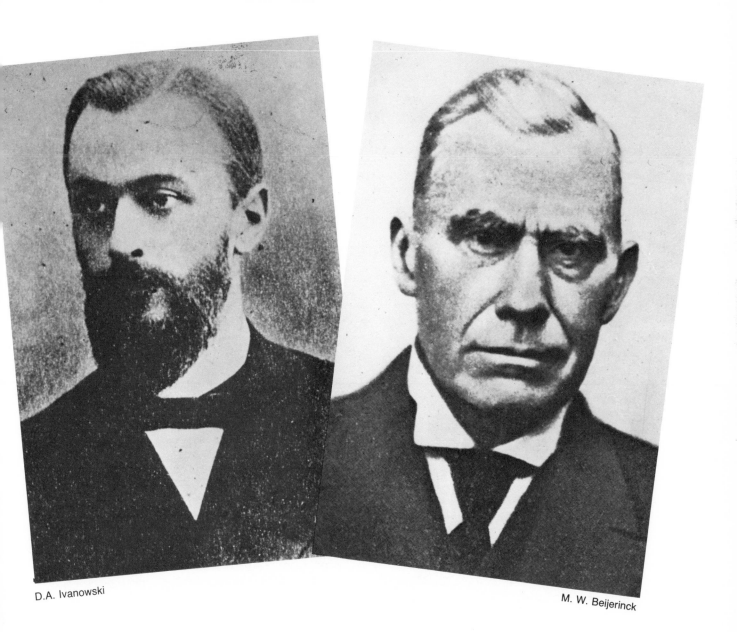

D.A. Ivanowski

M. W. Beijerinck

M. W. Beijerinck. Ueber ein Contagium Vivum Fluidum als
Ursache der Fleckenkrankheit der Tabaksblätter. **Centralbl.
f. Bakt. Abt. Jena II**, 5: 27-33, 1899.

Ludwik Gross. **Oncogenic Viruses**, ed. 2. New York:
Pergamon Press, 1970.

D. Ivanowski. Über die Mosaikkrankheit der Tabakspflanze.
Bull. Acad. Imp. Sci. St. Petersburg, n.s. 3(35): 67-70,
1894.

Preludes to the Next Century

VII-K-2. Ionizing radiation: Röntgen and Curies.

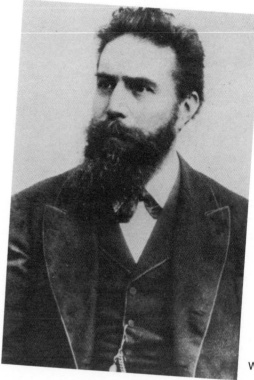

Wilhelm C. Röntgen

Röntgen, on a new kind of ray, 1895.

X-rays were discovered in 1895 by Wilhelm Conrad Röntgen (1845-1923), professor of physics at Würzberg. His brief report on a New Kind of Rays, which he called X-rays, is a landmark in science and medicine. Radiology became a scientific discipline and a sensation overnight. The story of the discovery has been told often; an excellent account was prepared by Glasser. Röntgen was the recipient of the first Nobel Prize in physics in 1901.

Early workers with X-rays noted that fluorescence of the glass of the vacuum tubes was a necessary condition for the formation of X-rays. This led to the study of other conditions for the formation of X-rays, and of other fluorescent sub-

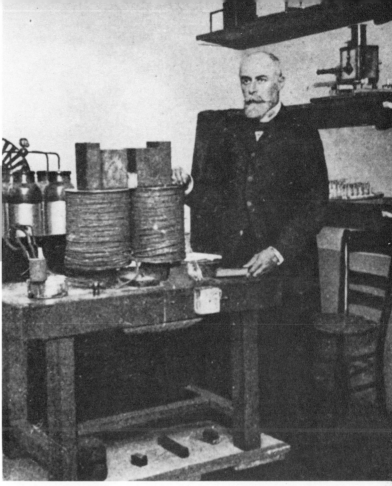

stances as possible sources of such rays. Antoine Henri Becquerel (1852-1908), a member of a renowned French family of scientists, in 1896-7 found that uranium compounds darkened photographic plates. The radiation thus revealed was given off by the substances and was similar to X-rays.

Marie Sklodowska (1867-1934), a Polish student in physics at the Sorbonne, and "a tall young man with dreamy eyes," Pierre Curie (1859-1906), a young physicist whom she married in 1895, extended Becquerel's experiments. They noted that pitchblende ore showed a higher radio-activity than could be accounted for by the content of uranium or thorium. Separation experiments led to the discovery of Polonium in the bismuth extract of the ore, and another substance with 2 million times as much radiation as uranium, which was called Radium. In 1903, the Nobel Prize in physics was shared by the Curies and Becquerel.

Eve Curie. **Madame Curie.** Garden City, N.Y.: Doubleday, Doran, 1937.

P. Curie and M. Curie. Sur la radioactivité provoquée par les rayons de Bécquerel. **Compt. rend. Acad. Sci.** (Paris), 129: 714-16, 1899.

L.. E. Etter. **The Science of Ionizing Radiation.** Springfield, Ill.: C. C. Thomas, 1965.

W. C. Röntgen. Ueber eine neue Art von Strahlen. **Sitzungsber. phys.-med. Gesellsch. Würtzb.**, 1895 (p. 132-141).

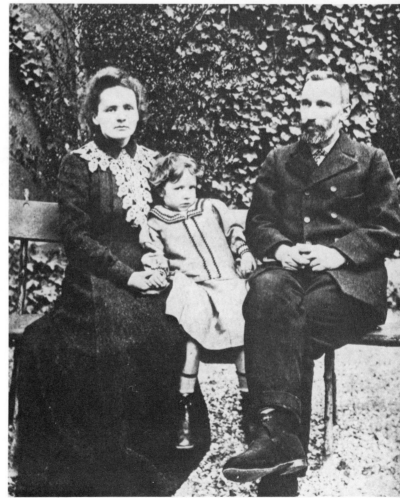

Marie and Pierre Curie with their daughter Irène, 1904.

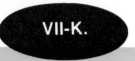

VII-K.

Preludes to the Next Century

VII-K-3. Genetics: Mendel and de Vries.

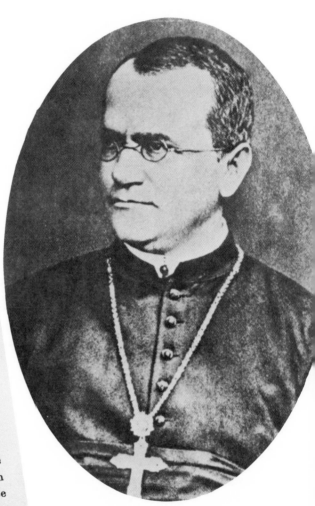

Gregor Johann Mendel

Versuche über Pflanzen-Hybriden.

Von

Gregor Mendel.

(Vorgelegt in den Sitzungen vom 8. Februar und 8. März 1865.)

Einleitende Bemerkungen.

Künstliche Befruchtungen, welche an Zierpflanzen desshalb vorgenommen wurden, um neue Farben-Varianten zu erzielen, waren die Veranlassung zu den Versuchen, die her besprochen werden sollen. Die auffallende Regelmässigkeit, mit welcher die-selben Hybridformen immer wiederkehrten, so oft die Befruch-tung zwischen gleichen Arten geschah, gab die Anregung zu weiteren Experimenten, deren Aufgabe es war, die Entwicklung der Hybriden in ihren Nachkommen zu verfolgen.

Dieser Aufgabe haben sorgfältige Beobachter, wie Köl-reuter, Gärtner, Herbert, Lecocq, Wichura u. a. einen Theil ihres Lebens mit unermüdlicher Ausdauer geopfert. Na-mentlich hat Gärtner in seinem Werke „die Bastarderzeugung im Pflanzenreiche" sehr schätzbare Beobachtungen niedergelegt, und in neuester Zeit wurden von Wichura gründliche Unter-suchungen über die Bastarde der Weiden veröffentlicht. Wenn es noch nicht gelungen ist, ein allgemein giltiges Gesetz für die Bildung und Entwicklung der Hybriden aufzustellen, so kann das Niemanden Wunder nehmen, der den Umfang der Aufgabe kennt und die Schwierigkeiten zu würdigen weiss, mit denen Versuche dieser Art zu kämpfen haben. Eine endgiltige Ent-scheidung kann erst dann erfolgen, bis Detail-Versuche aus den verschiedensten Pflanzen-Familien vorliegen. Wer die Ar-

Mendel, report on plant hybridization, 1866.

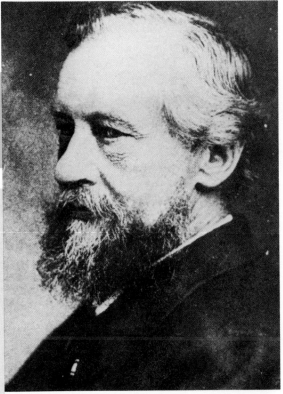

Hugo deVries

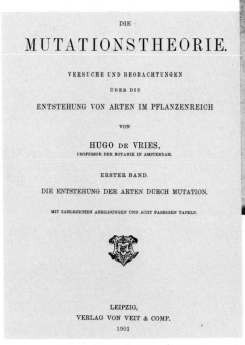

DIE

MUTATIONSTHEORIE.

VERSUCHE UND BEOBACHTUNGEN

ÜBER DIE

ENTSTEHUNG VON ARTEN IM PFLANZENREICH

VON

HUGO DE VRIES,

PROFESSOR DER BOTANIK IN AMSTERDAM.

ERSTER BAND.

DIE ENTSTEHUNG DER ARTEN DURCH MUTATION.

MIT ZAHLREICHEN ABBILDUNGEN UND ACHT FARBIGEN TAFELN.

LEIPZIG,

VERLAG VON VEIT & COMP.

1901

deVries, *Die Mutationstheorie,* 1901. Title page.

There are few major discoveries in science that can be as clearly attributed to a single source as the principles of heredity elucidated in 1866 by Gregor Johann Mendel (1822-1884). Mendel's report was forgotten until, in 1900, three botanists independently rediscovered his principles. One of these, Hugo de Vries (1848-1935), formulated the theory of mutations. A new science was born, which in 1906 was given the name of Genetics by William Bateson (1861-1926).

Genetics is one of the hubs of the biological sciences. It illuminated the processes of evolution, established by Darwin in 1859, blossomed in its biomedical applications during the early part of the 20th Century, and continues in a key role on the molecular biological level. The majestic sweep of its contributions is well told by Dunn.

The genetic factors in neoplasia were soon encountered in the work on transplanted and spontaneous tumors in animals that also commenced at the turn of the century.

L. C. Dunn. **A Short History of Genetics.** New York: McGraw-Hill Book Co., 1965.

Gregor Mendel. Versuche über Pflanzenhybriden. **Verh. Naturforsch. ver. Brünn** 4: 3-47, 1866.

Hugh de Vries. **Die Mutations Theorie.** Leipzig: Veit u. Co., 1901.

VIII. 20th Century: To World War II

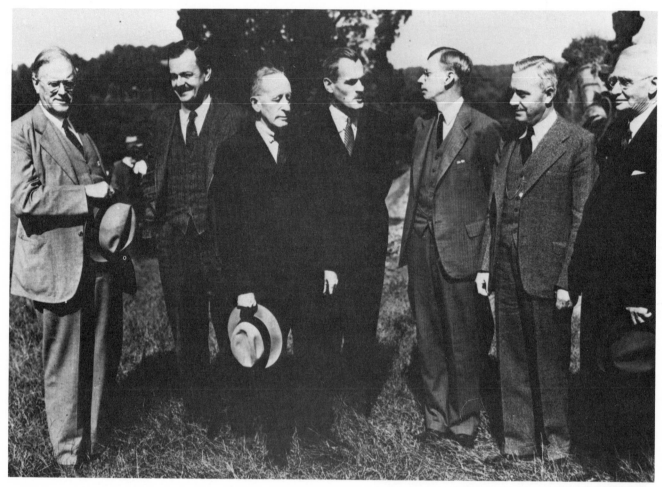

First National Advisory Cancer Council, at groundbreaking ceremonies of the National Cancer Institute, Bethesda, Maryland, 1938.
Left to right: Francis Carter Wood (1869-1951), director, Institute for Cancer Research, Columbia University, New York City; C.C. Little (1888-1971), director, Jackson Laboratory, Bar Harbor, Maine; James Ewing (1866-1943), director, Memorial Hospital for Treatment of Cancer and Allied Diseases, New York City; Arthur H. Compton (1892-1962), professor of physics, University of Chicago, Chicago, Ill.; James B. Conant (1893-   ), president, Harvard University, Cambridge, Mass.; Thomas Parran (1892-1968), Surgeon General, U.S. Public Health Service, member ex-officio and chairman; Ludvig Hektoen (1863-1951), professor emeritus of pathology, Rush Medical College, Chicago, Ill.

The National Cancer Institute Act, August 5, 1937.

The 20th Century is bisected by World War II, scientifically as well as politically. Scientifically, the first half may be typified by Einstein and the discoveries in physics and chemistry that led to the explosion of the atomic bomb in 1945. Scientific leadership during this period shifted from Germany to the United States.

In the biomedical sciences, the first half of the 20th Century is noted for the introduction of ionizing radiation in the diagnosis and treatment of disease, through the discoveries of Röntgen and of the Curies just before the century; for chemotherapy, introduced by Ehrlich and culminating in the discovery of synthetic and natural antibiotics; for quantitative physiological and biochemical determinations in clinical practice, and for accelerated studies in psychology and psychiatry.

Oncology became an experimental science at the turn of the century. Its first useful material was the transplanted tumor in rodents, to which soon were added the tumors induced in animals by viral and by chemical agents. Ionizing radiation was applied meaningfully to cancer treatment by 1930, and the surgical procedures for cancer were extended. Special institutions and journals arose for the study of cancer. In 1937, the United States made the resolution of the problem a national objective with the passage of the National Cancer Act. This law was a landmark for subsequent developments in oncology, not only in the United States but throughout the world.

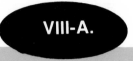

Pathology

VIII-A-1. Histologic oncology matures: Borst.

The histologic period of oncology began with Johannes Müller in 1838, and was developed during the latter half of the 19th Century by Rudolf Virchow and his illustrious students and contemporaries. Virchow's own views on neoplasia, and its derivation from connective tissue, required revision; he seemed to compromise for neoplasia his own aphorism, Omnis cellula e cellula. The work of Thiersch, Remak and Waldeyer, among others, oriented the taxonomy and pathologic understanding of neoplasia along histogenesis. A tumor received a name and position according to the organ and tissue which it most resembled, and from which it presumably arose.

Anaplasia, the histologic evidence of departure from normal cell appearance and organizational patterns, was the basis for determining the degree of differentiation. Von Hansemann in 1890 was among the first to develop the concept of grading tumors by their differentiation of appearance, a characteristic that correlated with the aggressiveness of the neoplasm and its sensitivity to radiotherapy.

Thus, the pathologist became the final arbiter in the diagnosis and classification of neoplasms. His task, in the surgical laboratories or the anatomical museums, was to establish the organ and tissue origin of the tumor, its extent or stage, and its differentiation, or grade.

The histologic period matured by the early 20th century. The 1902 text by Maximilian Borst (1869-1946), of Würzburg, is an excellent presentation of the knowledge regarding cancer up to that time.

The authoritative text on tumors in English, following the systematic patterns developed by German pathologists, was James Ewing's **Neoplastic Diseases**, which appeared in 1919. From then on, single-author, single-volume works became replaced by encyclopedic compilations, such as those of F. Henke and O. Lubarsch.

Max Borst. **Die Lehre von den Geschwülsten, mit einem mikroskopischen Atlas** (2 vols.). Wiesbaden: Bergmann, 1902.

D. von Hansemann. Ueber asymmetrische Zelltheilung in Epithelkrebsen und deren biologische Bedeutung. **Virchows Arch.** 119: 299-326, 1890.

F. Henke and O. Lubarsch (eds). **Handbuch der Speziellen Pathologischen Anatomie und Histologie**, 13 vols. Berlin: Julius Springer, 1926-55.

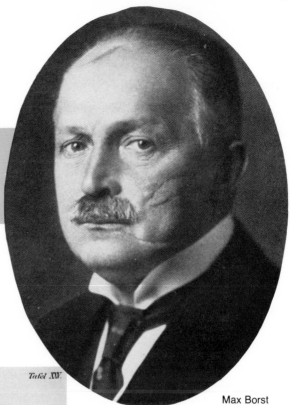

Max Borst

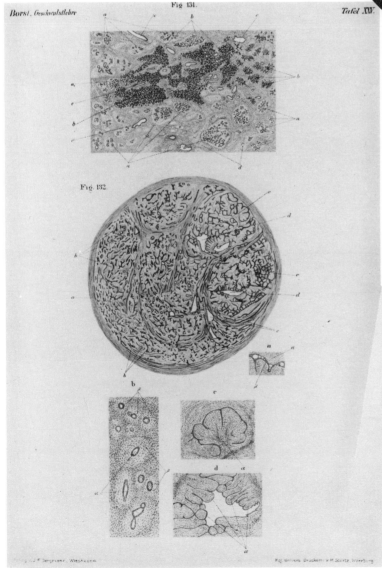

Histologic details of tumors. Drawings from Borst, 1902.

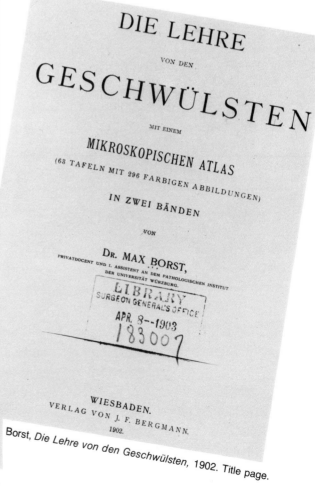

Borst, *Die Lehre von den Geschwülsten*, 1902. Title page.

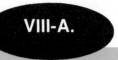

VIII-A.

Pathology

VIII-A-2. Oncologic pathology: Ewing and Willis.

James Ewing (1866-1943), American pathologist, was a commanding figure in oncology in the United States for four decades, and is remembered as the director of research at the Memorial Hospital for Cancer and Allied Diseases in New York City, as the author of **Neoplastic Diseases**, and for the eponymic Ewing's sarcoma.

Ewing was selected in 1899 to head the department of pathology at Cornell University Medical College. His association with the Memorial Hospital began in 1908, in connection with the Collis P. Huntington Fund that supported cancer research there, and continued until his retirement as director in 1940. **Neoplastic Diseases** first appeared in 1919, and continues to be an important scholarly treatise on the pathology of tumors.

Ewing was an effective teacher, and was an influential participant in national and international organizations in cancer. He was the first president of the American Association for Cancer Research (1907-9) and again thirty years later; he was a member of the original National Advisory Cancer Council. His life and the flavor of his times were engagingly presented by his successor in pathology, Fred W. Stewart.

Ewing in 1921 described 7 non-osteogenic tumors of bone, which occurred in young subjects, began with symptoms suggesting osteomyelitis, and affected the shafts of the small bones of the extremities. The tumors permeated through the periosteum and widened the shaft and invaded the soft tissues, without bone formation. The tumors "melt down under heavy radiation" but generally recurred.

Rupert A. Willis (1898-   ), an Australian pathologist, in 1934 made a signal contribution by his book on metastases, entitled **The Spread of Tumours in the Human Body**. The original was based upon several hundred autopsies, a critical review of the literature, and astute pathologic deductions. Willis moved to London; the book went through 3 revised editions.

James Ewing. **Neoplastic Diseases.** Philadelphia: W. B. Saunders, 1919.

James Ewing. Diffuse endothelioma of bone. **Proc. New York Path. Soc.** 21: 17-24, 1921.

F. W. Stewart. Obituary of James Ewing. **Arch. Path.** 36: 325-30, 1943.

F. W. Stewart. Retirement in New York: Prognosis and Reminiscences of a non-optimist. **Bull. New York Acad. Med.** 47: 1342-9, 1971.

R. A. Willis. **The Spread of Tumours in the Human Body.** London: J. & A. Churchill, 1934.

James Ewing

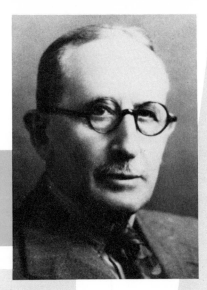

NEOPLASTIC DISEASES

A TEXT-BOOK ON TUMORS

By

JAMES EWING, A. M., M. D., Sc. D.
Professor of Pathology at Cornell University Medical College
New York City

WITH 479 ILLUSTRATIONS

UNIV OF CALIF
MEDICAL SCHOOL

PHILADELPHIA AND LONDON
W. B. SAUNDERS COMPANY
1919

Ewing, *Neoplastic Diseases*, 1919. Title page.

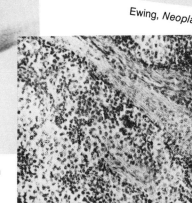

Ewing's sarcoma. Radiologic and histologic appearance (from
Ewing, Proc. N.Y. Path Soc., 21: 17-24, 1921).

Willis, *Spread of Tumours in the Human Body*, 1934. Title
page.

MONOGRAPHS OF THE BAKER INSTITUTE
OF MEDICAL RESEARCH

No. 2

THE SPREAD OF TUMOURS
IN THE HUMAN BODY

By
RUPERT A. WILLIS
M.D., B.S., D.Sc., Melbourne
Pathologist to the Alfred Hospital and to the
Austin Hospital for Chronic Diseases, Melbourne

WITH 103 ILLUSTRATIONS

LONDON
J. & A. CHURCHILL
40 GLOUCESTER PLACE
PORTMAN SQUARE
1934

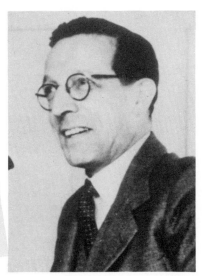

R.A. Willis

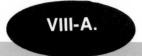

VIII-A.

Pathology

VIII-A-3. Mouse pathologists: Tyzzer, Wells and Slye.

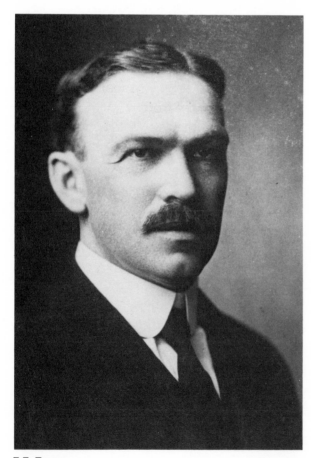

E.E. Tyzzer

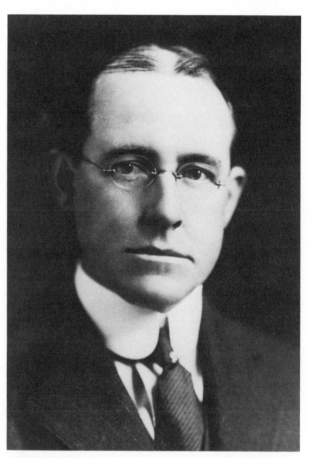

H. Gideon Wells

The early investigators using transplantable tumors had to establish that the rodent tumors, usually adenocarcinomas arising from the breast, were indeed neoplasms that resembled neoplasms in

man. During the first two decades of the century, pathologists in Germany, England and the United States described the development of metastases, recurrent growth, infiltration, and morphologic evidence of neoplastic behavior.

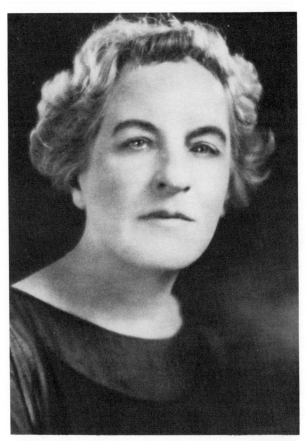

Maud Slye

E. E. Tyzzer. A series of spontaneous tumors in mice with observations on the influence of heredity on the frequency of their occurrence. **J. Med. Res.** 21: 479-518, 1909.

H. G. Wells, M. Slye and Harriet F. Holmes. The occurrence and pathology of spontaneous carcinoma of the lung in mice. **Cancer Res.** 1: 259-61, 1941.

C. C. Little. Evidence that cancer is not a simple Mendelian recessive. **J. Cancer Res.** 12: 30-46, 1928.

Maud Slye. The relation of heredity to cancer, with regard to the communication of President C. C. Little of the University of Michigan. **J. Cancer Res.** 12: 83-133, 1928.

Among the pioneer pathologists in Europe who concerned themselves with mouse and rat tumors were H. Apolant and L. Michaelis in Germany, M. Haaland, who worked with Borrel in France and J. A. Murray at the newly established Imperial Cancer Research Fund in England. Among American pathologists were E. E. Tyzzer of Harvard and H. Gideon Wells of Chicago.

Ernest Edward Tyzzer (1875-1965) "was a large, kindly man, who spoke slowly, softly, simply and succinctly." As professor of comparative pathology at Harvard, he devoted his talents to a wide range of problems, particularly viral and parasitic diseases of birds. His interests in cancer research were paramount during 1905 to 1916, when he was director of the Harvard Cancer Commission. He wrote 15 articles on spontaneous and transplantable tumors in mice and on genetic factors in neoplasia.

Harry Gideon Wells (1876-1943) had a distinguished career in pathology and clinical biochemistry at the University of Chicago where he was professor and head of the department of pathology. Wells's participation in cancer research spanned 30 years, from 1911 to 1942, and started with the historical controversy between Maud Slye (1879-1954) and Clarence C. Little (1888-1971) on cancer inheritance, which Slye claimed was a recessive trait. An exchange of articles in 1928 indicates the depth of this historic disagreement. Wells championed Slye but eventually admitted that she was in error.

The basic material for the investigations of Slye and of Little were mice, and the role of Wells was in the pathologic examination of all animals from Slye's colony. In a long series of papers between 1914 and 1941, by Maud Slye, Harriett F. Holmes and H. Gideon Wells, neoplasms of practically every organ and tissue from 143,132 mice were meticulously recorded and described. These pathologic descriptions of the neoplastic spectrum in mice remain unmatched for completeness and thoroughness.

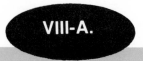

VIII-A.

Pathology

VIII-A-4. Plant tumors: E. F. Smith.

Erwin Frink Smith (1854-1927) was a plant pathologist who received his doctorate from the University of Michigan in 1889. His career was with the U.S. Department of Agriculture, and he occupied an important place in botany, rising to membership in the National Academy of Science.

In 1907 Smith and Townsend described crown gall, a cellular abnormality eventuating in a tumor in many plant species, and isolated a bacterium, **Agrobacterium tumefaciens** as the causative organism. Smith insisted that the bacterium had to be present for continued growth, in contrast with transplantable tumors in animals, and tried to extrapolate his plant findings to animal species. It was only in 1942 that P. R. White and A. C. Braun established that the crown gall of plants was truly autonomous.

The full potentials of the plant tumors as an experimental model remain to be exploited, as pointed out by Braun.

E. F. Smith and C. O. Townsend. A plant-tumor of bacterial origin. **Science** 25: 671-3, 1907.

A. C. Braun. **The Cancer Problem.** New York: Columbia Univ. Press, 1969.

L. R. Jones. Erwin Frink Smith. **Nat. Acad. Sci. Biogr. Mem.** 21: 1-71, 1941.

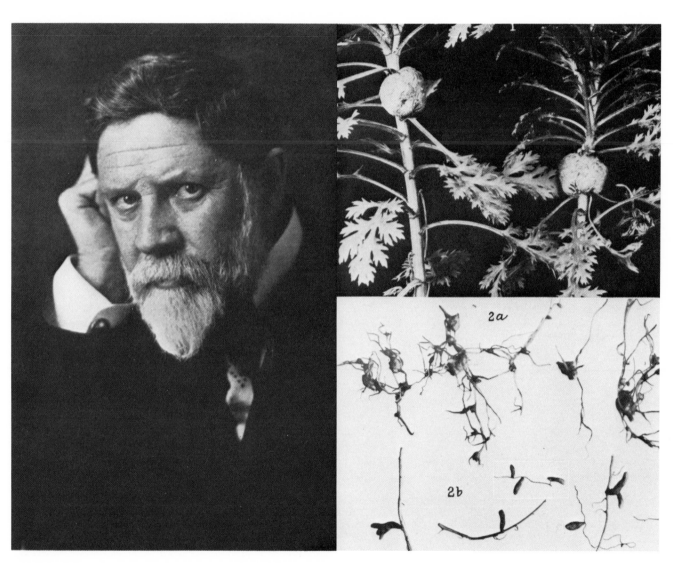

Erwin F. Smith

Crown gall on daisy plants (from Bulletin of U.S. Dept. Agriculture No. 213, 1911, from Dr. Jacques Lipetz of Manhattan College).

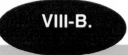

Transplantation of Tumors

VIII-B-1. Tumors in rats: Loeb.

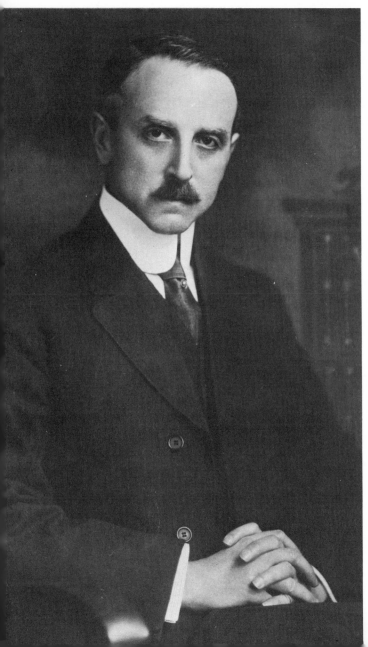

Leo Loeb

ON TRANSPLANTATION OF TUMORS.[1]

LEO LOEB, M.D., Chicago.

A few transplantations of a carcinoma of a cow and a carcinoma of a mouse were made into the same animals respectively, in which, if the pieces healed in, only connective tissue was found after a few weeks. More successful was a series of consecutive transplantations of a sarcoma found in the thyroid gland of a white rat. This work extended over a period of fifteen months, 360 pieces being transplanted into about 150 animals. The original tumor was a cystic sarcoma with rather small cells. The cysts were produced through a gelatinous softening of the tumor cells. The adjoining sarcoma cells arranged themselves in a regular way around the cyst, forming an almost epithelial-like lining. The tumor tissue was rich in blood-vessels, but the cells did not show any definite relation to the vessels. The original tumor was about the size of a nut. After extirpation it recurred and made, in the course of a few weeks, local metastases, little nodules near the primary tumor. No general metastases were found when the animal, a short time later, died during an operation.

From this tumor pieces were transplanted into the subcutaneous tissue or into the peritoneal cavity at each operation, about five to eight pieces being inserted into three to four other animals. At various periods after the operation, from six hours until more than three months, pieces which had been transplanted were taken out for microscopical examination. To avoid accidental findings usually more than one piece, often four or five, of the same period were investigated microscopically.

The main result of this part of my investigations is that the largest part of the transplanted piece became necrotic.

[1] An almost complete review of the literature on this subject is given by Sailer in the "Journal of the Medical Sciences," 1900.

from Journal of Medical Research, 1:28, 1901.

Cancer research started with transplanted tumors in animals, which provided the first reproducible and controllable material for investigations.

During the 19th Century, beginning with Novinsky in 1876, no less than ten other investigators reported the successful transplantation of tumors within the same species. As tabulated by Triolo, almost half of these experiments involved the transplantation of the transmissible venereal lymphosarcoma in dogs, and for the rest, mice and rats were the species employed.

Leo Loeb (1869-1959) at the turn of the century reported the most extensive work with rats. He transplanted a spindle cell sarcoma through 40 generations, and a thyroid carcinosarcoma through 7 generations. Microscopic observations indicated that the tumors grew from the peripheral cells of the transplants; tumor juice passed through filter paper did not produce tumors, and heating the tumors to 43°C retarded their growth. In a series of studies with Abbie E. C. Lathrop, who maintained a commercial mouse colony in Granby, Massachusetts, he also established that in mice mammary cancers had familial distribution, were increased by pregnancies, and reduced by ovariectomy.

Loeb came from Germany to the United States at the age of 28, following his older brother, Jacques Loeb, to Chicago. Between 1902 and 1910 he held posts in pathology at Johns Hopkins, McGill, Pennsylvania, and finally settled in St. Louis, where from 1915 he was professor of pathology in the School of Medicine at Washington University. His contributions to cancer research and investigative pathology spanned 50 years; he was a pioneer worker in genetic and hormonal aspects of tumors in mice as well as in transplantation. His classic work is considered to be **The Biological Basis of Individuality**.

Loeb's work on tumor transplantation failed to interest extension to other laboratories. His tumor lines were not continued although they were made available to the New York State Cancer Laboratory in Buffalo. From some of the Lathrop mouse families, however, were developed homozygous strains still used in cancer research.

Leo Loeb. Autobiographical notes. **Perspect. Biol. Med.** 2: 1-23, 1958.

Leo Loeb. Further investigations in transplantation of tumors. **J. Med. Res.** 8: 44-73, 1902.

Leo Loeb. On transplantation of tumors. **J. Med. Res.** 6: 28-39, 1901.

M. B. Shimkin. A. E. C. Lathrop: Mouse woman of Granby. **Cancer Res.** 35: 1597-98, 1975.

V. A. Triolo. Nineteenth century foundations of cancer research. Origins of experimental research. **Cancer Res.** 24: 4-27, 1964.

VIII-B.

Transplantation of Tumors

VIII-B-2. The transplanted tumor period: Jensen.

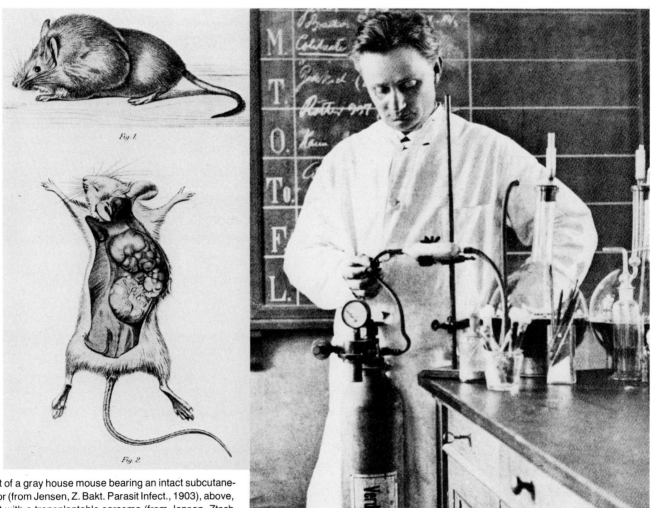

Woodcut of a gray house mouse bearing an intact subcutaneous tumor (from Jensen, Z. Bakt. Parasit Infect., 1903), above, and a rat with a transplantable sarcoma (from Jensen, Ztsch. Krebskrsch., 1909).

Carl Jensen

Carl Oluf Jensen (1864-1934), a Danish veterinary scientist of the Institute for Agricultural and Veterinary Research at Copenhagen, was the starting point for the use of transplanted rodent tumors in cancer research.

Between 1901 and 1903 Jensen succeeded in propagating a subcutaneous alveolar carcinoma, probably of breast origin, through 19 generations of white mice. His first reports appeared in an obscure clinical journal, and subsequently received wide attention in a German publication. In 1909 Jensen reported an inoculable rat sarcoma which also became a standard tumor line throughout the world.

Jensen's data gave firm evidence of transplantation of malignant tissue by inoculation of cells, rather than being due to a transference of some infective factor. The obvious usefulness of the material was recognized by other laboratories in Germany and England, and his strains of tumor began to be widely propagated.

At the Berlin Cancer Research Institute, L. Michaelis by 1905 studied the growth and histologic patterns of the Jensen tumors in mice of different stocks. At the Institute for Experimental Therapy at Frankfurt, Paul Ehrlich by 1903 began to use the Jensen tumors, and by 1905 added 11 transplantable lines of his own. In England, the Imperial Cancer Research Fund under E. F. Bashford imported the Jensen tumors and also developed additional lines. By 1905 the Jensen and Ehrlich tumors were taken up by the New York State Cancer Laboratory in Buffalo and other laboratories in the United States. Many laboratories contributed new lines of transplantable tumors, usually attaching the names of the investigators for identification. A rabbit carcinoma, the Brown-Pearce tumor, was added to the list of mouse and rat tumors.

A compilation of transplantable tumors still available was made by Stewart et al. in 1959.

Carl O. Jensen. Experimentelle untersuchungen über Krebs bei maüsen. **Zent. Bakt. Parasit. Infect.** 34: 28-34, 122-43, 1903.

Carl O. Jensen. Uebertragbare Rattensarkome. **Ztsch. Krebsforsch.** 7: 45-54, 1909.

C. O. Jensen. **Selected Papers.** Copenhagen: Munksgaard, 1948.

H. L. Stewart et al. Transplantable and transmissible tumors of animals. Ser. 1, XII, fasc. 40, **Atlas of Tumor Pathology.** Washington, D. C.: Armed Forces Inst. Path., 1959.

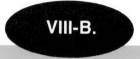
VIII-B.

Transplantation of Tumors

VIII-B-3. Tumor growth and regression: Murphy and Lynch.

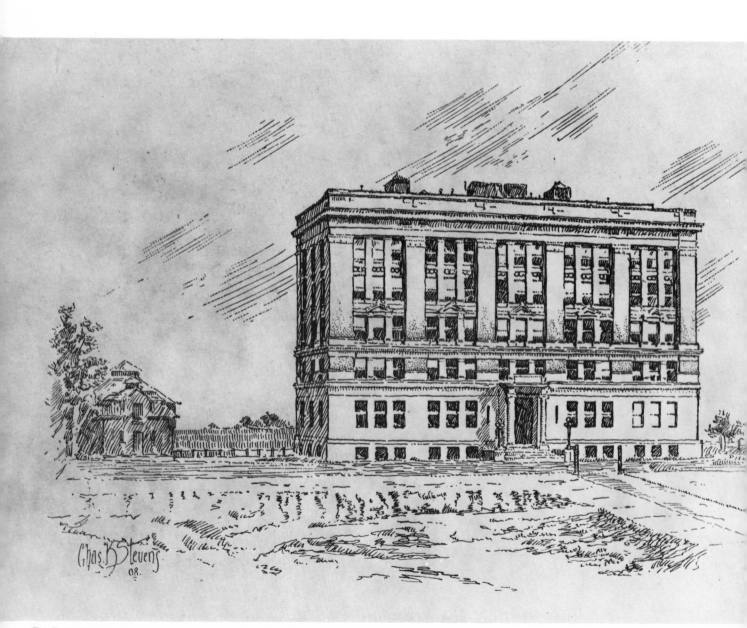

The Rockefeller Institute for Medical Research, New York City,
1908.

Clara J. Lynch

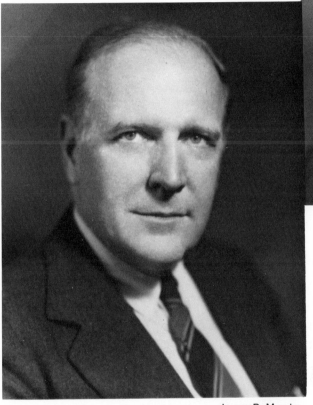

James B. Murphy

Murphy's long career involved many biological studies in cancer. He and E. Sturm in 1925 first described the appearance of primary lung tumors in mice painted with coal tar, which Clara J. Lynch (1882-) used in her pioneer studies on the relation of tumor susceptibility and heredity. Murphy was also an influential and firm councillor to the developing cancer activities in the United States, and was the chairman of the select committee that in 1938 drew up the plans in fundamental cancer research for the newly created National Cancer Institute.

James B. Murphy (1884-1950) of the Rockefeller Institute in New York in 1912 reported that malignant rat tumors grew in embryonated bird eggs, the first demonstration of tumor growth outside of homologous species.

He also demonstrated that induced tumor immunity, as evident in mice and rats in which tumor transplants were absorbed, could be disrupted by exposure of animals to X-rays. He was convinced that the lymphocyte was involved centrally in resistance to tumors, as well as in resistance to tuberculosis.

James B. Murphy. Transplantability of malignant tumors to the embryo of a foreign species. **J. Am. Med. Assn.** 59: 874-5, 1912.

James B. Murphy. **The Lymphocyte in Resistance to Tissue Grafting, Malignant Disease and Tuberculous Infection.** Monograph 21. New York: Rockefeller Inst. for Med. Res., 1926.

G. W. Corner. **A History of the Rockefeller Institute, 1901-1953.** New York: Rockefeller Institute Press, 1964.

C. J. Lynch. Studies on the relation between tumor susceptibility and heredity. **J. Exp. Med.**, 39: 481-95, 1924 to 54: 747-60, 1931.

Transplantation of Tumors

VIII-B-4. Tissue culture: Harrison, Carrel and Burrows.

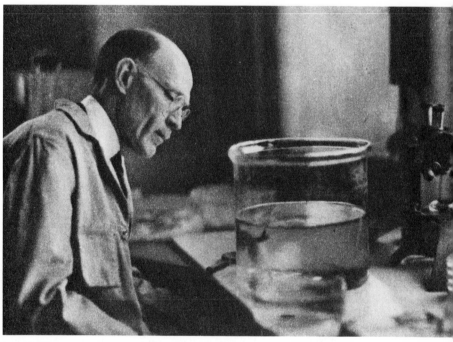

Ross G. Harrison

The growth of tumors and normal cells in nutrients in flasks was achieved during the first decade of the 20th Century.

Among the pioneers in these developments was Ross G. Harrison (1870-1959) of Yale University, New Haven, Connecticut, who used simple cover-slip preparations to observe nerve fibers; such preparations survived for "nearly four weeks."

True, long-term tissue culture was developed by Alexis Carrel (1873-1944) and Montrose T. Burrows (1884-1947), working at the Rockefeller Institute in New York. Burrows was sent to work with Harrison and then returned to develop the techniques under Carrel. The conditions were detailed in 1911, and Burrows coined the descriptive term, "tissue culture."

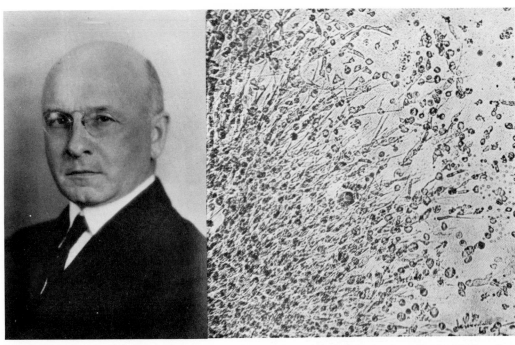

Alexis Carrel

Tissue culture of fibroblasts, showing active growth (from Carrel and Burrows, J. Exptl Med, 13: 387-96, 1911).

Carrel, a mystical yet flamboyant French scientist and winner of the Nobel Prize in 1912 for research in vascular surgery, was later involved in research on organ culture with Charles Lindbergh.

The techniques of tissue and cell cultures have been of inestimable value in research on cellular biology and virology, and represent one of the important contributions of cancer research to biomedical sciences.

A. Carrel and M. T. Burrows. Cultivation of tissues *in vitro* and its technique. **J. Exp. Med.** 13: 387-96, 1911.

A. Carrel and M. T. Burrows. Cultivation *in vitro* of malignant tumors. **J. Exp. Med.** 13: 571-75, 1911.

R. G. Harrison. Observations on the living developing nerve fiber. **Anat. Rec.** 116-18, 1907.

Kate Russel. Tissue culture—a brief historical review. **Clio Med.** 4: 109-19, 1969.

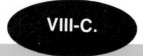

Genetics

VIII-C-1. Somatic mutation concept: Boveri.

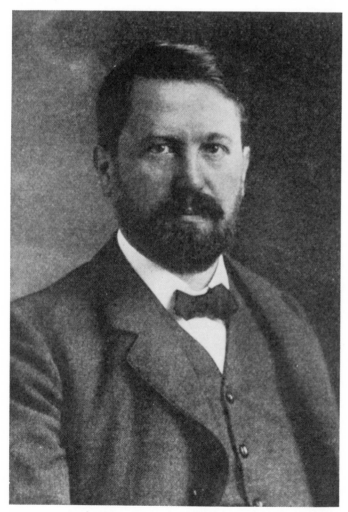

Theodor Boveri (from Fritz Baltzer, in Grosse Naturforscher, Bd. 25. Stuttgart: Wsch. Verlg. MBH, 1962. reproduced by permission)

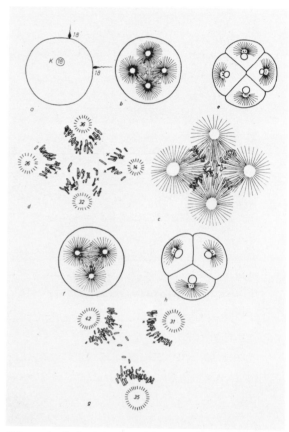

Schematized mitosis in sea urchin embryo, suggesting irregular tripolar and tetrapolar patterns as a model for neoplastic cells. (from Boveri, Zellenstudien, Hft 6, Jena: Fischer, 1907).

Theodor Boveri (1862-1915), professor of zoology at Würzberg, Germany, was one of the founders of the gene concept in the science of genetics that arose during the first decade of the 20th Century. He was the author of a hypothesis that cancer was due to abnormal chromosomes, which became known as the somatic mutation theory of cancer. Boveri's hypothesis, first reported in a 1902 study of cellular division in sea urchin embryos, especially the experimental induction of irregular mitoses, suggested a model for atypical chromosome combinations observed in neoplasms. He subsequently elaborated his analogy by extensive observations of mitoses in tumors.

Boveri's somatic mutation theory of cancer for several decades was an alternate to the infectious virus theory espoused by Borrel. Contemporary views appear to blend these seemingly divergent proposals in suggesting virus participation in the genome of cells as a mechanism leading to neoplasia.

The development of Boveri's theory through 1955 was reviewed by Burdette.

Fritz Baltzer. Theodor Boveri. Leben und Werk eines grossen Biologen. In, **Grosse Naturforscher**, Bd. 25. Stuttgart: Wssch. Verlagsgesch. MBH, 1962.

T. Boveri. **Zur Frage der Entstehung maligner Tumoren.** Jena: Fischer, 1914. Translated as **The Origin of Malignant Tumors.**

Walter J. Burdette. The significance of mutation in relation to origin of tumors. A review. **Cancer Res.** 15: 201-26, 1955.

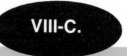

Genetics

VIII-C-2. Mammalian genetics: Little and Wright.

Clarence Cook Little (1888-1971) was a commanding figure in oncology in the United States during most of his long life. He was an organizer and an administrator as well as a research scientist in his own right. Little began to inbreed mice as a student at Harvard, foreseeing the need for homozygous animals for future rigorous work in genetics. He became president of the University of Michigan at the age of 36, and in 1929 founded the Roscoe B. Jackson Memorial Laboratory in Bar Harbor, Maine, for studies on mammalian genetics and cancer.

Little was a perennial director of the American Society for the Control of Cancer and the American Cancer Society into which it evolved, and a member of many cancer research councils. He also became the first director of the Tobacco Research Institute, probably because he preferred to receive research support from rich merchants rather than from the government.

Sewall Wright (1889-), Professor of Genetics at the University of Wisconsin, made basic contributions to population genetics. His studies of inbreeding and crossbreeding in guinea pigs contributed to the understanding of these process-

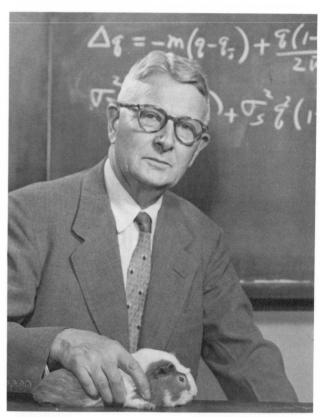

Sewall Wright

es in terms of Mendelian heredity. He derived coefficients of inbreeding and relationship applicable to any system of mating. These are generally accepted as expressing best the theoretical consequences of the Mendelian mechanism.

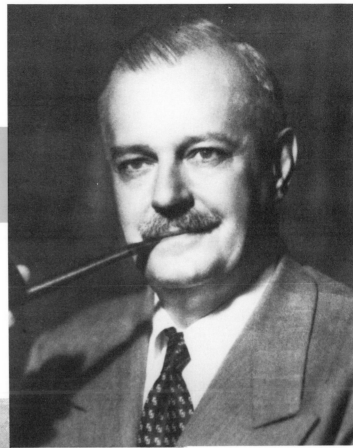

Jackson Laboratory, Bar Harbor, Maine, 1929. (from The
Jackson Laboratory, 35th Annual report, 1963-64)

Clarence Cook Little

Polydactyly in guinea pig substrans of strain 35, illustrating
segregation of slightly different tendencies even in rather late
generations of brother-sister mating. (from S. Wright, Proc.
First Natl. Cancer Conf., 1949).

W. E. Heston. Obituary of Clarence Cook Little. **Cancer
Res.** 32: 1354-56, 1972.
C. C. Little. The relation of genetics to the problems of
cancer research. **Harvey Lectures** 17: 65-88, 1921-22.
Sewall Wright. Differentiation of strains of guinea pigs
under inbreeding. **Proc. Nat. Cancer Conf.** 1: 13-27, 1949.

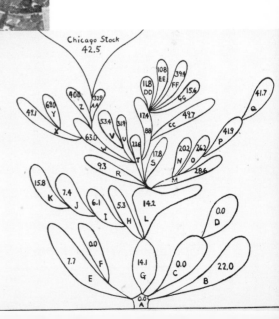

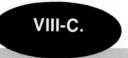

Genetics

VIII-C-3. Inbred mouse strains: Strong.

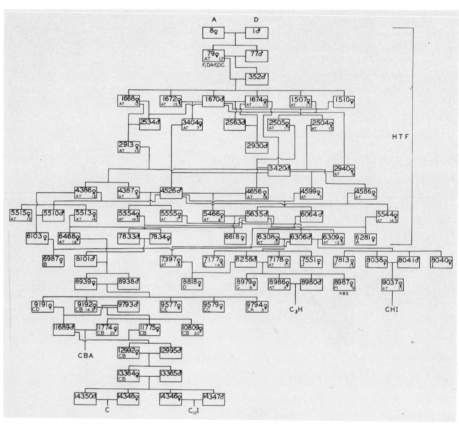

Chart of the progeny and derivation of some inbred strains of mice.

Leonell Clarence Strong (born 1894 in Renova, Pennsylvania), former Research Professor at Yale University School of Medicine, and Director of the Springville Laboratories of Roswell Park Memorial Institute, was the originator of many inbred strains of mice used in cancer research. The now famous A and C or High Tumor Family (HTF) of inbred mice were started in July 1921 at St. Stephen's College (now Bard College), Annandale, New York. The original un-

Leonell C. Strong

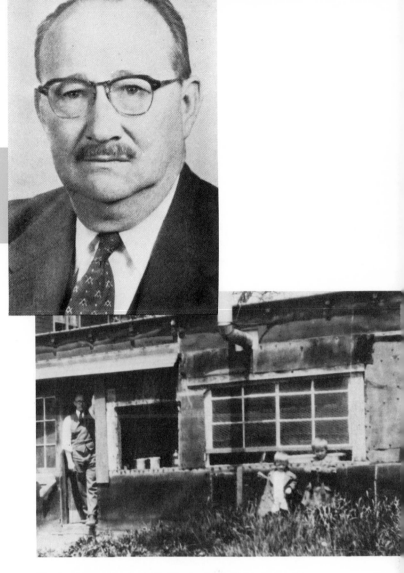

The tar paper shack at St. Stephen's College, Annandale, New York, origin of many inbred mouse strains, 1921-25

pedigreed mice and their descendants were housed from 1921 to 1925 in a tar paper shack. This building, shown with Strong and his two sons, was heated by a potbelly stove. Tar paper was added for warmth in the winter and removed during the summer. The mice were maintained in wooden boxes and fed a diet of bread, milk, and mixed seed.

The original matings of unpedigreed mice, obtained from various sources, were represented by a letter of the alphabet. From the original letters, only the F, I, and N strains exist today. The A and B lines, both albino, were mated and from this cross arose the A strain. The A line was crossed also to the D line, a dilute brown; the offspring were selected for high rates of spontaneous tumors. As shown in the pedigree, the descendants of this cross produced the C, CeH, CHI, and CBA strains. The letters on the bottom left side of the pedigree squares represent the line; the numbers on the right, the age when a spontaneous tumor first appeared in the mouse. The pedigree represents the direct descent of the first few generations of the C Family. Hundreds of collateral lines were not maintained or shown in the pedigree.

With the exception of a few father-to-daughter matings in the early pedigrees, all matings were strictly brother-to-sister, for over 100 generations. In terms of human generations, a comparable genealogy would span over 3500 years.

The strains, once developed, were disseminated among many investigators. Today there are hundreds of sublines scattered throughout the world. In a 17-month period, from December 1966 to April 1967, approximately 840 publications appeared in the world literature using mice as a research tool. Of these papers, 43% depended on the use of one or more strains of mice first developed in the old tar paper shack.

L. C. Strong. The establishment of the C_3H inbred strain of mice for the study of spontaneous carcinoma of the mammary gland. **Genetics** 20: 586-91, 1935.

L. C. Strong. The origin of some inbred mice. **Cancer Res.** 2: 531-39, 1942.

Earl L. Green (ed), **Biology of the Laboratory Mouse.** Ed. 2. New York: McGraw-Hill, 1966.

VIII-C.

Genetics

VIII-C-4. The extrachromosomal milk factor: Bittner and Korteweg.

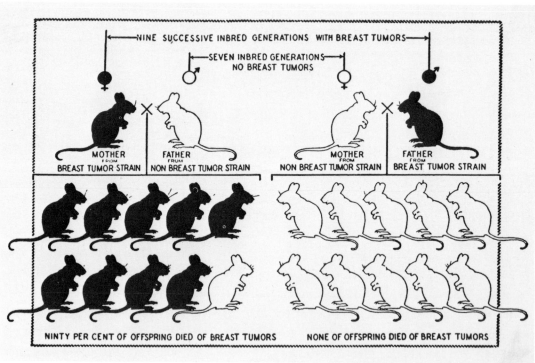

Maternal inheritance of mammary tumors in mice (from Symposium on Mammary Tumors in Mice, 1945, p. 125).

One of the most important contributions from genetic studies on cancer in homozygous mice was the discovery of the extrachromosomal transmission of their mammary tumors. Breast tumors were determined by the mother in reciprocal crosses between high and low-tumor strains, indicating that this extrachromosomal influence was through the cytoplasm of the ovum, during intra-uterine life, or during the postpartum period.

The basic discovery was made by the staff of the Jackson Memorial Laboratory in Bar Harbor, Maine, and, independently, by Remmert Korteweg (1884-1961) of Amsterdam.

John J. Bittner (1904-1961), a member

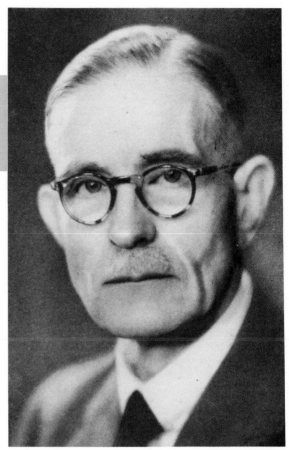

R. Korteweg

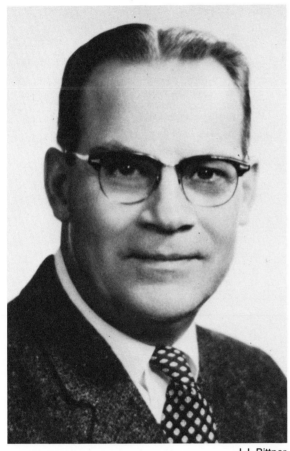

J.J. Bittner

strain females increased the occurrence of such tumors. Thus genetics reintroduced an infectious agent in the etiology of mammary cancers in mice. For years the obvious interpretation of this agent as a virus was disguised by such terms as "influence" or "factor" because scientific dogma held that cancer was not an infection.

of the Jackson Laboratory staff, undertook the exploration of the possible role of mother's milk in the extrachromosomal transmission. He soon established that foster-nursing of high-tumor strain offspring by low-tumor strain females reduced the occurrence of eventual mammary tumors, and that foster-nursing of low-tumor strain offspring by high-tumor

Staff, Roscoe B. Jackson Memorial Laboratory. The existence of nonchromosomal influence in the incidence of mammary tumors in mice. **Science** 78: 465-6, 1933.

R. Korteweg. On the manner in which the disposition to carcinoma of the mammary gland is inherited in mice. **Genetica** 18: 350-71, 1936.

J. J. Bittner. Some possible effects of nursing on the mammary gland tumor incidence in mice. **Science** 84: 162,1935.

Staff, National Cancer Institute. **A Symposium on Mammary Tumors in Mice.** Washington, D.C.: Amer. Assoc. Advanc. Sci., 1945.

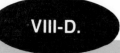

VIII-D.

Oncogenic Viruses

VIII-D-1. Virus hypothesis: Borrel and Oberling.

Amédée Borrel (1867-1936), was professor of bacteriology and hygiene at the University of Strasbourg, and was involved with Calmette of the Pasteur Institute in Paris in developing a plague vaccine. He presented his strong views on the viral etiology of cancer in a series of papers in 1907. This was several years before any neoplasm had actually been demonstrated to be transmitted by cell-free filtrates. Thus, Borrel took the French position for external agents as causes of disease, rather than the German cellular alteration hypotheses such as formulated by Boveri.

Charles C. Oberling (1895-1960) was a product of the University of Strasbourg and a convert to Borrel's theory, becoming eventually a strong advocate for the virus etiology of cancer. Oberling was a pathologist with broad interests. He traveled widely, and for several years (1939-1949) was dean of the medical school in Teheran, Iran. He then became director of the Institut de Recherches sur le Cancer of the Université de Paris in Villejuif. In 1943 Oberling wrote the book **Le Cancer** which W. H. Woglom translated into English as **The Riddle of Cancer**, and which is a masterpiece of its kind.

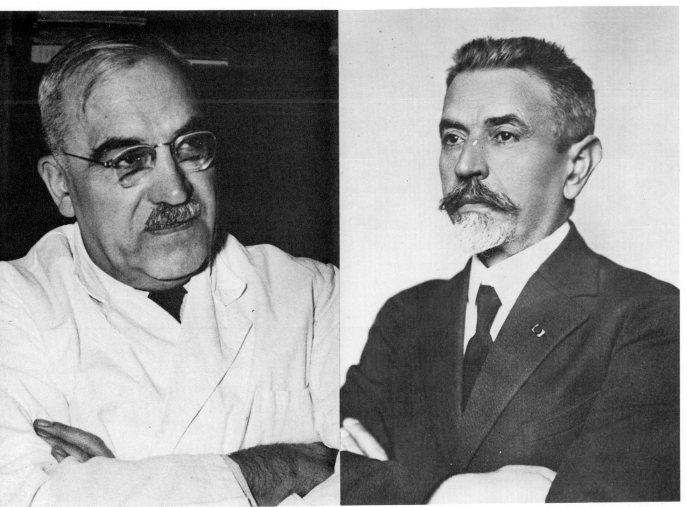

C.C. Oberling

A. Borrel

A. Borrel. Le Problème du cancer. **Bull. Inst. Pasteur**
5: 497-512, 545, 593-608, 641-662, 1907.

C. Oberling. **The Riddle of Cancer.** Transl. by W. H.
Woglom. New Haven, Conn.: Yale Univ. Press, 1952.

Ludwik Gross. **Oncogenic Viruses.** Ed. 2. New York:
Pergamon Press, 1970.

Oncogenic Viruses

VIII-D-2. Tumors with filtrates: Ellermann and Bang.

In 1908, Vilhelm Ellermann (1871-1924) and Oluf Bang (1881-1937), of Copenhagen, Denmark, succeeded in transmitting by cell-free filtrates the erythro-myeloblastic form of chicken leukemia. They postulated that the disease was due to an "ultravisible virus."

The recognition of this work was obscured by the fact that leukemia was not considered as a neoplastic disease at the time. As a matter of fact, the viral nature of a tumor-like condition of rabbits, myxomatosis, was recorded by G. Sanarelli in Montevideo in 1898, although actual filtration experiments were not carried out until 1911. Rabbit myxomatosis, however, remains outside the neoplastic categories.

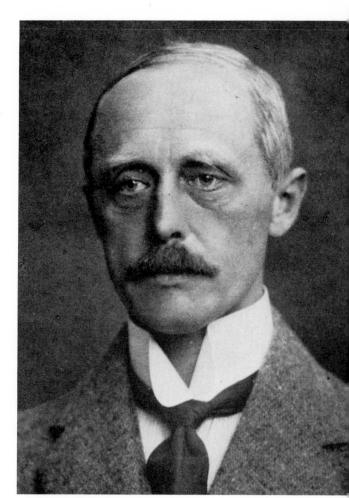

Vilhelm Ellermann

V. Ellermann and O. Bang. Experimentelle Leukämie bei Hühnern. **Centralbl. f. Bakteriol.** 46: 595-609, 1908 and **Z. f. Hyg. und Infectkrht.** 63: 231-73, 1909.

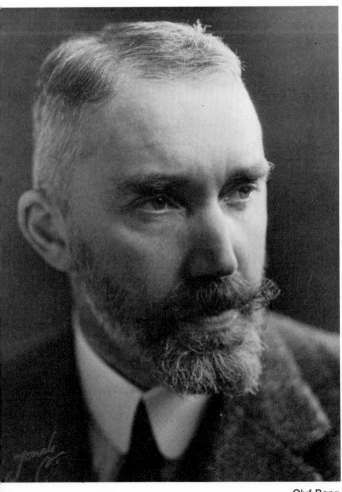

Oluf Bang

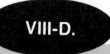

VIII-D.

Oncogenic Viruses

VIII-D-3. Chicken sarcomas: Rous.

In 1910, at about the time that scientific consensus was reached as to a non-infectious nature of cancer, a young investigator at the Rockefeller Institute in New York, Peyton Rous (1879-1970), began his classical studies on chicken sarcomas. Rous transplanted the tumors to other chickens, and passed the material from the tumor through filters that were impermeable to cells and bacteria. On injection into chickens the filtrate produced sarcomas.

Rous was born in Baltimore, Maryland, and obtained his doctorate from Johns Hopkins University School of Medicine in 1905. He joined the Rockefeller Institute in 1909 and remained there for his long, fruitful career.

Despite the incontrovertible, repeatable nature of his observations, they conflicted with evidence from other experimental tumors, primarily the transplantable tumors in rodents. The Rous sarcoma was considered a unique exception, or a granuloma with neoplastic morphology. For two decades Rous undertook other research, returning to cancer when Shope added the rabbit papilloma-carcinoma to virally-induced cancers.

In 1966 Rous was awarded the Nobel Prize for physiology or medicine, sharing it with Charles Huggins.

Peyton Rous. A sarcoma of the fowl transmissible by an agent separable from the tumor cells. **J. Exp. Med.** 13: 397-411, 1911.

Peyton Rous. The virus tumors and the tumor problem. **Harvey Lectures** 31: 74-115, 1935-36.

J. S. Henderson. Peyton Rous (obituary). **Arch. Path.** 90: 189-90, 1970.

Peyton Rous, 1912, at the time of his discovery of filterable chicken sarcomas.

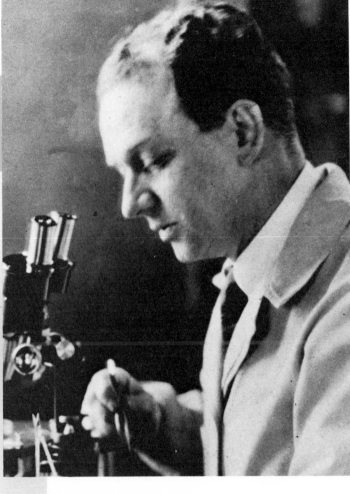

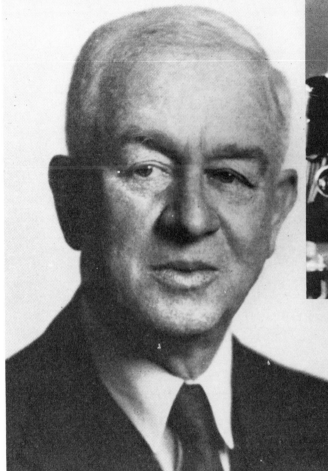

Peyton Rous, circa 1955.

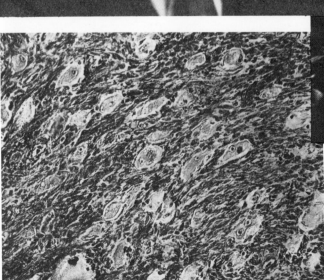

Fowl with a tumor, and the histology of a successful transplant is from Rous, J. Exptl. Med., 12: 696-705, 1910).

Oncogenic Viruses

VIII-D-4. Rabbit papilloma-carcinoma: Shope.

Richard Edwin Shope (1901-66), of the Rockefeller Institute station in Princeton, New Jersey, in 1933 found that the common papillomas of the skin of wild rabbits in Kansas and Iowa were caused by a filterable agent. Papillomas could be easily transmitted by rubbing the filtrate on the scarified skin of rabbits. Gross has published Shope's record of the discovery.

Shope was born in Iowa and obtained his doctorate from the University of Iowa School of Medicine in 1924. He joined the Rockefeller Institute the following year and remained there for his whole career.

The filtrates from papillomas also produced lesions in domestic rabbits, but in the resultant papillomas virus could not be demonstrated. Filtrates of papillomas from domestic rabbits failed to transmit papillomas, yet such filtrates would immunize against the active wild rabbit preparations. Moreover, Rous and Beard soon established that the papillomas had malignant potential; especially in the domestic rabbits and upon transplantation subcutaneously, the tumors became invasive squamous cell carcinomas.

These findings spanned a wide gap in viral oncogenesis that separated avian and mammalian species. Shope added to the roster of transmissible tumors a fibroma in deer. The main oncologic laboratory work with his rabbit material was continued by Rous and his co-workers.

R. E. Shope. Infectious papillomatosis of rabbits. **J. Exp. Med.** 58: 607-24, 1933.

R. E. Shope. Immunization of rabbits to infectious papillomatosis. **J. Exp. Med.** 65: 219-31, 1937.

P. Rous and J. W. Beard. The progression to carcinoma of virus-induced rabbit papillomas (Shope). **J. Exp. Med.** 62: 523-48, 1935.

Ludwik Gross. **Oncogenic Viruses.** Ed. 2. New York: Pergamon Press, 1970. (p. 49-51).

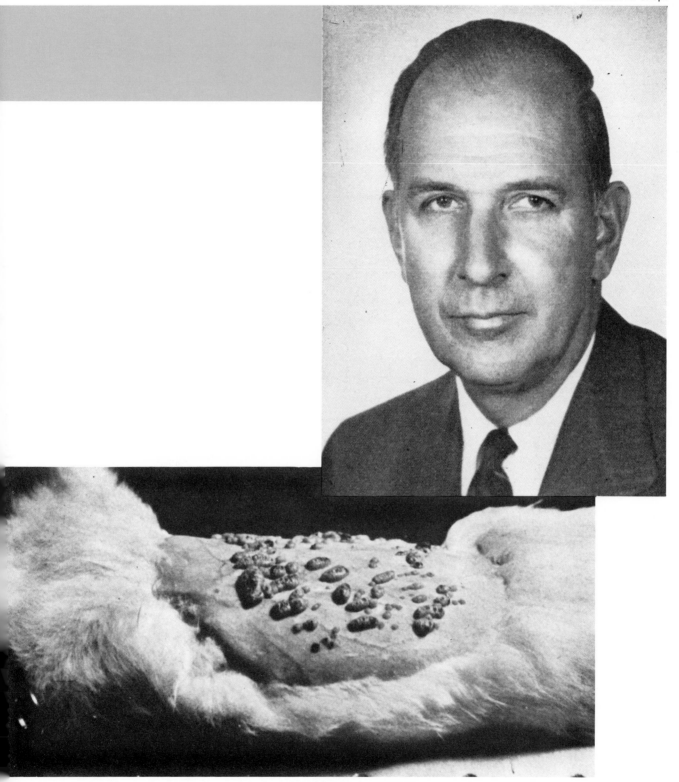

Richard E. Shope

Cutaneous papillomas in a rabbit (from Shope, J. Exptl. Med., 58:607-24, 1933)

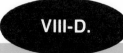

VIII-D.

Oncogenic Viruses

VIII-D-5. Frog kidney tumor: Lucké

Baldwin Lucké (1889-1954), professor of pathology at the University of Pennsylvania in Philadelphia, in 1934 described the occurrence of carcinoma of the kidney in the leopard frog (Rana pipiens) of the New England area.

Lucké was born in Germany, and graduated in 1912 in medicine from the Medical-Chirurgical College of Philadelphia. Two years later he joined the faculty of the University of Pennsylvania for a life-long association.

Dessicated or glycerinated tumor tissue inoculated into frogs increased the frequency of kidney tumors. On this basis, Lucké concluded in 1938 that the causative agent was a virus. Actual filtration experiments replicating the effect were performed by W. R. Duryee in 1956, and the DNA virus particles were photographed under the electron microscope by D. W. Fawcett the same year.

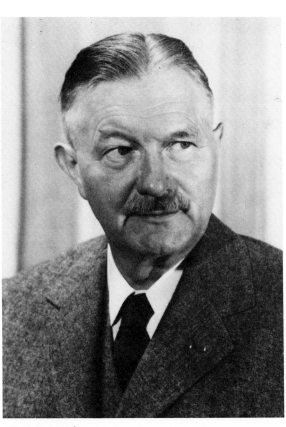

Baldwin Lucké

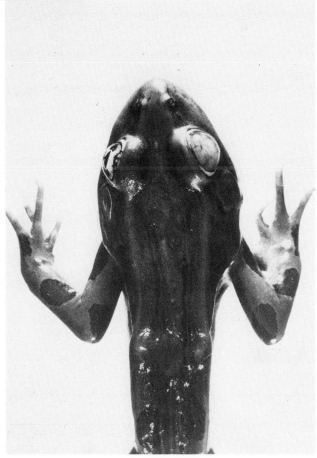

Frog with a transplant of the Lucké renal carcinoma into the anterior chamber of the right eye (from Shirley Hill Smith, Univ. of Pennsylvania School of Medicine).

B. Lucké. A neoplastic disease of the kidney of the frog, *Rana pipiens*. **Am. J. Cancer** 20: 352-79, 1934.

B. Lucké. Carcinoma in the leopard frog. Its probable causation by a virus. **J. Exp. Med.** 68: 457-68, 1938.

L. Gross. **Oncogenic Viruses.** Ed. 2. New York: Pergamon Press, 1970. (p. 82-94).

VIII-D.

Oncogenic Viruses

VIII-D-6. Transmission between species: Andrewes and Duran- Reynals.

Experiences with transplantable tumors indicated that such transplantation could be achieved only within the species of origin. The same species specificity was considered to be a characteristic of tumor viruses, which until the 1930s were limited to those of chickens.

Christopher Howard Andrewes (1896-   ), English pathologist working at the National Institute of Medical Research in London, in 1932 transmitted chicken sarcoma to pheasants, by means of filtrates. This was an early indication that species barriers of oncogenic viruses could be overcome.

Francisco Duran-Reynals (1899-1958), a Spanish medical investigator at Yale University, in 1942 extended the investigations, transmitting Rous sarcoma virus from chickens to ducklings, turkeys and guinea fowl. Newly-hatched recipients were used for successful attenuation of the virus in the new species, where it produced different types of sarcoma, such as of bone, as well as hemorrhagic lesions.

C. H. Andrewes. The transmission of fowl-tumours to pheasants. **J. Path. & Bact.** 35: 407-13, 1932.

F. Duran-Reynals. The reciprocal infection of ducks and chickens with tumor-inducing viruses. **Cancer Res.** 2: 343-69, 1942.

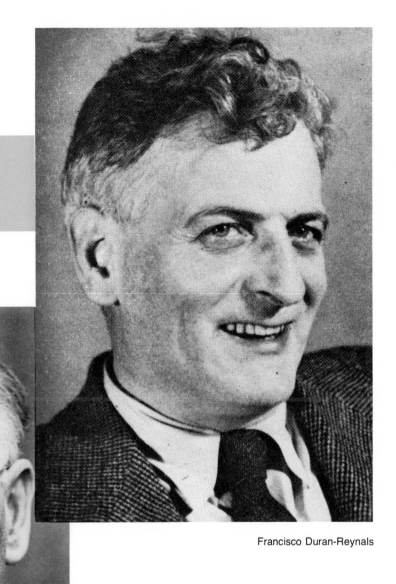

Francisco Duran-Reynals

C.H. Andrewes

VIII-E.

Chemical Carcinogens

VIII-E-1. Tar tumors: Yamagiwa and Ichikawa.

Katsusaburo Yamagiwa (1863-1930) and Koichi Ichikawa (1888-1948) opened the field of experimental chemical carcinogenesis by producing carcinoma of the skin of ears of rabbits by applications of coal tar. The experiments were reported at a special meeting of the Tokyo Medical Society on September 25, 1915, and published (with a dedication to Rudolf Virchow) in German in a Japanese journal. An extended account appeared in English three years later.

Crude coal tar dissolved in benzene was applied to the ears of 137 rabbits every 2 or 3 days. "Folliculoepitheliomas" arose in nearly all ears after a period longer than 100 days. Within a year, 7 cases of fully developed invasive carcinoma occurred, with regional lymph node metastases in 2 cases. Yamagiwa recorded this success with a Japanese haiku:

Cancer was produced!
Proudly I walk a few steps.

Yamagiwa, the third son of a Samurai, Seisaka Yamamoto, was adopted by a physician, Yoshiya Yamagiwa of Tokyo. He graduated from the Medical School of the Tokyo Imperial University in 1888.

The Japanese government sent him to Germany in 1891, where he studied under Virchow until 1894. The following year, at the age of 32, he was appointed full professor at the Tokyo Imperial University, where he remained until his retirement in 1923.

Yamagiwa was the father of cancer research in Japan. He was a founder of the Japanese Pathological Society and the Japanese Association for Cancer Research. In 1907 he initiated **Gann**, the Japanese Journal of Cancer Research. Yamagiwa received many honors, but the 1925 Nobel Prize escaped him and was awarded to Fibiger, as charmingly recounted by Henschen.

On 9 of Yamagiwa's papers on cancer the co-author is Koichi Ichikawa, a doctor of veterinary medicine, identified in the key report as a voluntary assistant at the Pathologic Institute of Tokyo.

Tar-painting became the favorite experimental method for inducing cancer, because of its simplicity, until polycyclic hydrocarbons derived from tar were isolated in 1930. A student of Yamagiwa, H. Tsutsui, extended the model by showing that mice were also susceptible.

Photomicrograph of one of the first carcinomas of the skin induced by repeated paintings of tar on an ear of a rabbit (from Yamagiwa, *Collected Papers*).

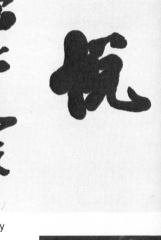

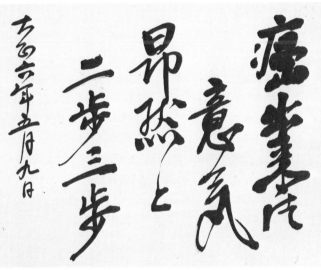

"Cancer was produced! Proudly I walk a few steps." (written by Yamagiwa on a silk scroll in 1917. In possession of Dr. Tadayoshi Kobayashi, through courtesy of Miss Dorothy U. Mizoguchi).

Katsusaburo Yamagiwa

Katsusaburo Yamagiwa and Koichi Ichikawa. Experimentelle Studie über die Pathogenese der Epithelialgeschwülste. **Mitteilungen Med. Facultat Kaiserl. Univ. Tokyo** 15(2): 295-344, 1915.

Katsusaburo Yamagiwa and Koichi Ichikawa. Experimental study of the pathogenesis of carcinoma. **J. Cancer Res.** 3: 1-29, 1918.

Katsusaburo Yamagiwa. **Collected Papers on Artificial Production of Cancer.** Tokyo, Japan: Maruzen Co., Ltd., 1965.

F. Henschen. Yamagiwa's tar cancer and its historical significance. **Gann** 59: 447-51, 1968.

H. Tsutsui. Über das künstlich erzeugte Cancroid bei der Maus. **Gann** 12: 17-21, 1918-9.

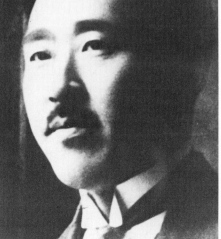

Koichi Ichikawa

VIII-E.

Chemical Carcinogens

VIII-E-2. Kangri cancer: Neve and Neve.

In 1900, Arthur Neve (1858-1919) of the Kashmir Mission Hospital recorded the occurrence of epitheliomas of the abdominal skin among the people of Kashmir. "The cause of this is not far to seek. During the severe winters and indeed for a great part of the year, every Kashmiri man, woman or child carries a portable charcoal brazier under the loose gown which constitutes his or her only garment . . . Slight burns frequently occur . . ."

Ernest F. Neve (1861-1946) in 1886 joined his older brother in Kashmir. In 1923 he reported that 2491 operations for epithelioma were performed and of these approximately 2000 or 84 percent, were kangri cancers. The primary factor was considered to be the heat and recurrent burns, "but it is possible that the volatile substances resulting from the combustion of the wood play a secondary part."

Cancer of the oral cavity is a common affliction in India, and has been associated with both smoking of tobacco and chewing betel-nut preparations. One exotic form of tobacco-induced cancer is the Chutta cancer, associated with the habit of reverse smoking of a cigar with the burning end being held inside the mouth. The high frequency of cancer of the palate in Andhra was attributed to this habit by B. R. Khanolkar. It is also seen among washerwomen of Panama, where reverse-smoking is practiced in order to keep the cigarette from being extinguished by spattering of water.

These are examples of cancer induced by environmental exposure to carcinogens.

A. Neve. Kangri-burn epithelioma in Kashmir. **Indian Med. Gaz.** 35: 81-3, 1900.

E. F. Neve. Kangri-burn cancer. **Brit. Med. J.** ii: 1255-6, 1923.

V. R. Khanolkar. Cancer in India in relation to habits and customs. In, R. W. Raven (ed), **Cancer** 3: 272-85. London: Butterworth, 1958.

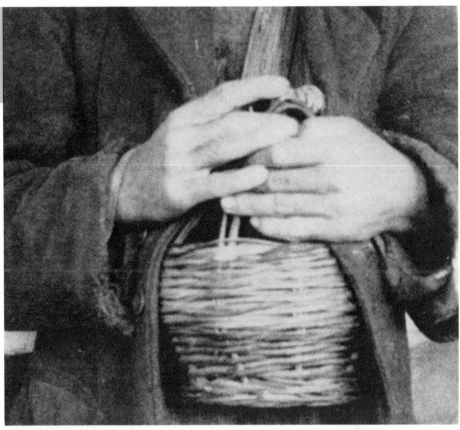

Kangri basket with live coals as used for warmth by Kashmir people (from E.F. Neve, 1923).

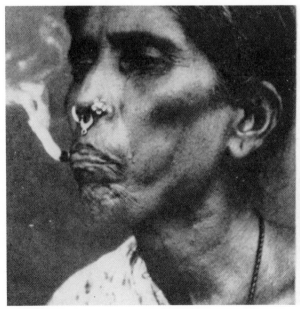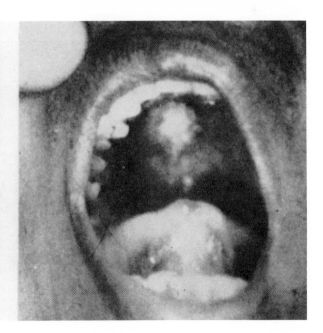

Chutta cancer from reverse smoking of tobacco (from V.R. Khanolkar, 1958).

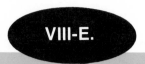

VIII-E.

Chemical Carcinogens

VIII-E-3. Occupational cancer: Hueper.

OCCUPATIONAL TUMORS
AND
ALLIED DISEASES

By

W. C. HUEPER, M.D.

ASSISTANT DIRECTOR AND PRINCIPAL PATHOLOGIST
WARNER INSTITUTE FOR THERAPEUTIC RESEARCH
NEW YORK CITY

1942

CHARLES C THOMAS · PUBLISHER

SPRINGFIELD · ILLINOIS   BALTIMORE · MARYLAND

Hueper, Occupational Tumors and Allied Diseases, 1942.
Title page.

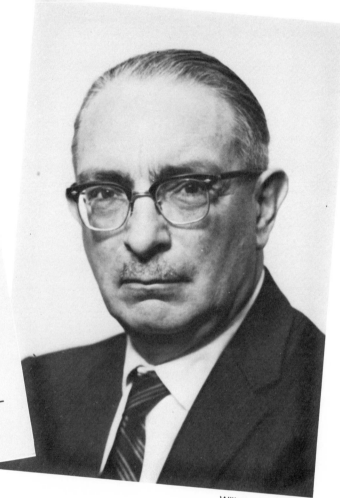

Wilhelm C. Hueper

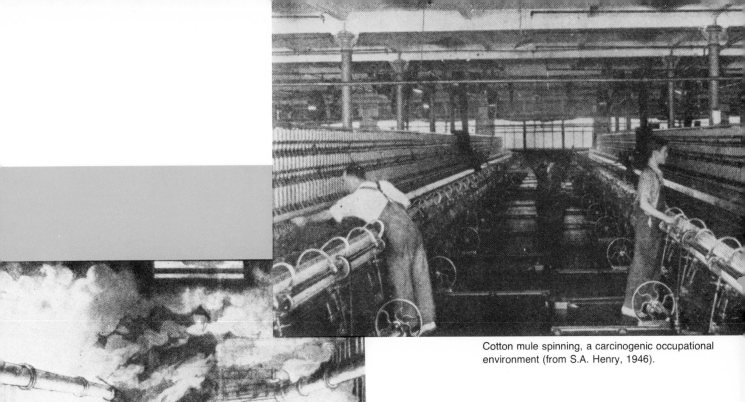

Cotton mule spinning, a carcinogenic occupational environment (from S.A. Henry, 1946).

Drawing the retorts at the Great Gas Light Establishment, Brick Lane, London (from a print by W. Read, 1821, reproduced by Henry, 1946).

The chimney sweep's cancer of the scrotum was a forerunner of descriptions of many other cancers induced by occupational exposures to carcinogenic materials. Skin cancers were seen in workers exposed to a wide variety of coal tars, oils and petroleum products. Richard von Volkmann of Germany and Henry Butlin of England made important contributions to the field of occupational cancer during the latter part of the 19th Century.

Wilhelm Carl Hueper was among the more intense students of the subject, and his book of 1942 was a definitive summary of occupational cancer. Hueper was born in 1894 in Germany, and obtained his medical doctorate from the University of Kiel in 1920. He emigrated to the United States in 1923, and con-

tinued his work in experimental pathology in Delaware and New York. He was on the staff of the National Cancer Institute in Bethesda, Maryland, from 1948 until his retirement in 1964. In 1962 he shared with L. M. Shabad of Moscow a United Nations award for investigations of environmental carcinogenesis.

Two examples illustrating environmental, occupational exposures associated with increased risk to cancer are from S. A. Henry's book of 1946.

Thus, industrial occupational exposures were among the important environmental causes of cancer in man. Such exposures, of course, extended to surrounding populations sharing the environments.

W. C. Hueper. **Occupational Tumors and Allied Diseases.** Springfield, Ill.: C. C. Thomas, 1942.

S. A. Henry. **Cancer of the Scrotum in Relation to Occupation.** London: Oxford Univ. Press, 1946.

VIII-E.

Chemical Carcinogens

VIII-E-4. Polycyclic hydrocarbon carcinogens: Kennaway, Hieger and Mayneord.

Ernest Laurence Kennaway (1881-1958) and his team of investigators at the Chester Beatty Institute for Cancer Research in London identified and isolated the carcinogenic polycyclic hydrocarbons in coal tar. Kennaway obtained his education in chemistry and in medicine at the University of London and at Oxford, and was professor of experimental pathology at the University of London as well as director of the Chester Beatty Institute. His contributions were recognized by fellowship in the Royal Society and a knighthood. Among his associates were J. W. Cook, I. Hieger and W. V. Mayneord, as well as Mrs. Kennaway.

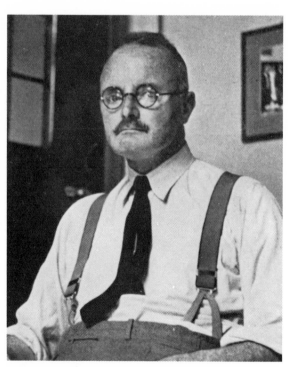

E.L. Kennaway

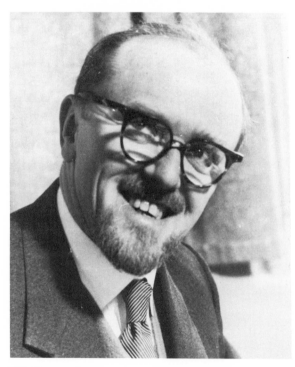

W.V. Mayneord

The first carcinogenic compound, reported in 1930, was recognized by its fluorescent spectrum; this was 1,2,5,6-dibenzanthracene. The isolation from coal tar and synthesis of 3,4-benzpyrene was achieved in 1932.

The effort was comparable with the isolation of radium from pitchblende. The parallel of radium and benzpyrene extends even further: radioactivity was the property that facilitated the isolation of radium, and the fluorescence spectrum was the single thread that led through the labyrinth of coal tar.

Kennaway's historical recollections of 1955, written when he was racked with paralysis agitans, are notable for their clarity, completeness and graciousness.

E. L. Kennaway and I. Hieger. Carcinogenic substances and their fluorescence spectra. **Brit. Med. J.** i: 1044-6, 1930.

J. W. Cook, I. Hieger, E. L. Kennaway and W. V. Mayneord. The production of cancer by pure hydrocarbons. Part I. **Proc. Roy. Soc. B.** III: 455-84, 1932.

I. Hieger. The fluorescence spectrum of 3,4-benzpyrene. **Am. J. Cancer** 29: 705-14, 1937.

E. L. Kennaway. The identification of a carcinogenic compound in coal-tar. **Brit. Med. J.** ii: 749-52, 1955.

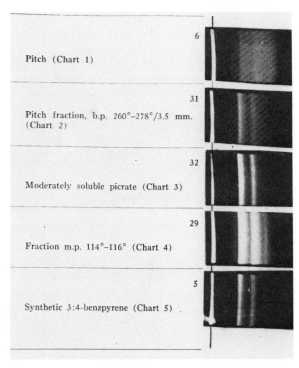

Pitch (Chart 1)

Pitch fraction, b.p. 260°–278°/3.5 mm. (Chart 2)

Moderately soluble picrate (Chart 3)

Fraction m.p. 114°–116° (Chart 4)

Synthetic 3:4-benzpyrene (Chart 5)

Fluorescence spectra of 3,4-benzpyrene and several fractions of pitch (from I. Hieger, 1937).

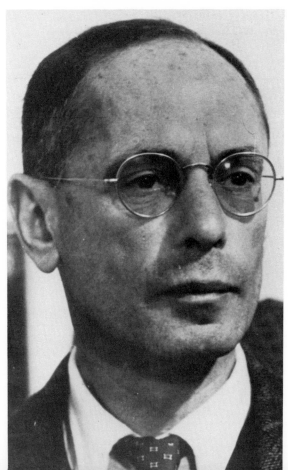

I. Hieger

Chemical Carcinogens

VIII-E-5. Hydrocarbon chemistry: Cook, Fieser and Buu-Hoi.

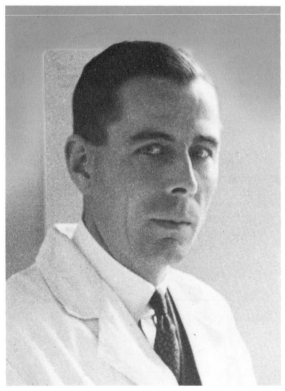

James W. Cook

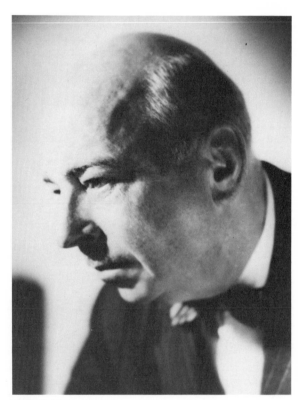

Louis F. Fieser

The isolation of 3,4-benzpyrene from coal tar introduced a decade of active chemical exploration of the analogues for carcinogenic activity, with the aim of eliciting a chemical structure relationship to cancer.

The two most important endeavors were centered in London and in Cam-

bridge, Massachusetts, where two organic chemists and their associates synthesized the chemicals.

James Wilfred Cook (1900-   ) was the chief organic chemist at the Royal Cancer (now Royal Marsden) Hospital in London and a member of E. L. Kennaway's group in the isolation of 3,4-

doctorate in chemistry from Harvard University in 1924. He joined the faculty at Harvard in 1930, and became professor of organic chemistry. He synthesized 20-methylcholanthrene in 1935, and many methyl-substituted benzanthracenes, introduced new reactions in steroid synthesis, and contributed to the chemistry of naphthoquinones. Fieser's polycyclic hydrocarbons were tested for carcinogenic activity at the Office of Cancer Investigations, a Public Health Service activity at Harvard.

Particular interest in carcinogenic hydrocarbons was aroused by the 1937 reports from both investigative groups of synthesis of 20-methylcholanthrene, an active carcinogen, from desoxycholic and cholic acids. This suggested the possibility of carcinogenesis being an inborn error of metabolism of cholesterol, a hypothesis that soon foundered in the wake of the discovery of the carcinogenic azo dyes.

The field of chemical structure relationships to carcinogenic activity, using the polycyclic hydrocarbons and related compounds as the models, was continued and expanded following World War II by Buu-Hoi.

Nguyen Phuc Buu-Hoi (1915-1972), a prince of Vietnam born in Hue, was educated in Hanoi in organic chemistry and moved to Paris in 1935. There he formed a fertile collaboration with A. Lacassagne at the Radium Institute which led to over a thousand publications.

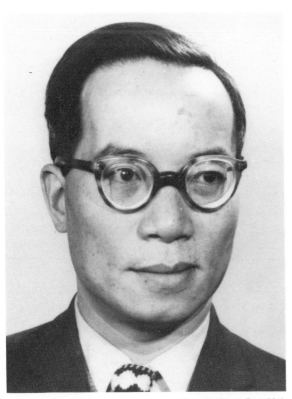

Nguyen Phuc Buu-Hoi

benzpyrene from tar. The studies established the extent of carcinogenic activity among hydrocarbons of the 1,2-benzanthracene and 3,4-benzphenanthrene groups. Cook was knighted for his contributions to chemistry.

Louis Frederick Fieser (1899-   ) was born in Ohio and received his

J. W. Cook et al. Chemical compounds as carcinogenic agents. **Am. J. Cancer** 29: 219-59, 1937.

J. W. Cook and E. L. Kennaway. Chemical compounds as carcinogenic agents. **Am. J. Cancer** 39: 381-428 and 521-82, 1940.

L. F. Fieser et al. Carcinogenic activity of the cholanthrenes and of other 1:2 benzanthracene derivatives. **Am. J. Cancer** 29: 260-8, 1937.

L. F. Fieser. Carcinogenic activity, structure, and chemical reactivity of polynuclear aromatic hydrocarbons. **Am. J. Cancer** 34: 37-124, 1938.

L. F. Fieser. Extensions in the use of plastic tetrahedral models. **J. Chem. Ed.** 42: 408-12, 1965.

Joseph C. Arcos. In memory of Nguyen Phuc Buu-Hoi, 1915-1972. **Cancer Res.** 32: 2856A-56, 1972.

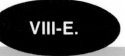

VIII-E.

Chemical Carcinogens

VIII-E-6. Azo dye carcinogens: Yoshida and Fischer-Wasels.

Tomizu Yoshida (1903-1974) professor of pathology at Tokyo University in Japan, in 1933-35 reported the induction of liver cancers in rats that ingested aminoazo compounds in their diet. The first compound, o-aminoazotoluene, was replaced by R. Kinosita by a more active chemical, 4-dimethylaminoazobenzene.

Liver tumors were a suitable material for biochemical studies of tissue changes during carcinogenesis and for comparisons of normal and neoplastic metabolism. It was soon found that the diet of the animals profoundly affected the carcinogenic response, with riboflavin being found by C. J. Kensler in 1941 to have the most marked effect. The mechanism of this retarding effect, however, was on the detoxification of the dyes, and was not related to carcinogenesis per se.

Without depriving Yoshida of well deserved recognition, it should be pointed out that Bernard Fischer-Wasels (1877-1941) in 1906 in Germany produced atypical epithelial proliferation in rabbits following injection of Scarlet Red, and that M. B. Schmidt, in 1924, reported the development of hepatomas in mice fed Scarlet Red. These were among the earlier discoveries of chemical activation of atypical growth, but Fischer's lesions receded when the stimulus was removed and Schmidt's hepatomas were interpreted as benign tumors.

Yoshida's report of 1935, with his mentor T. Sasaki as senior author, can be regarded as the starting point of the world-wide research on carcinogenic azo dyes that followed.

T. Sasaki and T. Yoshida. Experimentelle Erzeugung des Leberkarcinoms durch Fütterung mit o-Amidoazotoluol. **Virchows Arch. Path. Anat.** 295: 175-200, 1935.

J. A. Miller and E. C. Miller. The carcinogenic aminoazo dyes. **Adv. Cancer Res.** 1: 339-96, 1953.

M. B. Shimkin and V. A. Triolo. History of chemical carcinogenesis: some prospective remarks. **Progr. Exp. Tumor Res.** 11: 1-20, 1969.

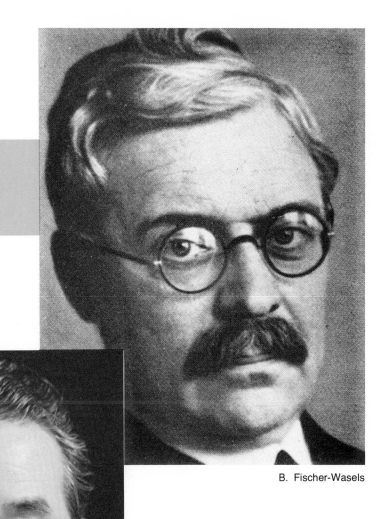

B. Fischer-Wasels

Tomizu Yoshida

VIII-F.

Hormones

VIII-F-1. Chemistry of estrogens: Doisy, Butenandt and Dodds.

Ovarian hormones were recognized by Marshall and Jolly in 1905, when they induced estrus in spayed dogs with extracts of ovary. Edgar Allen and E. A. Doisy in 1923 developed a bioassay procedure for measuring the activity of follicular fluid from sow ovaries by the cornification of the vagina in spayed rats.

Edward A. Doisy (1893-   ) and coworkers in St. Louis in August 1929 reported the preparation of a crystalline ovarian hormone "Folliculin," from the urine of pregnant women. Similar announcements followed in close succession from several investigators, the first by Adolph Butenandt (1903-   ), who in October 1929 introduced a nearly pure crystalline hormone "Progynon" from human pregnancy urine. In 1939 Butenandt shared a Nobel Prize in chemistry for his investigations on the sex hormones. Doisy shared a Nobel Prize in 1943 for his work on the chemistry of Vitamin K.

Highly active preparations of crystalline estrogens were also made available by Ernest Laqueur and his associates in Amsterdam. Guy Frederick Marrian of London also provided chemical data on a hormonal preparation called "Oestrin." The name Estrogen became applied to a series of steroids with a phenanthrene nucleus having estrogenic activity.

In a series of clever chemical manipulations and deductions, Edward Charles Dodds (1899-1974), of London, in 1938 introduced a highly active estrogenic synthetic compound, diethylstilbestrol.

H. Burrows. **Biological Actions of Sex Hormones,** Ed. 2. Cambridge: Cambridge University Press, 1949.

A. Butenandt. Über "Progynon." Ein krystallisiertes weibliches Sexualhormon. **Naturwissensch.** 17: 879, 1929.

E. C. Dodds, L. Goldberg, W. Lawson and R. Robinson. Oestrogenic activity of certain synthetic compounds. **Nature** 141: 247-48, 1938.

E. A. Doisy, C. D. Veler and S. Thayer. The preparation of the crystalline ovarian hormone from the urine of pregnant women. **J. Biol. Chem.** 86: 499-509, 1930.

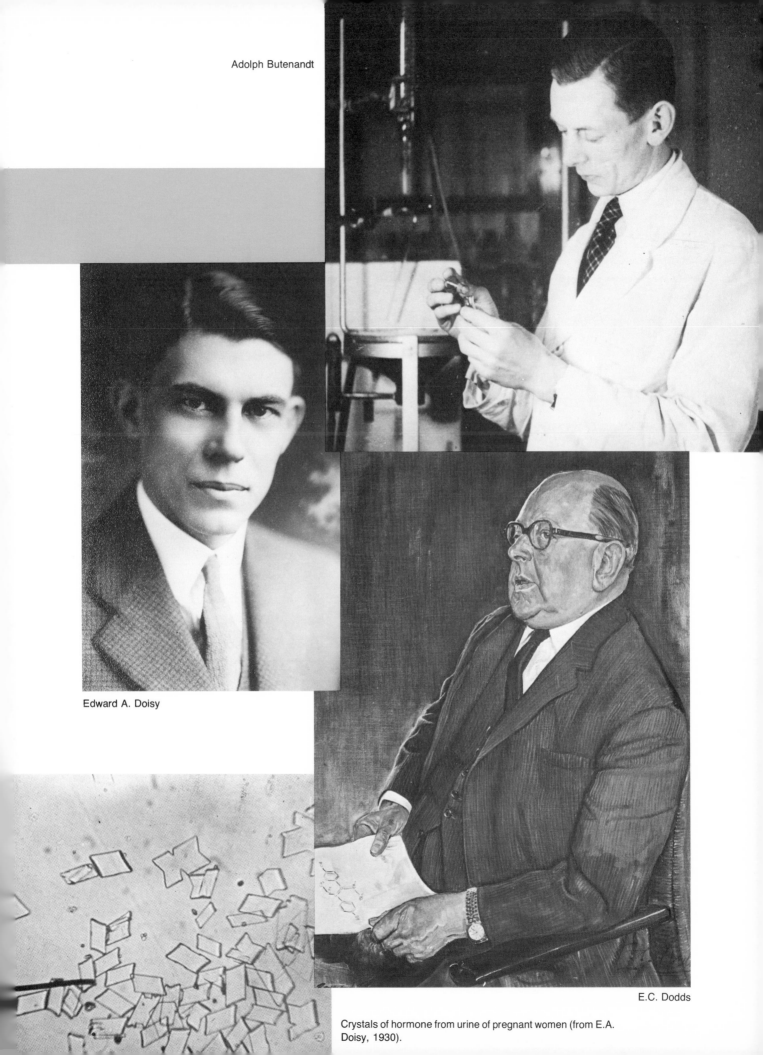

Adolph Butenandt

Edward A. Doisy

E.C. Dodds

Crystals of hormone from urine of pregnant women (from E.A. Doisy, 1930).

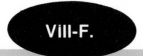

VIII-F.

Hormones

VIII-F-2. Hormone carcinogenesis: Lacassagne and W. S. Murray.

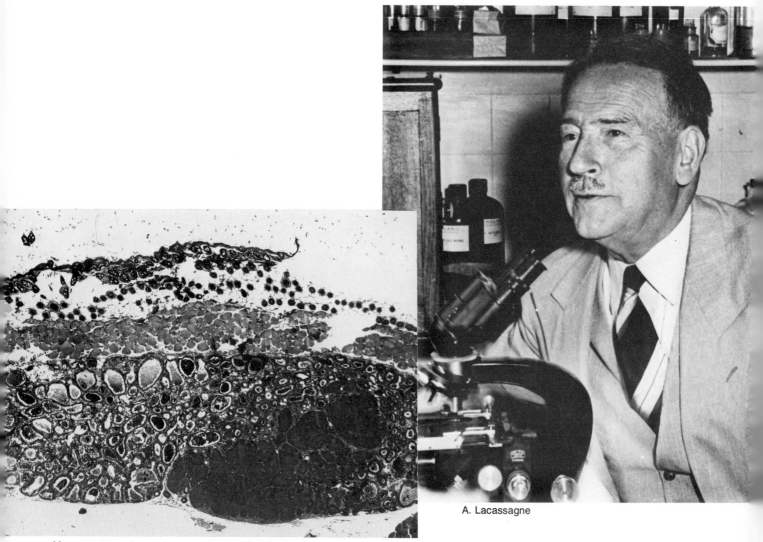

A. Lacassagne

Mammary tumor in a male mouse induced by injections of an estrogen (from Lacassagne, 1932).

Antoine-Marcellin-Bernard Lacassagne (1884-1971) of Paris, in 1932 reported the induction of mammary carcinoma in male mice that were injected weekly with a folliculin preparation. This was the first induction of a malignant neoplasm by exogenously administered female sex hormone. The mammary tumors appeared in males of strains with a high incidence of tumors among females, and Lacassagne concluded that the hormone permitted a latent hereditary predisposition to cancer to manifest itself. In 1938 Lacassagne demonstrated that the synthetic estrogen, diethylstilbestrol, also produced mammary tumors in male mice of susceptible strains.

The relationship of pregnancy and of ovariectomy to the occurrence of mammary tumors in mice was studied by several investigators between 1913 and 1927. Pregnancy increased the frequency of such tumors, whereas ovariectomy in young females reduced the frequency, suggesting a role of endocrine, ovarian factors. Loeb also grafted ovaries in castrated males, but obtained no tumors in a limited experiment.

In 1928, William S. Murray (1899-1971) grafted ovaries subcutaneously in 210 castrated male mice, and obtained mammary carcinomas in 15. The role of ovarian secretions in mammary carcinogenesis was thus established by this experiment.

The staff of the National Cancer Institute in 1945 summarized investigations on mammary tumors in mice, in which the etiologic factors include the complex of heredity, endocrines, and a milk-transmitted virus.

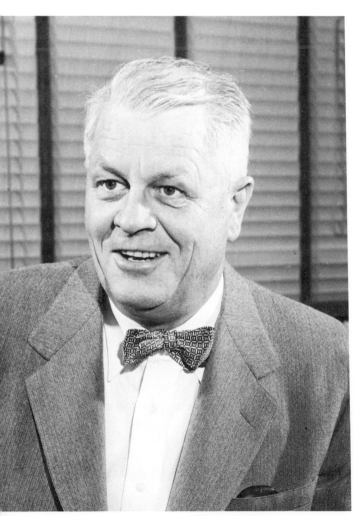

William S. Murray

A. Lacassagne. Apparition de cancers de la mamelle chez la souris mâle, soumise à des injections de folliculine. **Compt. Rend. Acad. Sci.** (Paris) 195: 630-32, 1932.

A. Lacassagne. Apparition d'adénocarcinomes mammaires chez des souris mâles, traitées par une substance oestrogène synthétique. **Compt. Rend. Soc. Biol.** 129: 641-3, 1938.

W. S. Murray. Ovarian secretion and tumor incidence. **J. Cancer Res.** 12: 18-25, 1928.

Staff, National Cancer Institute. **Mammary Tumors in Mice.** Washington, D.C.: Amer. Assoc. Advanc. Sci., 1945.

VIII-G.

Parasites

VIII-G-1. Bilharzial bladder cancer: Ferguson and Kuntz.

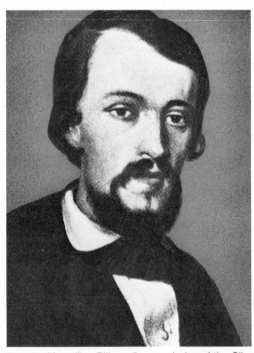

Theodor Maxmilian Bilharz (by permission of the Ciba Foundation, from Symposium on Bilharziasis, 1962)

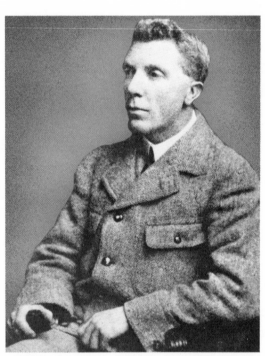

A.R. Ferguson (by permission from Mustacchi and Jassy, 1962).

Since the days of the pharaohs, the Egyptian peasants, wading in the waters of the Nile valley, have been afflicted with hematuria due to chronic cystitis.

In 1851 German parasitologist Theodor Maximilian Bilharz (1825-62) recovered flatworms from the mesenteric veins of an Egyptian peasant. He demonstrated that this worm and its terminal-spined eggs, which were discharged in the urine, were the cause of hematuria.

Schistosoma haematobium, the vesical fluke originally named after Bilharz, predominates in Africa, where it infects an estimated population of 10 to 25 million. Its reservoir is primarily man, who contaminates African waters with urine and feces. Eggs passed with excreta hatch into a free swimming stage (miracidium), which infects different species of the freshwater snail, **Bulinus**. Miracidia in the snail host give rise to many cercariae, which emerge from the snail, swim freely in water and, upon contact, penetrate the skin of man. Parasites, by way of the circulatory system, gain access to many parts of the body. **S. haematobium** has a tendency to reside

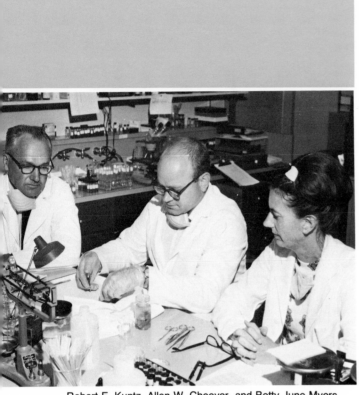

Robert E. Kuntz, Allen W. Cheever, and Betty June Myers.

in the vesical veins of man. The eggs are encysted in the bladder wall and are discharged through the urine to complete the life cycle.

Alexander Robert Ferguson (1870-1920), Scottish pathologist at the School of Medicine in Cairo, associated bilharziasis and carcinoma of the urinary bladder in 1911 on the basis of autopsy observations. This association was reported by previous pathologists, such as R. Harrison in 1889. Epidemiological studies in Egypt and West Africa substantiated the association. Nevertheless, bilharziasis as a cause of bladder cancer was not universally accepted since the pathogenesis was obscure and the situation had not been replicated in animals under experimental conditions.

Robert E. Kuntz (1916-   ) and Betty June Myers (1928-   ), of the Southwest Foundation for Research and Edu-

cation in San Antonio, Texas, and Allen W. Cheever (1932-   ), Laboratory of Parasitic Diseases of the National Institutes of Health, succeeded in infecting nonhuman primates with **S. haematobium**. Papillary transitional cell carcinomas of the urinary bladder were found in a talapoin monkey and a capuchin monkey, 21 and 53 weeks, respectively, after such infection. There were additional cases of proliferative epithelial lesions related to the presence of **S. haematobium** eggs in the lamina propria of the bladder. The evidence appears complete that **S. haematobium** causes cancer of the urinary bladder.

A. R. Ferguson. Associated bilharziasis and primary malignant disease of the urinary bladder, with observations on a series of forty cases. **J. Path. & Bact.** 16: 76-94, 1911.

R. E. Kuntz, A. W. Cheever and B. J. Myers. Proliferative epithelial lesions of the urinary bladder of nonhuman primates infected with *Schistosoma haematobium*. **J. Natl. Cancer Inst.** 48: 223-35, 1972.

Ciba Foundation. **Symposium on Bilharziasis.** Boston: Little, Brown & Co., 1962.

P. Mustacchi and L. Jassey. Alexander Robert Ferguson, M.D. On "The irritation cancer of Egypt." **Cancer** 15: 215-16, 1962.

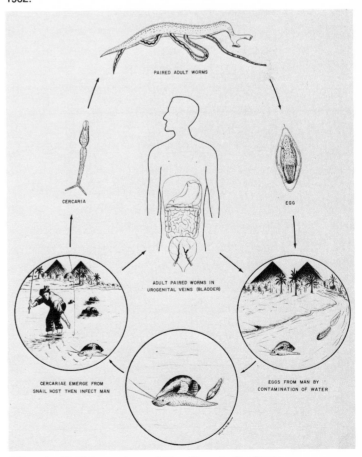

Life cycle of Schistosoma haematobium (drawn by Tao Cheng Huang)

VIII-G.

Parasites

VIII-G-2. Cysticercus sarcoma: Bullock, Dunning and Curtis.

Frederick D. Bullock (1878-1937) and Maynie R. Curtis (1880-1971), working at the Crocker Institute for Cancer Research at Columbia Univeristy in New York, demonstrated that sarcoma of the liver could be induced by the experimental infestation of young rats with the larval stage of the common tapeworm of the cat, **Cysticercus fasciolaris. Cysticercus** sarcoma in rats was first described by A. Borrel in 1907.

Several homozygous rat strains were developed in order to explain the observed differences in neoplastic incidence. Wilhelmina F. Dunning (1904-   ) joined the work in 1926. By 1933 data in **Cysticercus**-induced sarcoma were available on 3,669 rats and showed that the effective genetic factors were those that determined the susceptibility of the rat to the parasitic disease and resistance to common laboratory diseases. This was an early demonstration of a quantitative relationship between the stimulus and the response in experimental carcinogenesis.

Interest in **Cysticercus**-induced sarcomas continued in the demonstration that intraperitoneal injection of washed, ground larvae produced multiple intraperitoneal sarcomas in rats. Further attempts to isolate the active agent indicated that it was associated with the calcium carbonate fraction of the parasite. Thus, an unidentified chemical carcinogen must be elaborated by the parasite.

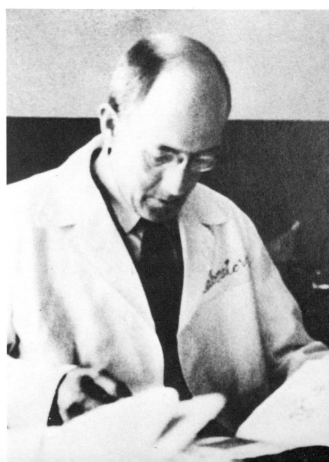

F.D. Bullock

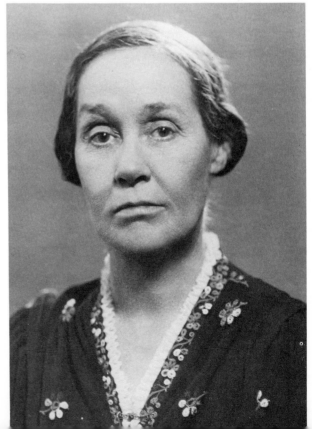

Afternoon sunshine and shadow on the building which was the home of the Institute of Cancer Research of Columbia University from 1913 to 1938.

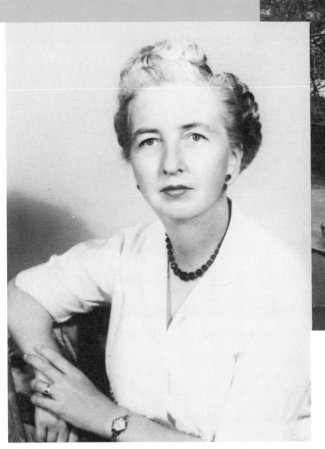

W.F. Dunning

F. D. Bullock and M. R. Curtis. *Cysticercus* sarcoma. **J. Cancer Res.** 8: 152-53, 1924.

M. R. Curtis, W. F. Dunning and F. D. Bullock. Genetic factors in relation to the etiology of malignant tumors. **Am. J. Cancer** 17: 894-923, 1933.

W. F. Dunning and M. R. Curtis. Attempts to isolate the active agent in *Cysticercus fasciolaris*. **Cancer Res.** 13: 838-42, 1953.

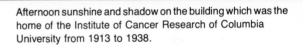

M. Curtis

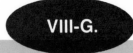

VIII-G.

Parasites

VIII-G-3. Cockroaches and rat cancer: Fibiger.

The history of science includes errors and false leads as well as successes, and no history of carcinogenesis can avoid the tale of Johannes Andreas Grib Fibiger (1867-1928). This Danish investigator in 1907 began his studies on the occurrence of neoplastic lesions of the stomach, which he interpreted as carcinoma, in rats at a sugar refinery. He associated the lesions with infestations of the rats by a nematode, the common cockroach serving as the intermediate host. The investigations attracted great attention in scientific circles, and in 1926 Fibiger was awarded the Nobel Prize, the first such accolade to cancer research.

Unfortunately, attempts to repeat the work were unsuccessful, and the neoplastic character of the lesions described by Fibiger was questioned. Vitamin A deficiency, together with "chronic irritation," became accepted as the explanation of the hyperplastic reactions observed by Fibiger. Yet it is to be wondered whether these explanations are final.

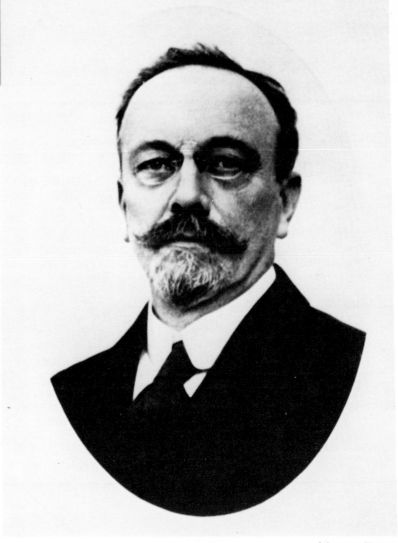

Johannes Fibiger

J. Fibiger. Untersuchung über eine Nematode (*Spiroptera* sp. n.) und deren Fähigkeit, papillomatöse und carcinomatöse Geschwulstbildungen im Magen der Ratte hervorzurufen. **Z. Krebsforsch.** 13: 217-80, 1913.

C. R. Hitchcock and E. T. Bell. Studies on the nematode, parasite, *Gongylonema neoplasticum* (*Spiroptera neoplasticum*) and avitaminosis A in the forestomach of rats: comparison with Fibiger's results. **J. Natl. Cancer Inst.** 12: 1345-87, 1952.

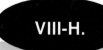

Physical Carcinogens

VIII-H-1. X-radiation cancer: Clunet and Feygin.

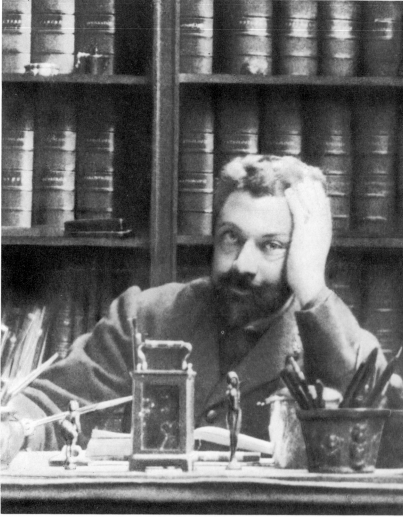

Clunet, *Tumeurs Malignes*, 1910. Title page.

J. Clunet

Skin burns and malignant epitheliomas were observed on the hands of radiologists and other users of X-ray devices and radium within a few years after their discovery in 1895 and 1898. By 1902 "radiation cancers" were recorded in case reports from Germany, England, and the United States. By 1914 a total of 104 cases were gathered and analyzed by Sophie Feygin. A list of radiological martyrs to the new form of energy has been compiled. Thus, the carcinogenic effects of ionizing radiation were first shown in man.

Pierre Edouard Jean Clunet (1878-1917) in 1908 exposed 4 white rats to X-rays, in doses sufficient to produce ulceration of the skin. One of the 2 survivors developed a sarcoma at the site. The limited finding was related to the effect of burn, as in the Kangri cancers, and was not expanded by other investigators. For laboratory research, tar painting was a much simpler method of inducing cancer.

It was not until 1930 that the leukemogenic effect of ionizing radiation was recognized in mice, by Krebs et al. The role of ionizing radiation in the causation of leukemia in man was shown in 1944, by March and by Henshaw and Hawkins.

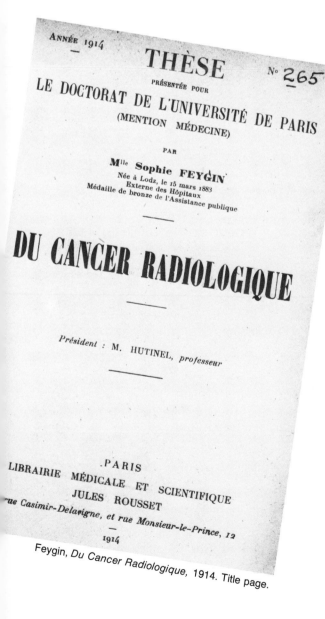

ANNÉE 1914

THÈSE

No 265

PRÉSENTÉE POUR

LE DOCTORAT DE L'UNIVERSITÉ DE PARIS

(MENTION MÉDECINE)

PAR

Mlle **Sophie FEYGIN**

Née à Lodz, le 15 mars 1883
Externe des Hôpitaux
Médaille de bronze de l'Assistance publique

DU CANCER RADIOLOGIQUE

Président : M. HUTINEL, *professeur*

.PARIS

LIBRAIRIE MÉDICALE ET SCIENTIFIQUE
JULES ROUSSET

rue Casimir-Delavigne, et rue Monsieur-le-Prince, 12

1914

Feygin, Du Cancer Radiologique, 1914. Title page.

J. Clunet. **Recherches Expérimentales sur les Tumeurs Malignes.** Paris: Steinheil, 1910.

S. Feygin. **Du Cancer Radiologique.** Paris: Rousset, 1915.

C. Krebs, H. C. Rask-Nielsen and A. Wagner. The origin of lymphosarcomatosis and its relation to other forms of leucosis in white mice. **Acta Radiol. Supp.** 10: 1-53, 1930.

P. S. Henshaw and J. W. Hawkins. Incidence of leukemia in physicians. **J. Nat. Cancer Inst.** 4: 339-46, 1944.

H. C. March. Leukemia in radiologists. **Radiology** 43: 275-8, 1944.

VIII-H.

Physical Carcinogens

VIII-H-2. Radium osteosarcoma: Martland.

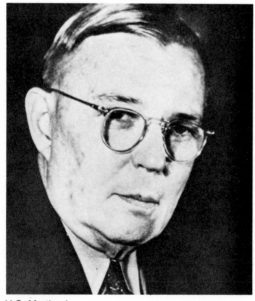

H.S. Martland

During the 1920s there occurred a historical industrial carcinogenic exposure in Orange, New Jersey. Watch dials were painted with a preparation containing radium and mesothorium, in order to make them luminescent. Some 800 young women, pointing the brushes with their tongue, were affected.

The true extent of the mortality from radioactive poisoning in this group will never be known, but Harrison Stanford Martland (1883-1954) eventually assembled 41 deaths during the first decade, of which 9 were from osteogenic sarcoma.

Martland was a physician and pathologist at the Newark City Hospital in New Jersey, and became chief medical examiner for Essex County during his dial-painter investigations.

An illustrative case was published by Martland and Humphries. A 25-year-old woman worked as a painter of dials, pointing the brushes with her lips. Eight years later she had pain in the right shoulder, and evidence of radiation osteitis of the right humerus and scapula.

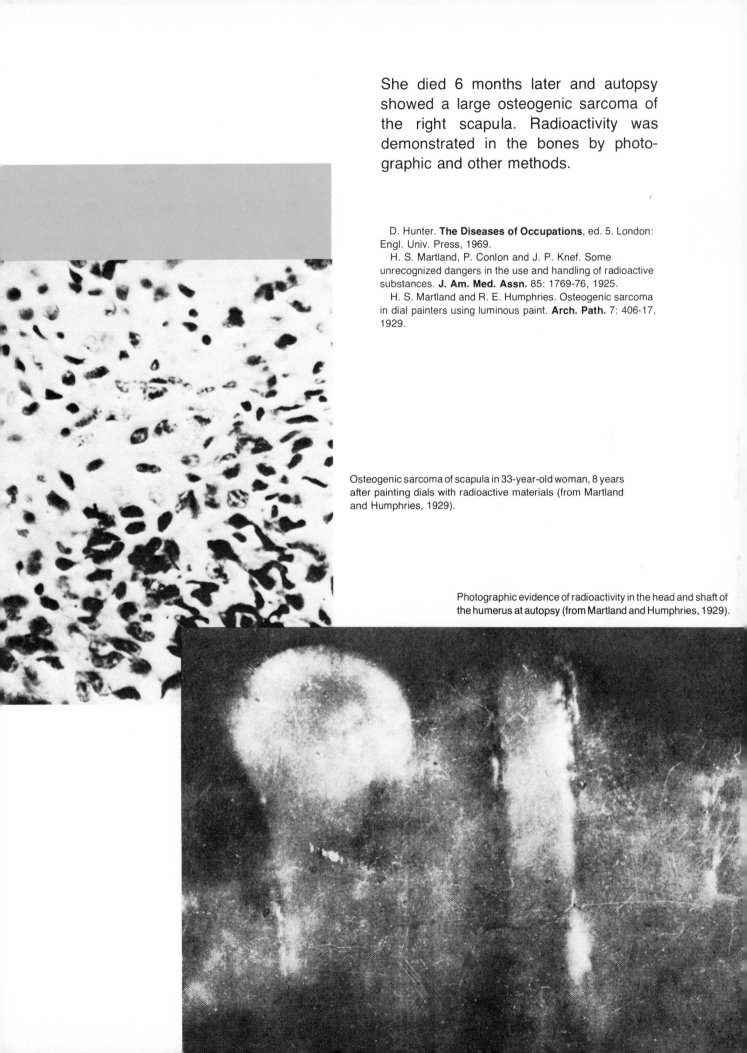

She died 6 months later and autopsy showed a large osteogenic sarcoma of the right scapula. Radioactivity was demonstrated in the bones by photographic and other methods.

D. Hunter. **The Diseases of Occupations**, ed. 5. London: Engl. Univ. Press, 1969.

H. S. Martland, P. Conlon and J. P. Knef. Some unrecognized dangers in the use and handling of radioactive substances. **J. Am. Med. Assn.** 85: 1769-76, 1925.

H. S. Martland and R. E. Humphries. Osteogenic sarcoma in dial painters using luminous paint. **Arch. Path.** 7: 406-17, 1929.

Osteogenic sarcoma of scapula in 33-year-old woman, 8 years after painting dials with radioactive materials (from Martland and Humphries, 1929).

Photographic evidence of radioactivity in the head and shaft of the humerus at autopsy (from Martland and Humphries, 1929).

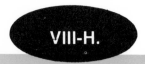

VIII-H.

Physical Carcinogens

VIII-H-3. Sunlight and skin cancer: Dubreuilh, Findlay and Roffo.

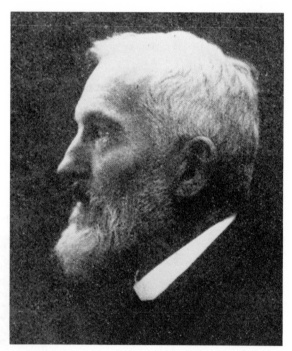

W. Dubreuilh

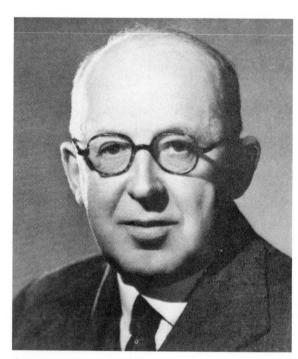

G.M. Findlay

The role of sunlight as an environmental hazard was suggested by dermatologists during the 19th Century. Paul Gerson Unna (1850-1915) indicated in 1894 a possible etiologic relationship between chronic dermatoses in sailors and their long exposures to solar radiation.

William Dubreuilh (1857-1935), a noted dermatologist of Bordeaux, France, in 1907 reported epidemiologic evidence of sunlight as a cause of skin cancer in man.

George M. Findlay (1893-1952), a British pathologist, published in 1928 an experimental verification, by inducing skin cancer in white mice exposed to ultraviolet radiation.

Angel H. Roffo (1882-1947), an outstanding figure in clinical and experimental cancer in Argentina, in 1934 reproduced the situation in white rats exposed to sunlight; the animals developed carcinomas and sarcomas of the skin. Roffo also reported in 1931 the appearance of carcinomas on the skin of rabbits painted with tobacco smoke condensates.

The field of ultraviolet carcinogenesis was surveyed and extended quantitatively by Blum.

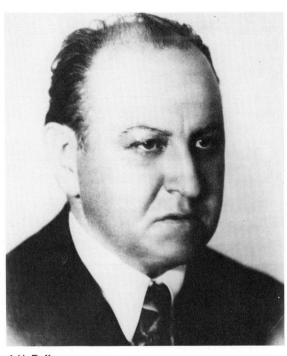

A.H. Roffo

P. G. Unna. **Die Histopathologie der Hautkrankheiten.** Berlin: A. Hirschwald, 1894.

W. Dubreuilh. Épithéliomatose d'origine solaire. **Ann. Dermat. Syphiliq.** 8: 387-416, 1907.

G. M. Findlay. Ultra-violet light and skin cancer. **Lancet** 2: 1070-3, 1928.

A. H. Roffo. Krebs und Sarkom durch Ultraviolett- und Sonnenstrahlen. **Ztschr. f. Krebsforsch.** 41: 488-67, 1935.

H. F. Blum. **Carcinogenesis by Ultraviolet Light.** Princeton, N.J.: Princeton Univ. Press, 1959.

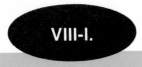

VIII-I.

Biochemistry of Cancer

VIII-I-1. Immunology of cancer: Woglom and Jones.

The early experiments of Loeb (1905), of Bashford, Murray and Cramer (1908) and many others showed that only a small proportion of rats and mice would allow the growth of inoculated tumors, demonstrating a natural immunity to such transplantation. Also, in animals showing temporary growth and subsequent regression, an acquired immunity developed. This immunity, however, was limited to the specific tumor and conferred no protection against other transplantable or spontaneous tumors.

The early observations, on non-inbred, genetically heterozygous animals, led to extensive investigations but equivocal results. William H. Woglom (1879-1953) of New York in 1929 reviewed some 600 papers dealing with resistance to transplantable tumors published since 1913. He concluded that "nothing may . . . be hoped for at present in respect to a successful therapy from this direction."

Woglom's authoritative, pessimistic analysis remained valid for over 2 decades, when cellular immune responses to tumors were demonstrated in homozygous animal systems, indicating the presence of tumor antigens. Until then, immune responses to tumors were considered to be as those to foreign tissue rather than any component specific for neoplasms.

Acquired resistance to individual tumors could be induced by a variety of procedures. One of the more novel and simpler ones was to inoculate the tumor into the tail of the mouse, and to snip off the tail after tumor growth was established, as described by H. B. Andervont. Acquired resistance could be inhibited by exposing the animal to ionizing radiation, or by blocking the reticulo-endothelial system with dyes. Tumor growth could be stimulated by the introduction of cotton fibers with the tumor inoculum, as found by E. Elizabeth Jones (1898-   ) of Wellesley, Massachusetts.

W. H. Woglom. Immunity to transplantable tumors. **Cancer Rev.** 4: 129-214, 1929.

E. Bashford, J. A. Murray and W. Cramer. The natural and induced resistance of mice to the growth of cancer. **3rd Sci. Rpt.**, Imperial Cancer Res. Fund. London: Taylor & Francis, 1908.

H. B. Andervont. The specificity of immunity elicited by mouse sarcoma 180. **Publ. Health Repts.** (USA) 48: 1472-6, 1933.

E. E. Jones. The breakdown of hereditary immunity to a transplantable tumor by the introduction of an irritating agent. **J. Cancer Res.** 10: 435-49, 1926.

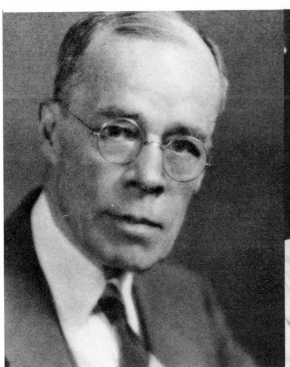

William H. Woglom

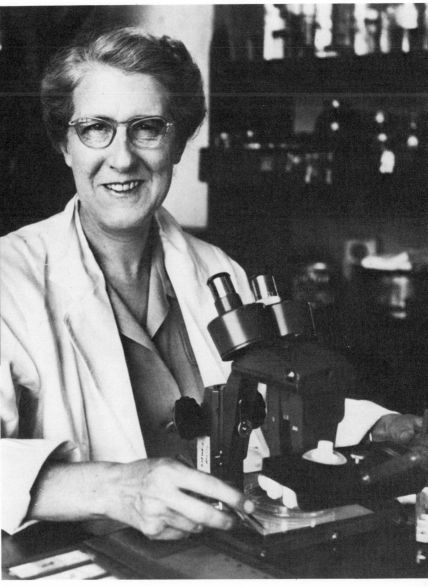

E. Elizabeth Jones

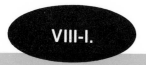

VIII-I.

Biochemistry of Cancer

VIII-I-2. Metabolism of cancer: Warburg.

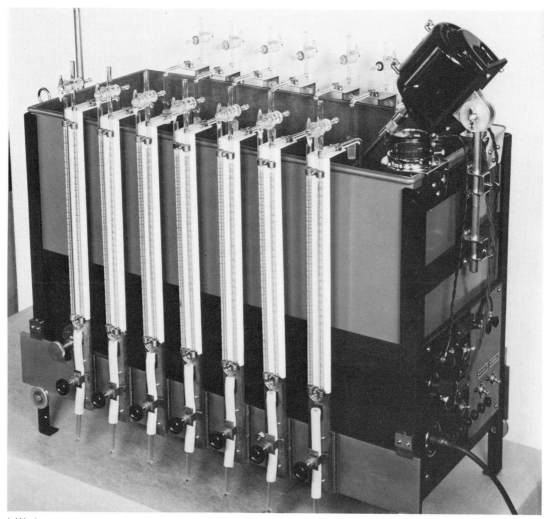

A Warburg apparatus for manometric studies of tissue
metabolism.

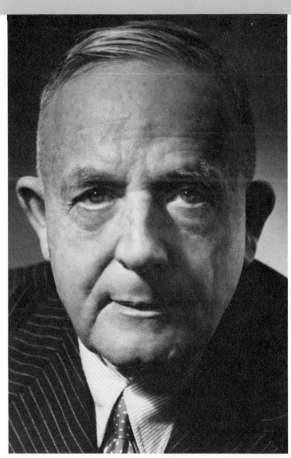

O. Warburg

K. Stern and R. Willheim in 1943 reviewed the subject of biochemistry of malignant tumors. The data on inorganic, organic, enzymatic or other characteristics led to no useful applications in the diagnosis or treatment of cancer. Indeed, much of such data was technically inadequate.

Otto Heinrich Warburg (1883-1970) was the most illustrious and colorful practitioner in the biochemistry of cancer up to the era of molecular biology. In his pursuits, cancer was but one of his contributions to biochemistry and cell physiology, for which he was the recipient of a Nobel Prize in 1931.

Warburg came from a family famous in science and commerce. He studied chemistry under the great Emil Fischer, and obtained his doctorate in 1911. From 1931 he was Director of the Kaiser Wilhelm Institute for Cell Physiology in Berlin.

The manometric apparatus for respiratory studies that bears his name has been used so widely as to have become virtually a symbol of biochemistry. Among his epoch-making discoveries are the respiratory pigments and their associated enzymes and the nicotinamide adenine dinucleotides. He described the anaerobic glycolysis of cancer tissue, and extrapolated the observations to a causation of cancer as a response to cell anoxia. His views were strongly presented and became controversial, but they were always important. His approach to research was authoritarian, allowing no deviation from his direction.

Chemical studies of tumors reflected the available technology of the time. Comparisons of tumors with normal tissues can be traced to Astruc in the 18th Century. According to Triolo, Delafond in 1855 summarized the morphology and chemical reactions of normal, embryonic and tumor cells, and failed to identify any characteristics typifying cancers.

V. A. Triolo. Nineteenth century foundations of cancer research. Advances in tumor pathology, nomenclature, and theories of oncogenesis. **Cancer Reș.** 25: 75-106, 1965.

K. Stern and R. Willheim. **The Biochemistry of Malignant Tumors.** Brooklyn, N.Y.: Reference Press, 1943.

O. Warburg. **Ueber den stoffwechsel der Tumoren.** Berlin: Springer, 1926.

O. Warburg. **The Metabolism of Tumors** (translated by F. Dickens). London: Arnold Constable, 1930.

VIII-I.

Biochemistry of Cancer

VIII-I-3. Chemotherapy of cancer: Ehrlich.

Paul Ehrlich (1854-1915) was the founder of modern chemotherapy, and his endeavors included experimental searches for agents useful against cancer.

The literature between 1906 and 1940 abounds with reports of inhibition of transplantable tumors in rodents. Salts of heavy metals, dyes, organic compounds and biological products were well represented. Helen Dyer's compilation of data lists 5031 substances that were tested for antineoplastic activity.

Among biological products, the tumor-damaging polysaccharide from **Serratia marcescens** was identified by M. J. Shear et al. as the possible active component of Coley's toxins. G. Roskin of the Soviet Union described an antitumor fraction from **Schistotrypanum cruzi**, which remained unconfirmed. More "rational" approaches were based on testing mitotic inhibitors such as colchicine, and chemicals affecting glycolysis, following the observations that cancer tissue slices produced lactic acid from glucose in the presence of oxygen, whereas most normal tissues did so only under anaerobic conditions.

Most of these investigations were unsuccessful in animals and were not pursued actively in the clinic. One of the few

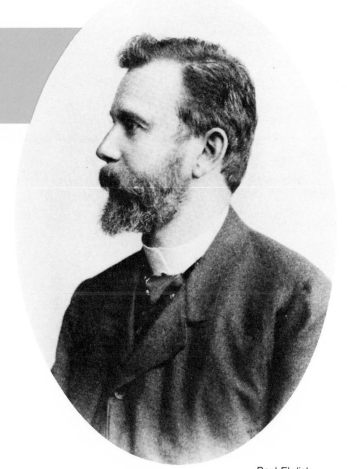

Paul Ehrlich

exceptions was the revival of lead therapy for cancer, advocated between 1924 to 1930 by W. Blair Bell of Liverpool, who claimed that 51 of the 566 patients with cancer so treated were "believed cured." The claims were not substantiated. Arsenic in the form of potassium arsenite (Fowler's solution) was revived by Forkner for leukemia, especially of the myelocytic type.

P. Ehrlich. Experimental Researches on Specific Therapeutics. **The Harben Lectures for 1907.** London: H. K. Lewis, 1908.

W. B. Bell. The present position of lead therapy in malignant disease. **Brit. Med. J.** 1: 431-37, 1929.

H. M. Dyer. **An Index of Tumor Chemotherapy.** Washington: U.S. Public Health Service, 1949.

Claude E. Forkner. **Leukemia and Allied Disorders.** New York: Macmillan, 1938.

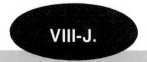

Surgical Treatment

VIII-J-1. Abdominal surgery: Miles and others.

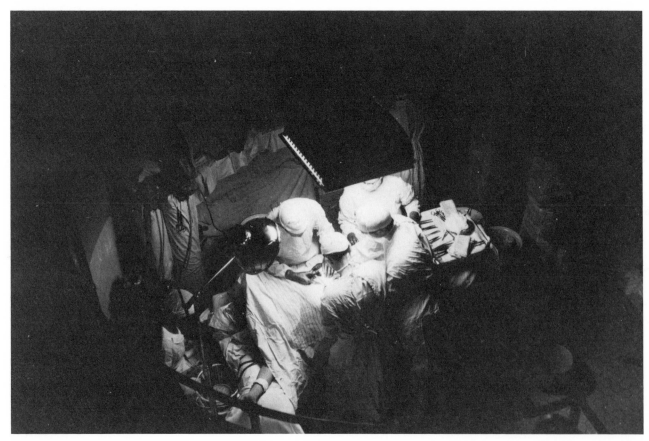

Surgery, San Francisco, 1935.

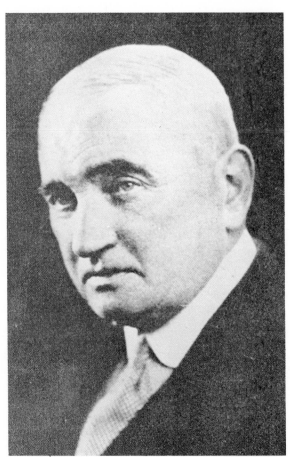

Ernest Miles

In cancer surgery, the giant figures of Theodor Billroth and his students and associates were preeminent at the turn of the century. Richard von Volkmann (1830-89), of Leipzig, who excised the rectum for cancer in 1878, and who described cancer among paraffin-workers, has a high place in the annals of oncology. Theodor Kocher (1841-1917) of Bern, Switzerland, known primarily for thyroid surgery for which he was recognized by a Nobel Prize in 1909, was an acknowledged master surgeon.

In abdominal surgery for cancer, among the better results were achieved eventually for cancer of the colon and rectum. The evolution of the procedures for the removal of the rectum has been told by Krolicki. An important figure during the early years of this century was William Ernest Miles (1869-1947), of London. He devised an abdomino-perineal resection in which the pelvic mesocolon as well as the rectum, anus, and a wide zone of adjacent tissue was removed. The operation was the result of careful studies of the lymphatic drainage of rectal carcinoma, and reduced the recurrence rate seen with more limited posterior resections.

The Miles operation became the preferred approach to cancer of the lower intestinal tract. Major later modifications were operations, described by W. Babcock and H. Bacon of Philadelphia, for cancers above the reflection of the peritoneum, in which colostomy could be avoided and the sphincter preserved.

R. H. Meade. **An Introduction to the History of General Surgery.** Philadelphia: W. B. Saunders, 1968.

T. A. Krolicki. History of cancer of the rectum and its surgical treatment. **J. Internat. Coll. Surg.** 25: 625-32, 1956.

W. E. Miles. A method of performing abdomino-perineal excision for carcinoma of the rectum and of the terminal portion of the pelvic colon. **Lancet** 2: 1812-3, 1908.

This is not the place for a history of surgery, in which cancer occupies an important but limited area. Surgery was the only curative method for cancer until ionizing radiation was developed during the first three decades of the 20th Century, and remains the most important single method by which a proportion of patients with cancer is salvaged.

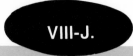

VIII-J.

Surgical Treatment

VIII-J-2. Gynecological surgery: Wertheim and Meigs.

The uterus, probably the most frequent site of cancer in women before the 20th Century, was unapproachable surgically until the advent of aseptic surgery. In 1878, W. J. Freund described a simple abdominal hysterectomy, and in 1895 E. Reis developed a more extensive resection to include regional lymph nodes.

Ernst Wertheim (1864-1920), of Vienna, in 1898 carried out his first radical hysterectomy, after careful histologic studies of the spread of cervical cancer reconstructed from surgical and autopsy specimens. In 1911 he published his experience in 500 patients. The operation, which became known by his name, included the removal of the uterus, tubes, ovaries, parametria, much of the vagina and paravaginal tissues as well as the pelvic nodes as high as the aorta. Wertheim was chief of the Second Gynecological University Hospital in Vienna and made many contributions to gynecology.

Although the mortality following operation was steadily reduced from its original 20 percent, the introduction of radium for uterine cancer offered an alternative to surgery and radium dominated the treatment for several decades.

During the 1930s, the role of surgery began to be re-evaluated, particularly for radiation failures and recurrences. Joe Vincent Meigs (1892-1963) of Boston was one of the important revivers of the surgical approach, which, with various modifications has remained paired with radiation therapy to improve the salvage rates.

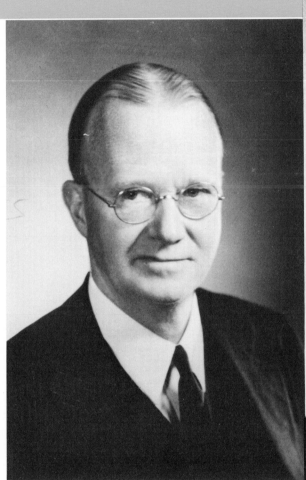

J.V. Meigs

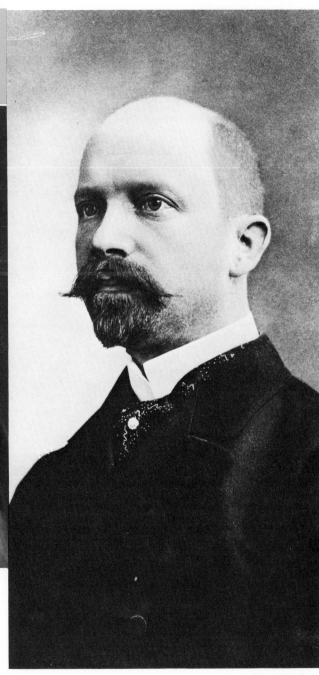

Ernst Wertheim

R. H. Meade. **An Introduction to the History of General Surgery.** Philadelphia: W. B. Saunders, 1968.

E. Wertheim. **Die erweitererte abdominale Operation bei Carcinoma Colli Uteri (auf Grund von 500 Fällen**). Berlin: Urban & Schwarzenberg, 1911.

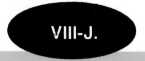

VIII-J.

Surgical Treatment

VIII-J-3. Thoracic surgery: Graham.

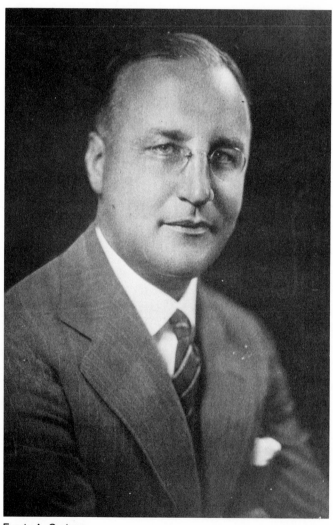

Evarts A. Graham

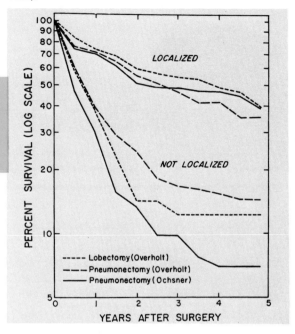

Survival of patients with lung cancer following pneumonectomy and lobectomy at the clinics of Alton Ochsner and Richard H. Overholt (from J. Thoracic and Cardiovasc. Surg., 44:503-19, 1962).

The contents of the chest were also invaded by surgeons with increasingly better results in terms of risk to the patient.

According to Meade, the first real lobectomy for cancer of the lung was performed by H. Morriston Davies (1879-1965) of London, in 1912. The patient, however, died of empyema. Lobectomies were attempted for bronchiectasis by F. Sauerbruch in Germany, Edward Churchill, and others in the United States, but the operative mortality was about 50 percent until Harold Brunn in 1929 introduced his one-stage procedure.

In April 1933, the first successful pneumonectomy for cancer of the lung was performed by Evarts Ambrose Graham (1883-1957) of St. Louis. A mass ligation of the hilum was carried out and the stump transfixed, followed by a thoracoplasty. The patient, a doctor, outlived the surgeon.

Graham, a native of Chicago and a graduate of Rush Medical College there, was appointed in 1919 professor of surgery at the Washington University School of Medicine. He and Warren Cole developed cholecystography for gall bladder disease in 1922. In 1951 he encouraged and participated in one of the early epidemiologic studies on the relation of cigarette smoking and lung cancer. He eventually stopped smoking, but not soon enough, and died of lung cancer.

Operative removal of the lung for cancer improved technically, but the salvage rates continued to be distressingly low. It was shown that lobectomy was as successful as more extensive resections through a comparison of results achieved by Alton Ochsner of New Orleans and Richard H. Overholt of Boston.

R. H. Meade. **A History of Thoracic Surgery.** Springfield, Ill.: C. C. Thomas, 1961.

E. A. Graham and J. J. Singer. Successful removal of entire lung for carcinoma of the bronchus. **J. Am. Med. Assn.** 101: 1371-4, 1933.

M. B. Shimkin *et al.* Pneumonectomy and lobectomy in bronchogenic carcinoma. **J. Thorac. Cardiovasc. Surg.** 44: 503-19, 1962.

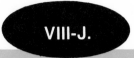

VIII-J.

Surgical Treatment

VIII-J-4. Urological surgery: Young.

Hugh Hampton Young (1870-1945), originally of Virginia and with a life-long association with Johns Hopkins Hospital, was the epitome of urology during the early decades of the 20th Century, at least in the United States. His students, starting with Frank Hinman, in turn headed many University departments of urology. His own institute at Johns Hopkins, the James Buchanan Brady Urological Institute, was endowed by the notorious "Diamond Jim" Brady in gratitude for successful treatment of his chronic prostatitis.

Young was interested in all aspects of urology, founded the **Journal of Urology** in 1917, and developed perineal prostatic surgery. Partial prostatectomy for carcinoma was performed by Billroth in 1867, and more complete operations were attempted by a number of European surgeons. In 1904, Young carried out a radical perineal prostatectomy for carcinoma, and by 1937 could report a 50 percent 5-year survival rate in cases of carcinoma treated by this method. Unfortunately, less than 10 percent of patients were suitable for a radical operation by the time a diagnosis was made.

A history of urology has been compiled by Murphy, and contains good descriptions of its oncologic aspects.

H. H. Young. The early diagnosis and radical cure of carcinoma of the prostate. **Bull. Johns Hopkins Hosp.** 16: 315-20, 1905.

H. H. Young. The radical cure of cancer of the prostate. **Surg., Gynec. and Obst.** 64: 472-84, 1937.

L. J. T. Murphy. **The History of Urology.** Springfield, Ill.: C. C. Thomas, 1972.

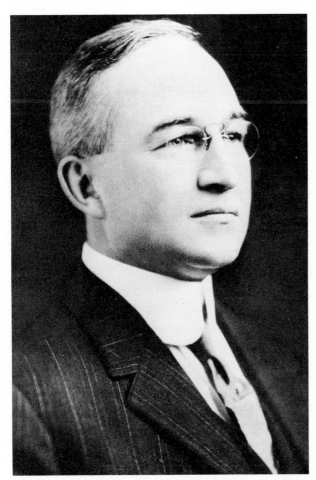

H.H. Young

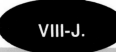

VIII-J.

Surgical Treatment

VIII-J-5. Neurological surgery: Godlee and Cushing.

In 1884, Alexander Hughes Bennett (1848-1901) diagnosed a brain tumor in a 25-year-old farmer with paralysis of the left hand and arm. He persuaded Rickman John Godlee (1859-1925) to perform a craniotomy and to remove a cerebral glioma. Unfortunately, the patient died of meningitis within a month after the operation. Despite criticisms, the field of neurological surgery had been opened.

Bennett was the son of John Hughes Bennett, professor at Edinburgh, who shared with Virchow the recognition of leukemia. He was physician to the Hospital for Epilepsy and Paralysis in London. Godlee was Lister's nephew, surgeon to the University College Hospital, and eventually a knighted surgeon to three royal British households.

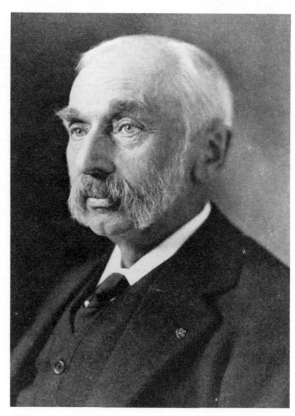

Rickman John Godlee

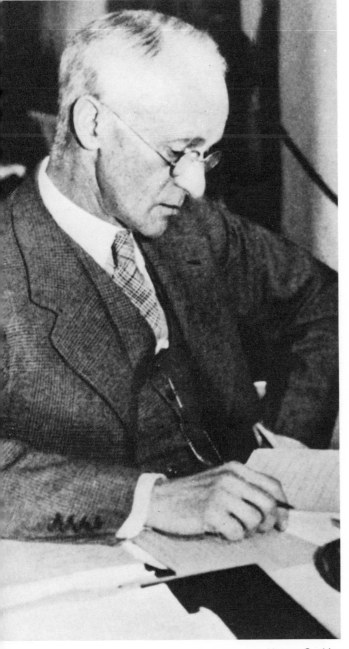

Harvey Cushing

William Macewen (1848-1924) and Victor Horsley (1857-1916) developed neurological surgery in England. The preeminent name in the field, however, is Harvey Cushing (1869-1939) of Cleveland, Ohio, professor of surgery at Johns Hopkins and at Harvard Universities. A meticulous operator, his experience included the removal of more than 2000 brain tumors. His studies on the pituitary gland culminated in an important monograph on the subject, and his name is eponymically associated with an adrenocortical syndrome. A graceful writer, his **Life of Sir William Osler** is an outstanding medical biography. He, in turn, was the subject of a biography by John Fulton.

A. Hughes Bennett. A case of cerebral tumor—the surgical treatment, by Rickman J. Godlee. **Roy. med. chir. Soc. Lond., Trans.** 68: 243-75, 1885.

H. Cushing. **The Pituitary Body and Its Disorders.** Philadelphia: Lippincott, 1912.

H. Cushing. **Intracranial Tumors: Notes upon a series of two thousand verified cases with surgical-mortality percentages pertaining thereto.** Springfield, Ill.: C. C. Thomas, 1932.

John F. Fulton. **Harvey Cushing. A Biography.** Springfield, Ill.: C. C. Thomas, 1946.

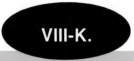

Radiotherapy

VIII-K-1. Radiobiology: Perthes and Bergonié.

X-rays were first medically directed to diagnostic applications. The pioneer workers soon discovered that exposure to X-rays and to radium produced damage to the skin, which led to trials in a variety of clinical conditions, including cancer. E. H. Grubbe of Chicago supposedly treated a patient with advanced breast cancer in 1896. Tage Anton Ultimus Sjorgen (1859-1939) of Sweden presumably cured an epithelioma of the cheek in 1899. Radium was introduced into the uterus for uterine cancer by Margaret Cleaves in 1903, and interstitially by Robert Abbe in 1905.

During this early period, without standardization of dose or knowledge of the biological effects, radiation therapy was used empirically as a destructive agent, with frequent disastrous consequences.

The first steps in radiobiology were taken when George Perthes (1869-1927) of Leipzig in 1903 noted a correlation of radiosensitivity of cells and their rate of reproduction. These basic facts were elaborated in further studies by Jean Alban Bergonié (1857-1925) and L. Tribondeau (1872-1914) of Paris, who summarized them in a descriptive law: "The effect of radiations on living cells is the more intense: (1) the greater their reproductive activity, (2) the longer their mitotic phase lasts, and (3) the less their morphology and function are differentiated." In a general way, this statement underlies the whole theory of radiation treatment of neoplasms.

Glasser has summarized the development and acceptance of dose and time measurements in radiotherapy, so essential for its intelligent use.

G. P. Perthes. Ueber den Einfluss der Röntgenstrahlen auf epitheliale Gewebe, inbesondere auf das Carcinom. **Arch. Klin. Chir.** 71: 955-1000, 1903.

J. Bergonié et L. Tribondeau. Interprétation des quelques résultats de la radiothérapie et essai de fixation d'une technique rationnelle. **Compt. Rend. Acad. Sci.** (Paris) 143: 983-5, 1906.

F. Buschke and R. G. Parker. **Radiation Therapy in Cancer Management.** New York: Grune & Stratton, 1972.

O. Glasser. The evolution of dosimeters in Roentgen ray therapy. **Radiology** 37: 221-27, 1941.

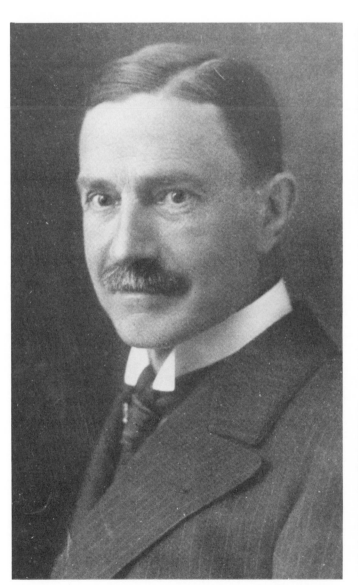

Georg Perthes

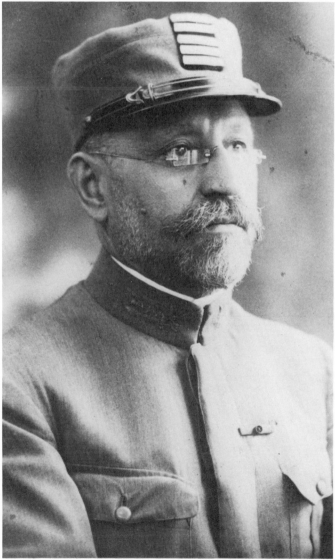

Jean Alban Bergonié

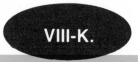

VIII-K.

Radiotherapy

VIII-K-2. Radium Centers: Roux and Marie Curie.

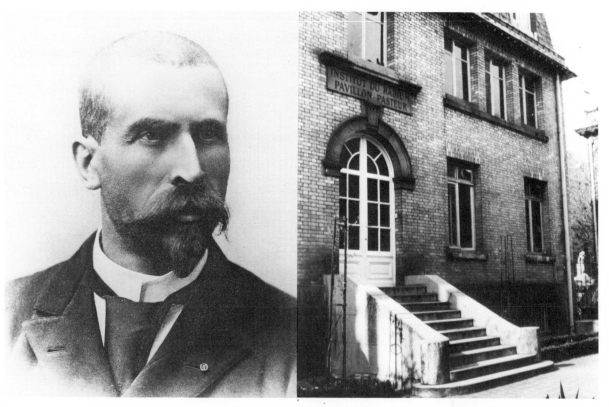

Emile Roux

Radium Institute of the Pasteur Institute, Paris, 1921.

Pierre Paul Émile Roux (1853-1933), one of the great bacteriologists of the Pasteur era, was director of the Pasteur Institute in Paris for 20 years, 1904-1925. He foresaw the need for studies on the physics, biology, and clinical applications of radium, and made a place for such studies at the Pasteur Institute. Soon after the tragic death of Pierre Curie in 1906, Roux appointed his widow to head the newly-organized Radium Institute. The development was interrupted by the war, but resumed in 1919, and the Radium Institute was formally dedicated in 1921. It was here, in a specialized cancer treatment and research center, that radiobiology and radiotherapy developed into scientific disciplines.

Marie Curie (1867-1934) traveled widely to distribute radium and radon to radium centers that were being set up all over the world. Particularly noteworthy were the Radiumhemmet, organized by the surgeon John Berg in 1910 in Stockholm, and the Holt Institute in Manchester. Her brilliant career won her a second Nobel Prize in chemistry in 1911. In 1926 her daughter, Irène, with her husband Frédérick Joliot, discovered artificial radioactivity and in 1935 were awarded the Nobel Prize for chemistry. Marie Curie's life is best told by her daughter, Eve, in a book first published in 1937.

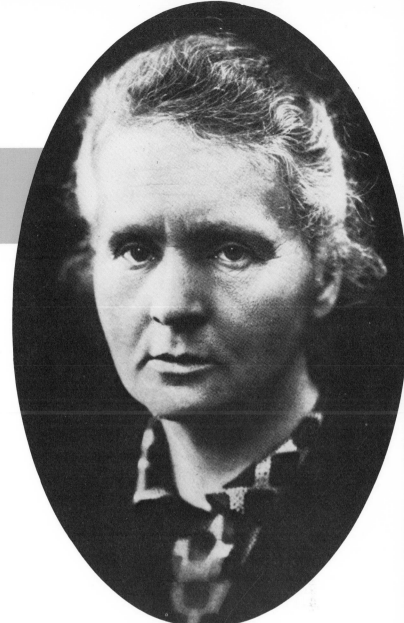

Marie Curie

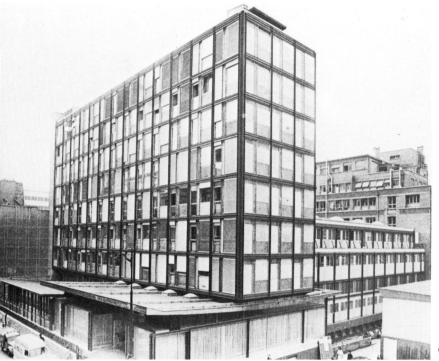

Maurice Lenz. The early workers in clinical radiotherapy of cancer at the Radium Institute of the Curie Foundation, Paris, France. **Cancer** 32: 519-23, 1973.

Stephen B. Dewing. **Modern Radiology in Historical Perspective.** Springfield, Ill.: C. C. Thomas, 1962.

Eve Curie. **Madame Curie.** New York: Doubleday, 1949.

Curie Foundation, Paris, 1970.

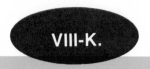

VIII-K.

Radiotherapy

VIII-K-3. Fractional radiotherapy: Regaud and Coutard.

Clinical radiation therapy was born in 1922, when Regaud, Coutard and Houtant presented evidence to the International Congress of Otology in Paris that advanced laryngeal cancer could be cured without disastrous, treatment-produced sequelae.

Claudius Regaud (1870-1940), professor of histology at the University of Lyon, was invited in 1906 to head the biological studies on radiation at the Institute du Radium in Paris. His first research was on the effect of ionizing radiation on various tissues, which showed the radiosensitivity of testicular tubular cells. He described moist radioepidermitis of irradiated skin, and developed an early system of radium dosimetry. Following the interruption of World War I, he recruited a group of colleagues, among them Lacassagne, Coutard, Ferroux, Monod and Roux-Berger. Using ram testes as the experimental model, he proved the advantage of a dose of radiation fractionated in ten days over a greater total dose administered in a single exposure. This observation on the time-dose relationship was an important radiobiological contribution to modern radiotherapy.

Henri Coutard (1876-1950) joined the Radium Institute in Paris in 1919. With a single piece of radiological equipment and interchangeable tubes, he studied experimental radiophysiology, radiodiagnosis, and clinical radiotherapy. In 1922 he described the mucous membrane reaction which he named radioepithelitis. He originated the radiographic study of the larynx. Refusing to accept the theoretical limitations of Regaud's fractionation, Coutard extended daily irradiations of patients to periods of several weeks. This method was named the protracted-fractional treatment. Coutard's contributions are now at the basis of the practice of clinical radiotherapy.

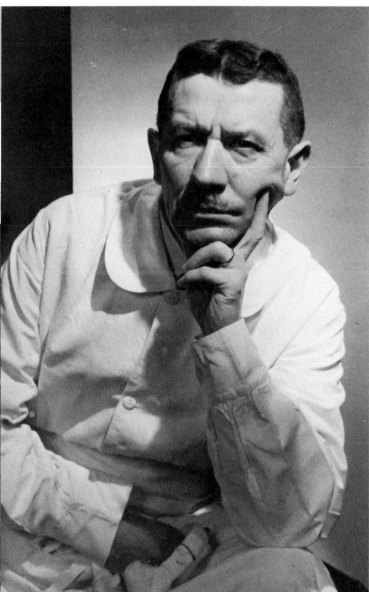

Henri Coutard

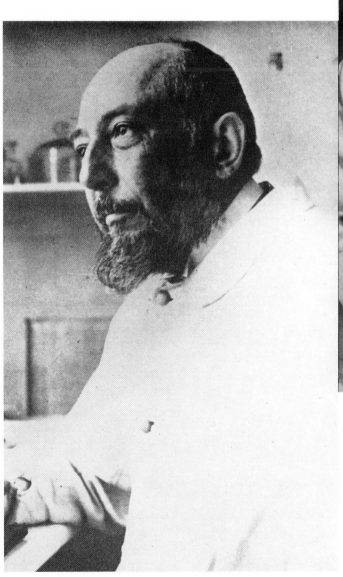

Claudius Regaud

C. Regaud, H. Coutard and A. Houtant. Contribution au traitèment des cancers endolarynges par les rayons-X. **Congr. Xe Internat. d'Otol.** 19-22 juillet, 1922.

H. Coutard. Principles of X ray therapy of malignant diseases. **Lancet** ii: 1-8, 1934.

F. Buschke and R. G. Parker. **Radiation Therapy in Cancer Management.** New York: Grune & Stratton, 1972.

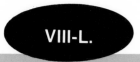

VIII-L.

Cancer Statistics

VIII-L-1. Cancer mortality: Hoffman and Schereschewsky.

The need for reliable statistics on the incidence and mortality of cancer became increasingly apparent during the first decade of the 20th Century.

Frederick L. Hoffman (1865-1946), German-born statistician for the Prudential Life Insurance Company, was an important instigator of statistical studies in cancer. He was one of the founders of the American Society for the Control of Cancer (ASCC) in 1913, being convinced that cancer mortality was increasing. In 1915 he issued a monumental compilation and analysis of cancer statistics available throughout the world.

As chairman of the statistical advisory committee of ASCC, Hoffman succeeded in having the U.S. Census Bureau prepare an analysis of cancer mortality in the registration area of the United States for 1914, using the International List of Causes of Death for its pattern, and having a widely representative advisory council to guide its work.

In 1922, Joseph W. Schereschewsky (1873-1940), of the United States Public Health Service, began to analyze national cancer mortality statistics. Numerically the disease was increasingly becoming a leading cause of death, and thus a public health problem. While better reporting and an aging population rendered dubious the conclusion that there was a true increase in risk to cancer, nevertheless Schereschewsky recommended a major national investment in cancer as a public health problem, wryly pointing out that the solution of the cancer problem would cancel out the increasing mortality from automobile accidents. He proceeded to organize the Office of Cancer Investigations in association with Harvard. This office, organized to perform basic research in cancer, was transferred and became part of the National Cancer Institute in Bethesda, Maryland, in 1939.

Mortality trends in cancer received further analyses by Mary Gover during 1939-1941, and were extended to field surveys of cancer incidence in 1937 by Harold Dorn.

Frederick L. Hoffman. **The Mortality From Cancer Throughout the World.** Newark, N.J.: Prudential Press, 1915.

J. W. Schereschewsky. **The Course of Cancer Mortality in the Ten Original Registration States for the 21-Year Period, 1900-1920.** U.S. Public Health Service, Public Health Bulletin No. 155. Washington, D.C.: U.S. Govt. Print. Off., 1925.

H. B. Andervont. J. W. Schereschewsky: an appreciation. **J. Nat. Cancer Inst.** 19: 331-3, 1957.

V. A. Triolo and M. B. Shimkin. The American Cancer Society and cancer research. Origins and organization: 1913-1943. **Cancer Res.** 29: 1615-40, 1969.

J. W. Schereschewsky

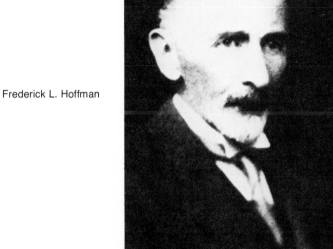

Frederick L. Hoffman

PUBLIC HEALTH REPORTS

VOL. 53   JUNE 17, 1938   NO. 24

THE PREVENTION AND CONTROL OF CANCER: A PLAN FOR NATION-WIDE ORGANIZATION*

By J. W. SCHERESCHEWSKY, Medical Director (Retired), United States Public Health Service

Without attempting to analyze the various causes which have led to a steady rise in the tide of cancer mortality, the fact remains that the annual increase in the number of deaths caused by cancer constitutes a major problem in public health and preventive medicine.

If we were without time-tried and effective means of opposing this increase, inaction might be excusable. This, however, is far from the case. A substantial reduction in the cancer mortality rate is not only possible, but the means to this end are susceptible of practical application. That the problem of organizing these means and of effectively resisting the increase in cancer mortality is difficult is freely admitted. Yet the rewards to be realized in the conquest of the fear of cancer, in the direct saving of human life, and in the mastery of the most relentless disease in the roster of human ills are so rich as fully to justify a supreme and coordinated effort to this end.

The Bone Act, establishing the National Cancer Institute, with its broad provisions for cooperation with the States, which are implicit in the act, the long-existing cooperative relations which obtain between the United States Public Health Service and the State departments of health, the commencing recognition by States, through legislative act, that the cancer problem is, in fact, a public health problem, all inspire the hope that a Nation-wide official organization to combat this disease should, commensurate with its degree of perfection, produce results, perhaps not so dramatic as has been the case in tuberculosis, but still amply repaying the efforts put forth to that end.

This campaign to be effective should be—

1. Nation-wide in its scope.
2. Constitute a preventive activity of each State department of health.
3. Enlist the cooperation of State medical societies and of State cancer commissions.
4. Bring about the achievement of certain specific ends, known to be effective against cancer, yet robbed of controlling power because of the lack of sufficient application.

* Presented at the Thirty-sixth Annual Conference of State and Territorial Health Officers with the Public Health Service, Washington, D. C., April 11, 1938.

66443°—38——1

Schereschewsky, Cancer control proposal, 1938.

THE MORTALITY
FROM CANCER THROUGHOUT
THE WORLD

BY

FREDERICK L. HOFFMAN, LL.D.,
F.S.S., F.A.S.A.

Statistician The Prudential Insurance Company of America; Chairman Committee on Statistics, American Society for the Control of Cancer; Member American Association for Cancer Research; Associate Fellow American Medical Association; Associate Member American Academy of Medicine, etc., etc.

NEWARK, NEW JERSEY
THE PRUDENTIAL PRESS
1915

Hoffman, *Mortality from Cancer Throughout the World*, 1915.
Title page.

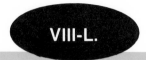

VIII-L.

Cancer Statistics

VIII-L-2. End-results in cancer: Winiwarter and Greenwood.

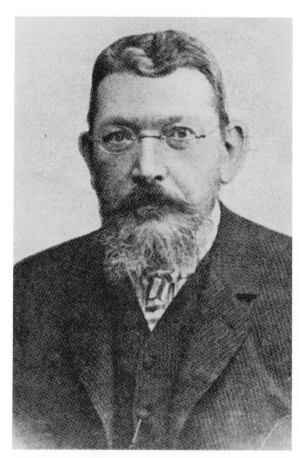

Alexandre von Winiwarter

Two essential components of oncology are the studies on the natural history of cancer, and on the effects of treatment on the course of the disease.

Alexandre von Winiwarter (1848-1916) of Belgium was a student and affiliate at Theodor Billroth's clinic in Vienna, and was given the task of examining the end results of his mentor's surgical experiences. He compiled these data into one of the first statistical reviews of operative results in cancer, especially of patients with mammary and gastric cancer.

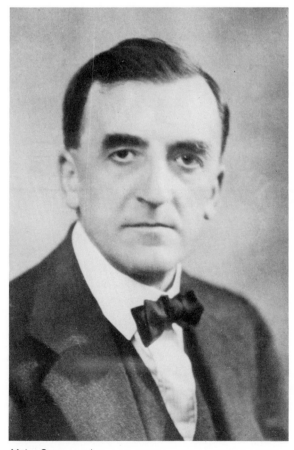

Major Greenwood

Major Greenwood (1880-1949), a noted British epidemiologist and statistician, analyzed data on survival in untreated patients with cancer, compiled by British hospitals between 1882 and 1924. His report remains useful in considerations of therapeutic results in cancer. Similar compilations were reported from Massachusetts, on data gathered from 1912 to 1935.

On the basis of clinical statistical considerations, there arose the conventions of considering the 5-year end results in cancer as indicating cure of the disease, and of considering all deaths within 30 days of operation as operative mortality.

A. von Winiwarter. **Beiträge zur Statistik der Carcinome.** Stuttgart: Enke, 1878.

M. Greenwood. **A Report on the Natural Duration of Cancer.** Ministry of Health Reports on Public Health and Medical Subjects No. 33. H. M. Stationer's Office, London, 1926.

M. B. Shimkin. Natural history of neoplastic disease. In F. Homburger (ed) Ed. 2 **The Physiopathology of Cancer.** New York: Hoeber-Harper, 1959. pp. 855-71.

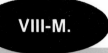

VIII-M.

Cancer Institutions

VIII-M-1. Memorial Hospital and Sloan-Kettering Institute.

A number of large specialized institutions for cancer were initiated at the turn of the 20th Century. Initially called laboratories or hospitals, they became Institutes by mid-century, and Centers by 1975, to reflect expansions in size and importance.

James Marion Sims (1813-1883), a South Carolina-born surgeon, has a secure place in medical history for the first successful operation for vesico-vaginal fistula in 1852. He was the founder of the New York Woman's Hospital (1854) and of the New York Cancer Hospital, opened in 1884. Sims' efforts to provide treatment for cancer victims received the endorsement of prominent New York City citizens, who raised funds for the construction of the first American hospital to regularly admit cancer patients.

In 1899 the New York Cancer Hospital became the General Memorial Hospital for the Treatment of Cancer and Allied Diseases. Research was initiated at the Memorial Hospital in 1902 through the Collis P. Huntington Fund for Cancer Research, established in conjunction with the Loomis Laboratory for Research in Experimental Pathology at the Cornell University Medical College. James Ewing (1866-1943) was appointed first Director of Research and Director of the Memorial Hospital in 1931. The Sloan-Kettering Research Institute was established at a new site provided for the Memorial Hospital in 1939. Ewing was succeeded by Cornelius Packard Rhoads (1898-1959) as second Director of the Memorial Hospital and its research affiliate.

One of the largest and most important cancer centers of the world, the Memorial-Sloan-Kettering Center has a long tradition of service toward the prevention and treatment of cancer. Its laboratories have pioneered in the development of cancer therapeutic agents, as well as in basic laboratory studies. Its president in 1975 was Lewis Thomas, and its research director, Robert A. Good.

Bob Considine. **That Many May Live: Memorial Center's 75 Year Fight Against Cancer.** New York: Memorial Center for Cancer and Allied Diseases, 1959.

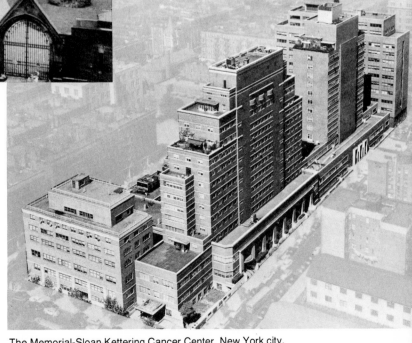

J. Marion Sims

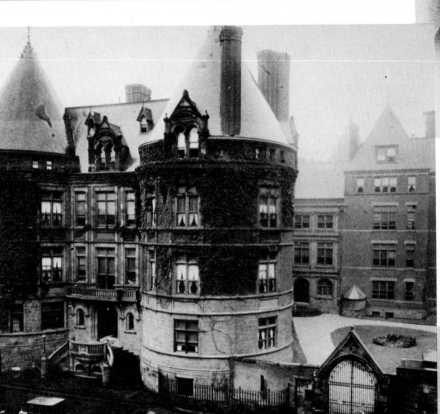

Memorial Hospital for the Treatment of Cancer and Allied Diseases, New York City, 1920. Built in 1899.

The Memorial-Sloan-Kettering Cancer Center, New York city, 1968.

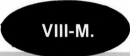

Cancer Institutions

VIII-M-2. Roswell Park Memorial Institute.

In the spring of 1898 the New York State legislature appropriated $10,000 for the purpose of "equipping and maintaining a laboratory to be devoted to the study of the causes, mortality rate and treatment of cancer." The New York State Pathological Laboratory of the University of Buffalo, opened the same year, was thus founded and became one of the earlier cancer research facilities organized under government auspices.

Roswell Park (1852-1914), Professor of Surgery at the University of Buffalo, was appointed first Director. In 1901 the laboratory was relocated in a separate building known as the Gratwick Research Laboratory in honor of a benefactor. The following year, the Gratwick Laboratory became affiliated with the New York State Department of Health, and in 1911 a fully official status was granted by a legislative act that created the New York State Institute for the Study of Malignant Diseases. In 1946 the Institute was reorganized and enlarged under the direction of George E. Moore. It was renamed the Roswell Park Memorial Institute, commemorating its founder and organizer.

The Institute now occupies an extensive site, comprising a clinical center with adjoining units for experimental research in central Buffalo. A biologic station at Springville, New York, was established in 1913. Research at the Roswell Park Memorial Institute traverses a full spectrum of laboratory and clinical problems: cancer epidemiology and statistics, the action of chemotherapeutic agents, chemical carcinogenesis, the role of viruses in tumor formation, cancer biology, and other approaches. It is one of the larger clinical and research facilities for cancer in the world. In 1975, now a cancer Center, it was directed by Gerald P. Murphy.

E. A. Mirand. **History of Roswell Park Memorial Institute.** Buffalo, N.Y.: Buffalo and Erie County Historical Society, 1961.

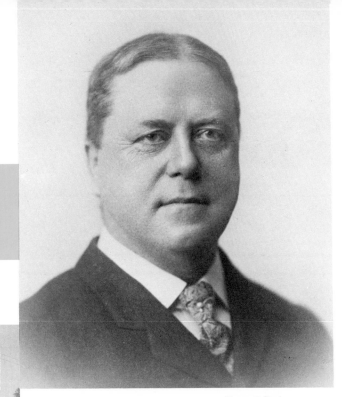

Roswell Park

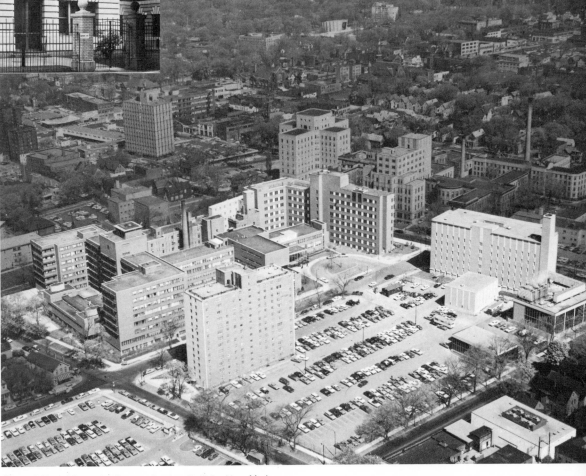

The Gratwick Building, housing the original laboratories of the
Roswell Park Memorial Institute, Buffalo, New York, 1901.

Roswell Park Memorial Cancer Center, Buffalo, New York,
1973

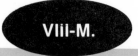

VIii-M.

Cancer Institutions

VIII-M-3. Imperial Cancer Research Fund.

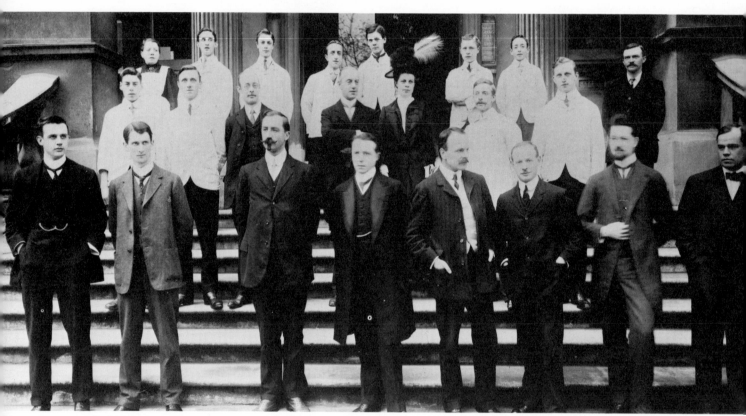

Staff of the Imperial Cancer Research Fund, London, 1909

The Imperial Cancer Research Fund was inaugurated as a conjoint enterprise of the Royal College of Physicians of London and the Royal College of Surgeons of England on July 4, 1902. The Fund ranks as the oldest continuous research institution devoted to cancer in Great Britain. A plan for the study of cancer, known as the "Draft Scheme,"

was devised by Dr. E. F. Bashford (1873-1923) the first director, 1902-1914. This Scheme outlined the aims of the program along statistical, experimental, and, to a lesser extent, clinical lines.

The pioneer laboratory investigators associated with the Fund in its initial period are shown in a 1909 group photograph. In the first row (left to right)

Imperial Cancer Research Fund laboratories, Lincoln's Inn Fields, London 1973.

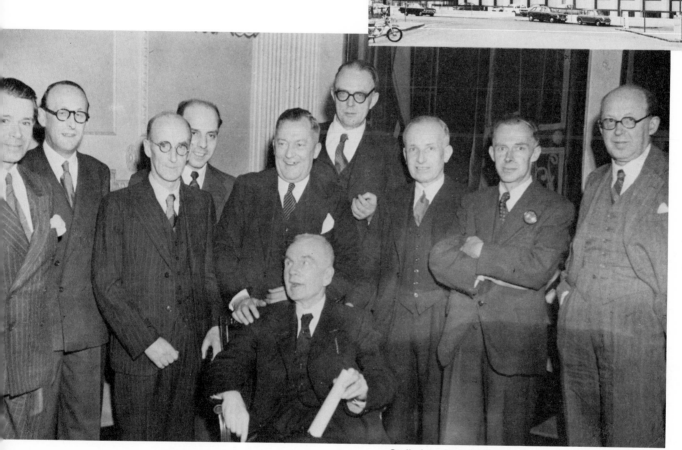

Staff of the Imperial Cancer Research Fund, ca. 1935.

are: W. H. Bowen, B. R. G. Russell, M. Haaland, E. F. Bashford, J. A. Murray, C. Da Fano, F. Medigrazianu, and W. H. Woglom.

J. A. Murray (1873-1950) succeeded Bashford in 1914 and continued as director until 1935. The group picture at the occasion shows Murray with, standing (left to right): E. S. Horning, F. R. Selbie,

A. M. Begg, E. Vasquez-Lopez, R. J. Ludford, H. G. Crabtree, A. F. Watson, Leslie Foulds and G. M. Findlay.

The Fund has occupied four quarters since 1902, and is now housed in the Institute at Lincoln's Inn Fields, London. The director in 1975 was M. G. P. Stoker.

Imperial Cancer Research Fund, 1902-1952. **Fifty Years of Cancer Research**, Supplement to Forty-Ninth Annual Report, April, 1952.

C. E. Dukes. The origin and early history of the Imperial Cancer Research Fund. **Ann. Roy. Coll. Surg. Engl.**, 36: 325-38, 1965.

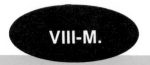

VIII-M.

Cancer Institutions

VIII-M-4. National Cancer Institute.

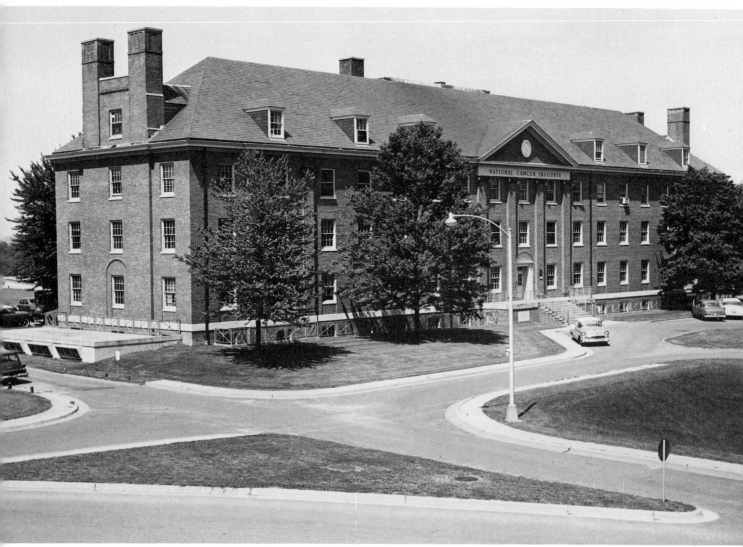

National Cancer Institute, Bethesda, Maryland, 1940.

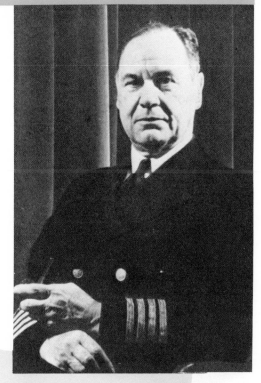

Carl Voegtlin

NATIONAL INSTITUTE OF HEALTH

JOURNAL OF THE
NATIONAL

CANCER

INSTITUTE

VOLUME I *August 1940–June 1941*

FEDERAL SECURITY AGENCY
UNITED STATES PUBLIC HEALTH SERVICE
WASHINGTON, D. C.

The National Cancer Institute (NCI) of the United States was established by an Act of Congress on August 5, 1937. In October 1939, a research facility at the National Institutes of Health was opened at Bethesda, Maryland, a suburb of Washington, D.C. The intramural program of the Institute was staffed by investigators from two pre-existing Public Health Service Research units: one was a group from the Pharmacology Laboratory of the National Institutes of Health, located in Washington, D.C., and the other a group associated with the U.S. Public Health Service's Office of Cancer Investigations in Boston, Massachusetts. From 1938 to 1943, Dr. Carl Voegtlin (1880-1960), a Swiss-born pharmacologist, served as the first Director. The NCI also administered a national grant-in-aid program, with the applications being reviewed by appropriate study sections selected from peer scientists, and then approved by the National Cancer Advisory Council. A program of research fellowships and traineeships also was organized.

The NCI initiated a periodical, the **Journal of the National Cancer Institute**, in 1940. The Institute grew steadily and expanded among the complex of other buildings of the National Institutes of Health and adjacent township's facilities.

J. R. Heller, *et al*. The National Cancer Institute. : A twenty-year retrospect. **J. Natl. Cancer Inst.** 19: 133-349, 1957.

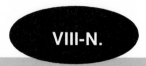

Organizations and Publications

VIII-N-1. Societies and Periodicals: Europe and Japan.

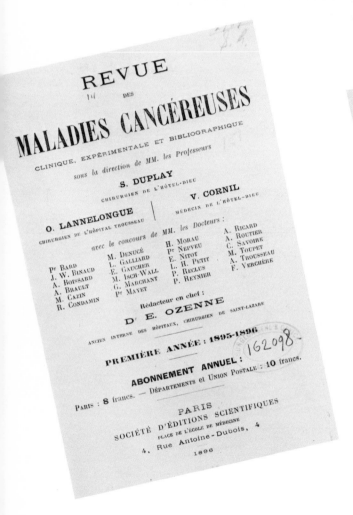

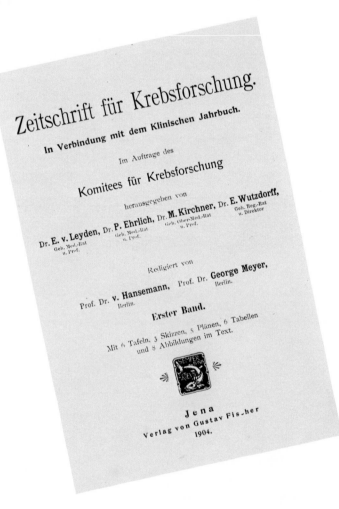

Professional societies and the periodicals they publish or sponsor have been important media for scientific communication since 1665, when the Paris Academy and the London Royal Society issued their first journals.

Communications regarding cancer during the 19th Century appeared in the many journals of medicine and its specialties. The first journal devoted to cancer was the **Revue des Maladies Cancéreuses**. It appeared in Paris in 1896, under the editorship of S. Duplay, surgeon at l'Hotel-Dieu. This periodical, however, lasted only 6 years. The French cancer society was formed in 1906, and began to publish its journal in 1911, under the title, **Bulletin de l'Association Française pour l'Etude du Cancer**, now shortened to **Bulletin du Cancer**.

A Zentral-Komitee für Krebsforschung was organized in Berlin in 1900, with the internist E. von Leyden as its chief instigator. He also was instrumental in starting, in 1904, the **Zeitschrift für Krebsforschung**. This is the oldest continuing cancer publication, although its publication was interrupted for 3 years following World War II.

Yamagiwa, on his return from Germany, in 1907 initiated the Japanese cancer journal, **Gann**. The word Gann is stone or cancer in Japanese. This periodical also has continued publication except for the interruption occasioned by World War II.

The Italian cancer journal, **Tumori**, began publication in 1911.

J. R. Porter. The scientific journal—300th anniversary. **Bact. Rev.** 28: 211-30, 1964.

Pauline M. Vaillancourt. **Bibliographic Control of the Literature of Oncology, 1800-1960.** Metuchen, N.J.: Scarecrow Press, 1969.

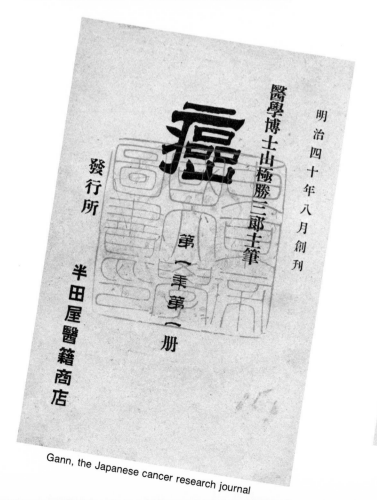

Gann, the Japanese cancer research journal

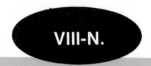

Organizations and Publications

VIII-N-2. Societies and Periodicals: America.

THE JOURNAL
OF
CANCER RESEARCH

Vol. XIV   AUGUST, 1930   No. 3

FRANCIS CARTER WOOD

Editor

PUBLISHED QUARTERLY
BY
THE INSTITUTE OF CANCER RESEARCH
OF
Columbia University

Subscription: Domestic, $5.00; Canada, $5.25;
All Other Countries, $5.50

THE AMERICAN
JOURNAL OF CANCER

Vol. XXXIX   MAY, 1940   No. 1

FRANCIS CARTER WOOD, *Editor*
COLUMBIA UNIVERSITY
NEW YORK

The Official Organ of
THE AMERICAN ASSOCIATION FOR CANCER RESEARCH
PUBLISHED AT PRINCE AND LEMON STREETS, LANCASTER, PA.

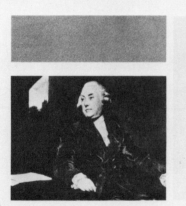

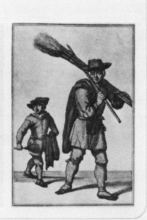

Cancer Research

The Official Organ of the American Association for Cancer Research, Inc.

VOLUME 26 / January 1966 / NUMBER 1

V. A. Triolo and I. L. Riegel. The American Association for Cancer Research, 1907-1940. **Cancer Res.** 21: 137-67, 1961.

Proceedings
of the
American Association for Cancer Research

VOLUME 1   APRIL 1953   No. 1

ABSTRACTS OF PAPERS PRESENTED
at the
44th ANNUAL MEETING

April 9-11, 1953
Chicago, Illinois

Published by THE UNIVERSITY OF CHICAGO PRESS

The American Association for Cancer Research was organized in 1907, with James Ewing as its first president. The Association has continued to grow in numbers and in importance. Its history, up to 1940, has been recorded by Triolo and Riegel.

The Association has had an official periodical since 1916, with the first issue of the **Journal of Cancer Research**. In 1931, it was replaced by the **American Journal of Cancer**, which started as Volume 15 and terminated in 1940 with Volume 40. **Cancer Research** appeared as a continuation in 1941. The annual **Proceedings** of the Association, recording abstracts of papers of its yearly conference, and of minutes of its meetings, was introduced in 1953.

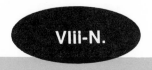

VIII-N.

Organizations and Publications

VIII-N-3. Public education: Winter and Childe.

Georg Winter (1856-1946), gynecologist of Königsberg, East Prussia, was a pioneer worker in cancer education. As early as 1891 Winter urged that women be informed of early symptoms in order to obtain prompt treatment for cancer of the uterus. Winter, at the beginning of 1903, undertook an unprecedented crusade to publicize the danger signals of cancer through a newspaper campaign launched within East and West Prussia.

Charles Plumley Childe (1858-1926), South African-born surgeon of Portsmouth, England, is one of the earliest writers of a treatise on cancer education. Childe opposed contemporary social taboos by encouraging early detection of cancer and prompt recourse to surgery. He devoted himself to erasing the popular notion that a diagnosis of cancer was equivalent to a death warrant. Childe also advocated the establishment of cancer control societies on a world-wide basis.

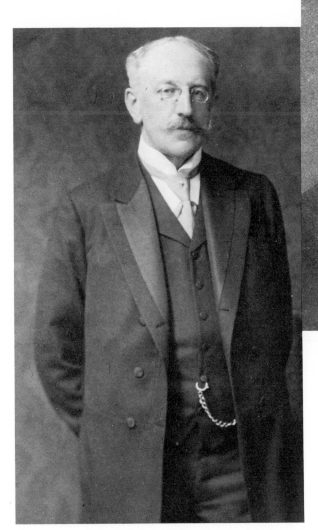

Charles Plumley Childe.

Georg Winter

G. Winter. **Die Bekämpfung des Uteruskrebses. Ein Wort an alle Krebsoperateure**. Stuttgart: Enke, 1904.

C. P. Childe. **The Control of a Scourge, or How Cancer Is Curable.** London: Methuen, 1907.

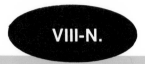

VIII-N.

Organizations and Publications

VIII-N-4. American Society for Control of Cancer.

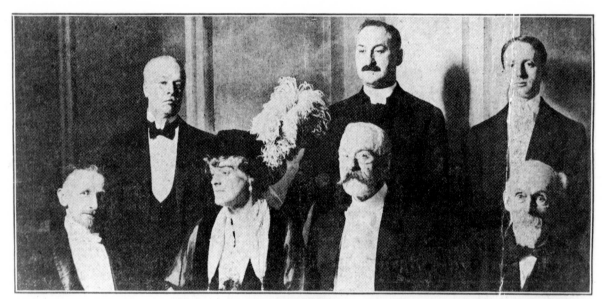

Standing, left to right—Edward A. Woods, Pittsburgh; Rabbi J. Leonard Levy, Curtis E. Lakeman, New York. Sitting, left to right—Dr. Frederick L. Hoffman, Newark; Mrs. Robert G. Mead, New York; Dr. Edward Reynolds, Boston; Dr. John A. Brashear.

Founding group of the American Society for the Control of
Cancer, 1913.

A grouping of volunteer professional and non-professional citizens for the purpose of alleviating the problems of cancer was organized in 1913, under the name of the American Society for the Control of Cancer.

Committees of the American Medical Association and the American College of Surgeons had urged that the public be educated about cancer to reduce the paralyzing effects of fear. Among the precipitating events in 1913 was a paper by Frederick L. Hoffman before the American Gynecological Society, indicating that cancer mortality was increasing and suggesting the establishment of a national society. The first article on cancer for the public, by Samuel Hopkins Adams, appeared in the May 1913 issue of the **Ladies' Home Journal**. He concluded, "Be careful of persistent sores or irritations, external or internal. Be watchful of yourself, without undue worry. At the first suspicious symptoms go to some good physician and demand the truth. . . . The risk is not in surgery but in delayed surgery."

The Society grew steadily, and chapters were established in other states, "Fight cancer with knowledge" became its slogan, and the radiant sword, with Caduceus intertwined, became its symbol in 1927. A cancer detection unit, the Strang Clinic, was founded in 1933 in New York by Elise l'Esperance (1879-1959). The Woman's Field Army was organized in 1935, to educate women to refer earlier upon the appearance of symptoms that might connote cancer.

While public education remained the main theme of the Society, the participation of many clinicians and research workers led to increasing involvement in research. The Society became a potent lobby for federal involvement in cancer, leading to the National Cancer Act of 1937.

In 1944, the American Society for the Control of Cancer was reorganized on a national basis as the American Cancer Society.

F. L. Hoffman. The menace of cancer. **Am. Gynec. Soc. Trans.** 38: 397-452, 1913.

S. H. Adams. What can we do about cancer? **The Ladies' Home Journal**, May 1913.

New York City Cancer Committee. **History of the American Society for the Control of Cancer**, 1913-1943. New York: N.Y. City Cancer Committee, 1944.

V. A. Triolo and M. B. Shimkin. The American Cancer Society and cancer research. Origins and organization: 1913-1943. **Cancer Res.** 29: 1615-40, 1969.

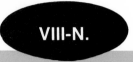

Organizations and Publications

VIII-N-5. International Union Against Cancer.

The necessity for international cooperation in the fight against cancer was recognized at the turn of the century when a group of experts decided to meet to exchange their ideas and information. Ultimately, this meeting formed the basis of the present International Union Against Cancer.

Three international congresses were held before the First World War: Heidelberg in 1906, Paris in 1910, and Brussels in 1913. Immediately after the war, with a revival of interest in the field of cancer, a great conference was held at Strasbourg in 1923 on the occasion of the centenary of Pasteur's birth.

The 1923 conference was followed by meetings which eventually led to the establishment of a permanent organization to promote the campaign against cancer. One was held in Lake Mohonk, New York, in 1926, and was sponsored by the American Society for the Control of Cancer. The other was held in London in 1928 under the sponsorship of the British Empire Cancer Campaign.

The first successful attempt to create an international organization was made during the First International Congress held in Madrid in 1933. At the conclusion of the Congress, a proposal was put forward calling for the establishment of the International Union Against Cancer. An organizing committee met in Paris in March 1934 to lay the foundations of the proposed organization. The Union was officially founded in Paris in May 1935. The Madrid Congress was followed by nine other International Congresses, which were held in Brussels (1936), Atlantic City (1939), St. Louis (1947), Paris (1950), São Paulo (1954), London (1958), Moscow (1962), Tokyo (1966), Houston (1970), and Florence (1974).

Among the many illustrious pioneer participants in the activities of the Union were Justin Godart (1871-1956) of France, a lawyer who became involved in medical affairs during World War I and in 1935 helped to found the organization. Another one was Henri-Fernand-Joseph Maisin (1893-1971) of Belgium, a physician with interests in pathology, radiobiology and oncology who in 1925 became director of the Cancer Institute in Louvain. He was, at various times, the Union's Secretary-General, President, and editor of **Acta**.

The Union published its **Acta** between 1936 and 1964, when it was replaced by the **International Journal of Cancer**, edited by E. Saxén of Finland.

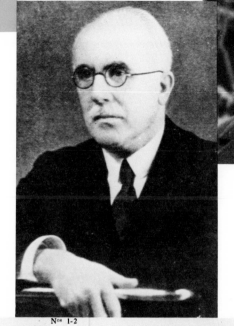

Justin Godart

Henri-Fernand-Joseph Maisin

VOL. I   N°s 1-2

UNIO INTERNATIONALIS CONTRA CANCRUM

ACTA

INTERNATIONAL
Journal of Cancer

JOURNAL INTERNATIONAL DU CANCER

SOMMAIRE

NOTE : L'Ordre des différentes langues est suivi d'après l'ordre alphabétique français.

Nous publierons dans les prochains numéros :
     1. Les articles sur la « Lutte Sociale contre le Cancer dans les divers pays », des Professeurs de Balogh,
         Gallenga, de Daranyi, du Docteur André Kubanyi, des Professeurs Mataro Nagayo, Alsknis, du
         Docteur Elliot, du Professeur Grégoire Singian, des Docteurs Marzynski, Athias et du Professeur Petroff.
     2. Les compte rendus des séances annuelles des Organismes anticancéreux.
     3. Les articles scientifiques du Professeur Blumenthal, du Docteur W. Cramer, du Professeur Fischer-Wasels,
         du Professeur E. Freund et du Docteur W. Woglom.

Editor-in-Chief: E. A. Saxén
Rédacteur en chef

Assistant Editor: J. J. Saukkonen
Rédacteur adjoint

Editorial Office: International Journal of Cancer,
Rédaction   Liisankatu 21 B, Helsinki, Finland

IX . 20th Century: Post World War II

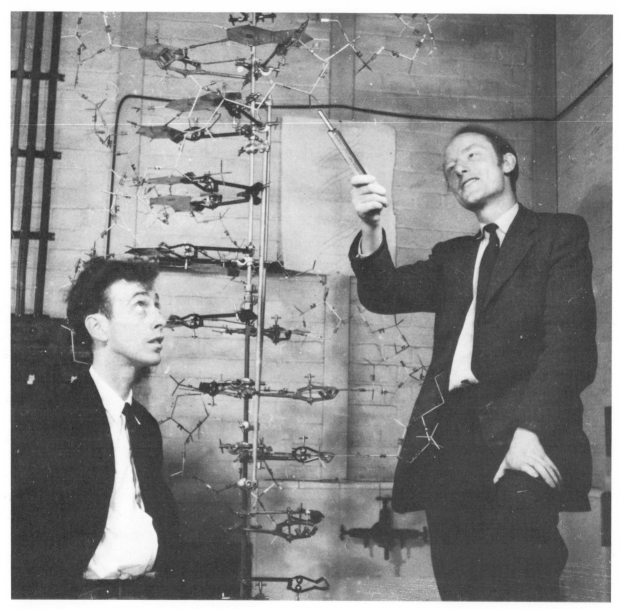

The structure of DNA was clarified by Watson (left) and Crick (right) in 1953 (J.D. Watson and F.H.C. Crick, Molecular structure of nucleic acids. A structure for desoxyribose nucleic acid. Nature, 171:737-8, 1953). (photograph from James D. Watson, *The Double Helix: A Personal Account of the Structure of DNA*, New York: Atheneum, 1968. Reproduced by permission).

Writing about contemporary events lacks the benefit of a distant view that provides perspective and detachment. The pace of progress in science continues to accelerate, with more subdivisions and specialization that make selection and synthesis increasingly more difficult.

In science, the second half of the century shows no deceleration in the pace of research in physics as it reaches further into elementary particles, antimatter, and the origins of our universe. Biomedical sciences also claim attention, as the new science of molecular biology delves into the very heart of genetic mechanisms and their interaction with environmental stimuli. The clarification of the structure of the deoxyribonucleic acid (DNA) molecule, achieved by Watson and Crick in 1953, well typifies the present period.

Oncology came of age during the 1960s, becoming a progressively more important source of new knowledge for biomedical sciences rather than being primarily an application of advances made in other fields of research. Neoplastic cells, as caricatures of the normal, help to define molecular cellular processes, as at one time the clinical caricatures of acromegaly helped to establish the hormonal role of the anterior pituitary.

Surgery and radiation as primary treatments of cancer are approaching their ultimate limits. Diagnosis of smaller, presumably earlier, lesions becomes essential if improvements in ablative therapy are to continue. On the other end of the scale, rehabilitation of successfully treated patients becomes of greater concern as their numbers become larger. But of even greater significance is the entry of systemic chemotherapy into oncology, with ever-improving yields in results as the number and variety of chemical agents with antineoplastic activity grows, and as the chemicals are used with maturing sophistication and in relation to biochemical and cytological guides.

The portents are now more than portents: neoplastic diseases will yield to man's insistent research queries. In the next century cancer will take its place with tuberculosis as a problem that has been controlled. Not eliminated, since man has not eliminated any disease from the earth, but driven to acceptably low levels and replaced by other problems. For problems there always will be. The next century will contend with social anthropology, the ethology and psychology of our species that may allow better interactions between individuals, groups of individuals, and all to their environment. In these endeavors oncology will continue to have a part, because the control of cancer requires prevention through better understanding of what causes it, as well as better knowledge of how to reverse its overt malignant characteristics.

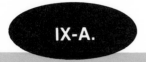

IX-A.

Tumor Pathology

IX-A-1. Armed Forces Institute of Pathology.

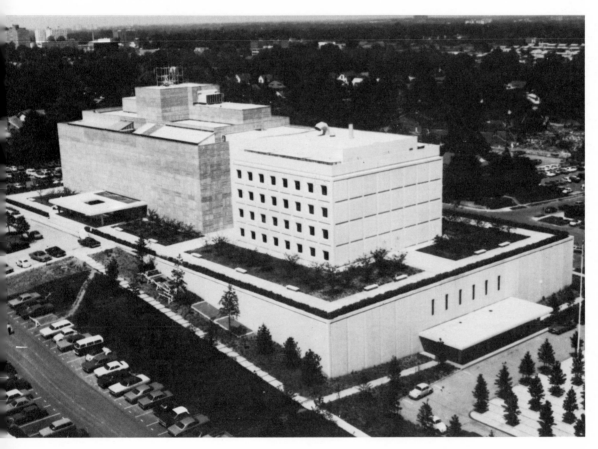

Armed Forces Institute of Pathology, 1965.

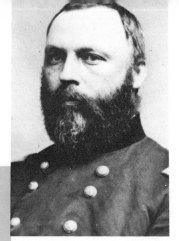

William A. Hammond

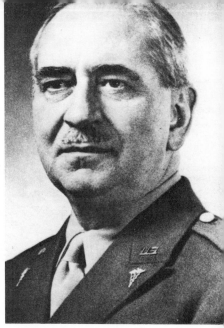

George R. Callender

Between Max Borst's 1902 textbook of oncologic pathology and World War II, single-author works on tumors were replaced by encyclopedic compilations. In 1949, the Armed Forces Institute of Pathology initiated the **Atlas of Tumor Pathology**, in which "fascicles" were written by experts on a special topic. By 1973, 40 such volumes appeared, profoundly affecting pathological criteria and nomenclature in neoplastic disease.

The Armed Forces Institute of Pathology, Washington, D. C., was established as the Army Medical Museum in 1862 by Surgeon General William A. Hammond (1828-1900). He issued a circular stating, "Medical officers are directed diligently to collect, and to forward to the Office of the Surgeon General, all specimens of morbid anatomy, surgical or medical, which may be regarded as valuable." The museum flourished, and became regarded as a National Medical Museum.

In 1920, Major George R. Callender (1884-1973), a trained pathologist, became the curator of the Museum, and supplemented the material by civilian sources, through a system of special registries. The American Academy of Ophthalmic and Otolaryngology in 1921 entered into an agreement with the Medical Museum whereby the Academy members would supply pathological material from operations on the eye which the Museum did not have, while the Museum would provide the professional and technical help needed for the study of the material. The Ophthalmic Pathology Registry was followed by the Lymphatic Tumor Registry (1924) and Bladder Tumor Registry (1926).

In 1944, the Museum became the Army Institute of Pathology and in 1948, the Armed Forces Institute of Pathology and the Central Laboratory of Pathology for Veterans Administration. It has become the repository of the largest collection of pathologic material and clinical data on neoplastic diseases in the world. The Institute has over 1,500,000 accessions, most of which are in cancer; e.g. 17,000 brain tumors, 20,000 eye tumors, 15,000 lung tumors, 15,000 bladder tumors, 7,000 testicular tumors and 30,000 soft tissue tumors. Its staff numbers more than 700 with over 100 pathologists. The Institute houses the World Health Organization International Reference Centers for Soft Tissue Tumors, for Tumors of Urogenital Organs, for Comparative Oncology and for Tumors of the Eye.

Max Borst. **Die Lehre von den Geschwülsten mit einem Atlas**. 2 vol. Wiesbaden: J. F. Bergmann, 1902.

F. Henke and O. Lubarsch (eds). **Handbuch der speziellen pathologischen Anatomie und Histologie**. 13 vol. Berlin: Julius Springer, 1926-1955.

R. S. Henry. **The Armed Forces Institute of Pathology. Its First Century, 1862-1962.** Washington, D.C.: U.S. Government Printing Office, 1964.

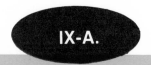

IX-A.

Tumor Pathology

IX-A-2. Experimental animal pathology: Stewart and Dunn.

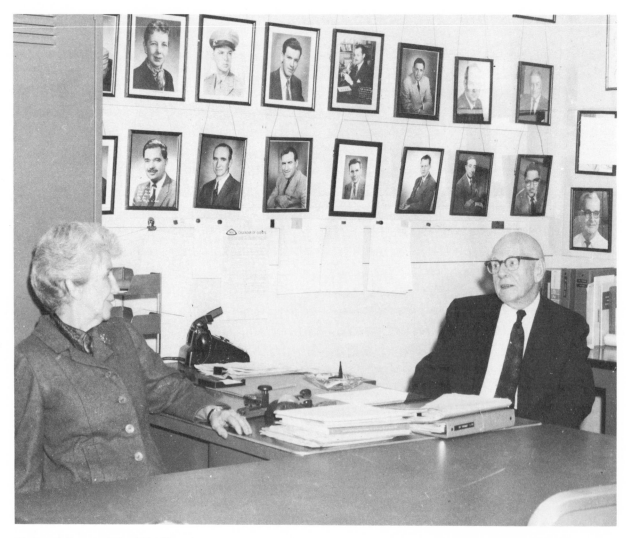

Thelma B. Dunn and Harold L. Stewart

Harold L. Stewart (1899-   ), chief of the Laboratory of Pathology of the National Cancer Institute, and Thelma Brumfeld Dunn (1900-   ), his associate, for over three decades until their retirement in 1969, were the authorities on tumors in experimental laboratory animals. Their own contributions include Stewart's studies on the induction and characterization of cancers of the alimentary tract in mice, and Dunn's analyses of hematopoietic and lymphoreticular neoplasms in mice.

Stewart and Dunn were strongly influential in national and international organizations of pathology and cancer research. Their role continued after retirement in the organization of a Registry of Experimental Cancers.

For almost 2 decades Stewart's office in the National Cancer Institute was an open house for informal lunch-time meetings. The meal itself became a tradition in frugality, but the intellectual fare was sufficient to lure visiting colleagues from laboratories everywhere. Stewart and Dunn were "pater-mater" to a family of cancer researchers and pathologists around the globe.

H. L. Stewart and E. Lorenz. Morbid anatomy, histopathology, and histopathogenesis of forestomach . carcinoma in mice fed carcinogenic hydrocarbons in oil emulsions. **J. Natl. Cancer Inst.** 10: 147-166, 1949.

T. B. Dunn. Normal and pathologic anatomy of the reticular tissue in laboratory mice, with a classification and discussion of neoplasms. **J. Natl. Cancer Inst.** 14: 1281-1433, 1954.

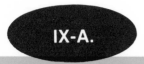

IX-A-3. Comparative oncology: Schlumberger.

Many animal species have yet to be investigated in the continuing search for information relating to cancer biology. Least explored of all are the invertebrate and cold-blooded vertebrate metazoans. Much of the information on neoplasia in these widely diversified groups is recorded in a monograph edited by Dawe and Harschbarger in 1969.

Three examples of poikilothermic animals bearing anomalous growths are pictured (top to bottom): (1) a Sydney rock oyster (**Crassostrea commercialis**) with an epithelioma of the mantle; (2) a coral colony (**Madrepora kauaiensis**) in which one corallite manifests anomalous growth reflected in the skeletal remains; and (3) a sea lamprey (**Petromyzon marinus**) with a melanoma with multiple subcutaneous, renal, and branchial metastases.

Hans George Schlumberger (1913-1967) was an outstanding comparative pathologist with an unbounded enthusiasm for studying neoplasia wherever they could be found in the animal kingdom. He was particularly interested in neoplasms in fish, amphibians, and reptiles, and bent his abilities with equal zest to studies of the response to methylcholanthrene in the cockroach **Periplaneta americana**. Schlumberger was born in Germany, educated at the Universities of North Carolina and Pennsylvania, and was professor and head of the Department of Pathology at the Arkansas University School of Medicine.

Tumor in an oyster

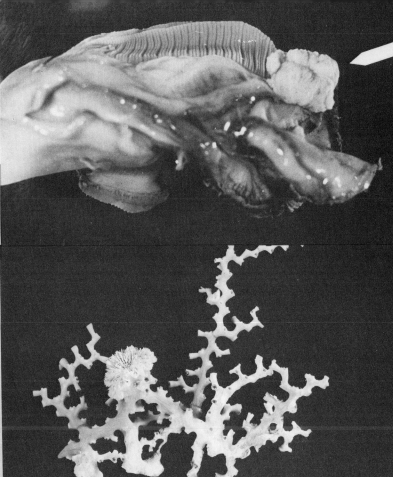

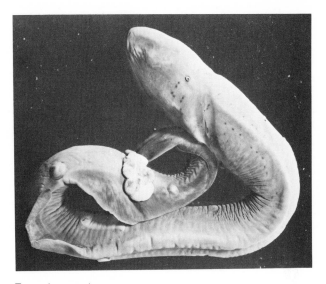

Tumor in a coral

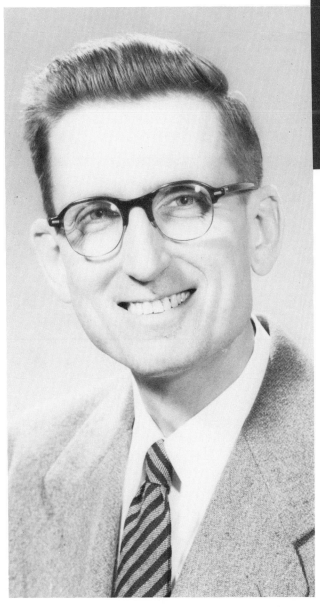

Hans G. Schlumberger

Tumor in a sea lamprey

H. G. Schlumberger and B. Lucké. Tumors of fishes, amphibians and reptiles. **Cancer Res.** 8: 657-753, 1948.

H. G. Schlumberger. Tumors characteristic for certain animal species: a review. **Cancer Res.** 17: 823-32, 1957.

C. J. Dawe and John C. Harschbarger. (eds). **Neoplasms and Related Disorders of Invertebrate and Lower Vertebrate Animals.** National Cancer Institute Monograph 31, July 1969.

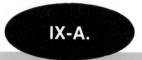

IX-A.

Tumor Pathology

IX-A-4. Tissue culture: Earle and Gey.

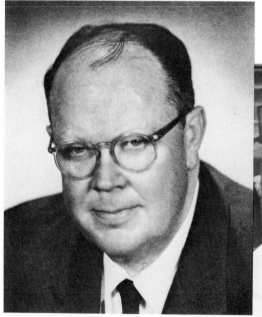

Wilton R. Earle

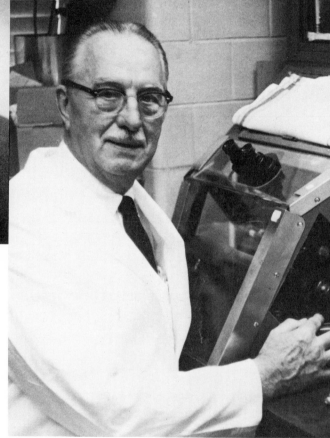

George O. Gey

Wilton Robinson Earle (1902-64), of the National Cancer Institute in Bethesda, Maryland, and George Otto Gey (1899-1970), of the Johns Hopkins University School of Medicine, were pioneer developers of tissue culture techniques for the long-term propagation of mammalian cells.

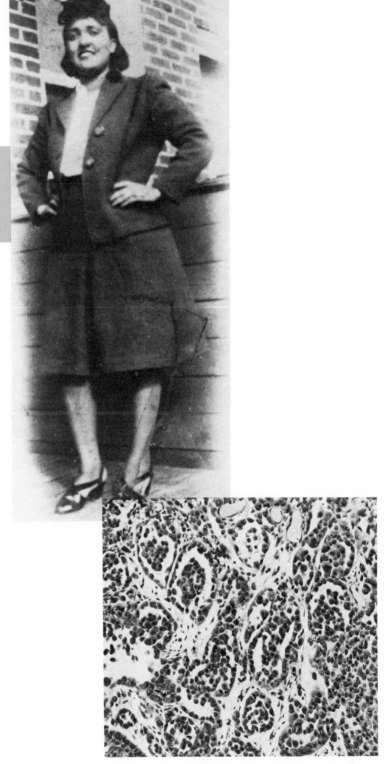

Henrietta Lacks (HeLa).

The goal of research conducted by Earle and his group was to convert mouse fibroblasts into sarcoma by exposure to 3-methylcholanthrene. Such conversion was observed, but probably was not due to the chemical carcinogen. The work did establish that carcinogenesis could take place under **in vitro** conditions, thus not requiring the participation of the host.

Gey also observed the appearance of sarcoma in rat fibroblast cultures, without intentional exposure to known exogenous carcinogens. In the propagation of many cultures on roller tubes, one was derived from an aggressive cancer of the cervix of Henrietta Lacks (or, perhaps, Helen Lane or Helen Larson). The cell line, called HeLa after its source, has been continued in laboratories throughout the world, outliving both the patient and the cytologist. For many years the HeLa line was considered to be an epidermoid carcinoma, but a review of the original specimen by Jones indicates that it was an adenocarcinoma.

Cell culture became a biological tool within the reach of most laboratories after the methodology was simplified and defined media became available through commercial sources. Extensive observations were then made of cells grown in culture and their transformation by viruses and chemicals.

Original biopsy from which HeLa cells were first cultured in 1951, showing adenocarcinoma of the uterus

Wilton R. Earle *et al*. Production of malignancy *in vitro*. **J. Natl. Cancer Inst.** 4: 131-248, 1943.

George O. Gey. Some aspects of the constitution and behavior of normal and malignant cells maintained in continuous culture. **Harvey Lectures** 50: 154-229, 1954-55.

H. W. Jones, Jr. *et al*. George Otto Gey. The HeLa Cell and a reappraisal of its origin. **Obst. & Gynec.** 38: 945-9, 1971.

Kate Russell. Tissue culture—a brief historical review. **Clio Med.** 4: 109-19, 1969.

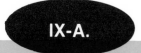

Tumor Pathology

IX-A-5. Electron microscopy: Dmochowski.

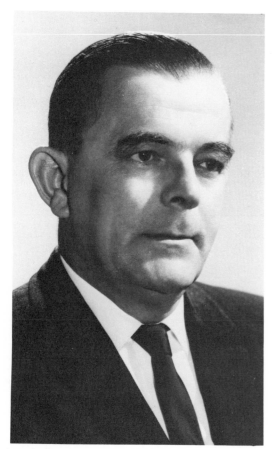

Leon L. Dmochowski

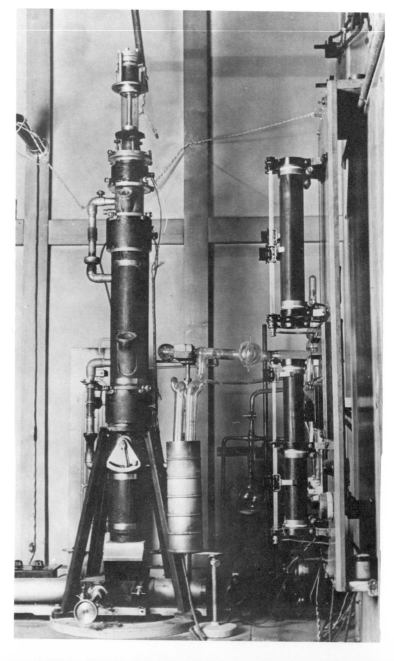

An early (1938) electron microscope developed by Prebus and Hillier in Toronto.

The electron microscope, an instrument that allows observations of objects beyond resolution by wave lengths of visible light, was developed through several steps of engineering since approximately 1930. The names of M. Knoll and E. Ruska of Berlin are prominent during the earlier phases. L. Marton of Brussels published the first electron micrograph of a biological specimen. The evolution of the instrument was described by Bradbury.

The electron microscope was applied to experimental oncology soon after commercial instruments became available. Leon Dmochowski's studies, beginning in 1947, are among the more intense systematic explorations of tumors and tumor viruses by electron microscopy.

Leon L. Dmochowski was born in Poland in 1909, and obtained his doctorate at the University of Warsaw in 1937. From 1939 to 1953 he worked at the University of Leeds, England, and in 1954 joined the faculty of Baylor University College of Medicine, and then the University of Texas Postgraduate School of Medicine, and the M. D. Anderson Hospital and Tumor Institute, Houston.

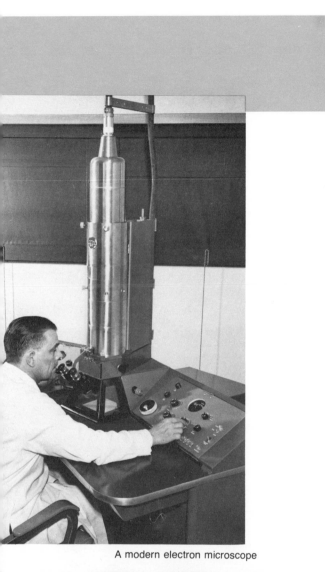

A modern electron microscope

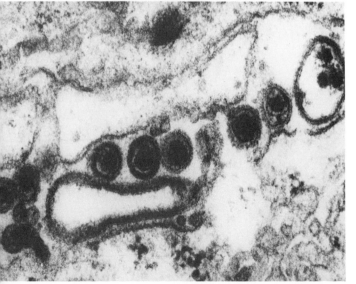

Virus particles in a spontaneous mammary cancer in a mouse, x 150,000.

S. Bradbury. **The Evolution of the Microscope.** New York: Pergamon Press, 1967.

R. D. Passey, L. Dmochowski, W. T. Astbury, and R. Reed. Electron microscope studies of normal and malignant tissues of high- and low-breast-cancer strains of mice. **Nature** 160: 565, 1947.

L. Dmochowski. Viruses and tumors in the light of electron microscope studies. A review. **Cancer Res.** 20: 977-1015, 1960.

IX-B.

Cancer Biology

IX-B-1. Biology of experimental cancer: Andervont and Furth.

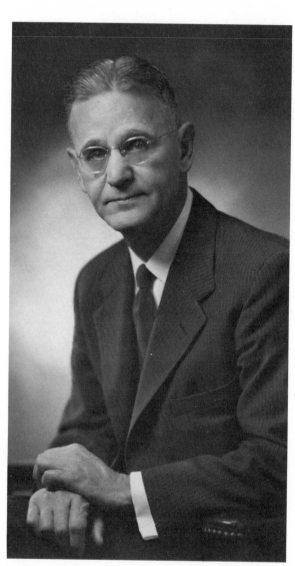

Howard B. Andervont

Among the generalists in experimental cancer research over several decades during mid-century were H. B. Andervont and J. Furth.

Howard Bancroft Andervont was born in 1898, in Ohio, and received his Doctor of Science degree from Johns Hopkins University in 1926. He joined Schereschewsky's cancer investigations group at Harvard in 1930, being its first professional staff member. The group moved as a nucleus of the National Cancer Institute to Bethesda in 1939, and he remained with the Institute until his retirement in 1968.

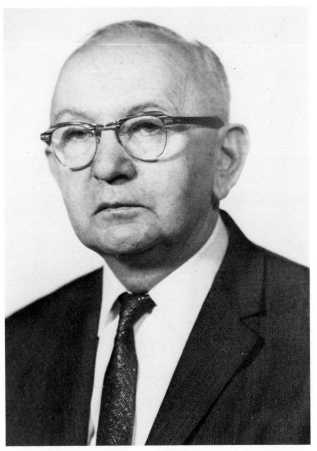

Jacob Furth

Jacob Furth was born in 1896, in Hungary, and obtained his doctorate at the German University of Prague in 1921. He came to the United States in 1924, and joined the faculty of Cornell University Medical College in New York in 1932, where he remained in the department of pathology until 1949. He served with the Atomic Energy Commission between 1949 and 1953, was at the Children's Cancer Research Foundation in Boston between 1954 and 1959, at the Roswell Park Institute between 1959 and 1961, and returned to Columbia University in New York in 1961, being on emeritus status since 1967.

Furth's research has ranged over carcinogenesis and growth of tumors induced with a variety of agents, including hormones, radiation and chemicals. He developed the concept of conditioned neoplasms, and emphasized the pituitary cybernetics in carcinogenesis. Tumors of the ovary and leukemia in mice were to him of particular interest.

Andervont's research ranged over transplanted, chemically and virally induced tumors, and genetics in mice; he made particularly noteworthy contributions in his studies on mammary, hepatic and pulmonary tumors in mice. He was used widely as a consultant on the biology of cancer, and was editor of the **Journal of the National Cancer Institute**.

H. B. Andervont. Pulmonary tumors in mice. **Pub. Health Rep.** 52: 212-21; 304-15; 347-55; 1584-9, 1937.

H. B. Andervont. Influence of environment on mammary cancer in mice. **J. Natl. Cancer Inst.** 4: 579-81, 1944.

H. B. Andervont. Biological background for experimental work on tumors. **Canad. Cancer Conf.** 1: 2-24, 1955.

M. B. Shimkin. Howard B. Andervont: an appreciation. **J. Natl. Cancer Inst.** 40: xiii-xxv, 1968.

J. Furth. Conditioned and autonomous neoplasms: a review. **Cancer Res.** 13: 477-92, 1953.

J. Furth and J. L. Tullis. Carcinogenesis by radioactive substances. **Cancer Res.** 16: 5-21, 1956.

J. Furth. Pituitary cybernetics and neoplasia. **Harvey Lectures** 63: 47-71, 1967-68.

J. Furth. The making and missing of discoveries: an autobiographical essay. **Cancer Res.** 36: 871-80, 1976.

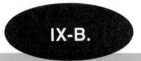

IX-B.

Cancer Biology

IX-B-2. British cancer biologists: Horning, Foulds and Bonser.

The cancer laboratories and clinics of London, Leeds and others in the British Isles continued to add important information to our knowledge of cancer. Among the many names in the biology category were Harold Burrows (1875-1955) and Georgiana Bonser (1898-   ), E. S. Horning (1899-1959) and Leslie Foulds (1902-1974).

Bonser, of the Manchester University Medical School, contributed many investigations on carcinogenesis, especially with hormones.

Horning, with Burrows, contributed a book on estrogens and neoplasia, an extension of Burrows' previous comprehensive treatise on sex steroids.

Foulds synthesized his thoughtful observations on the carcinogenic process in a book entitled **Neoplastic Development**, issued in 1969.

The British Journal of Cancer began publication in 1947, a late comer to specialized oncologic periodicals. Ronald W. Raven, a surgeon in London, edited a 6-volume compilation, **Cancer**, between 1957 and 1959.

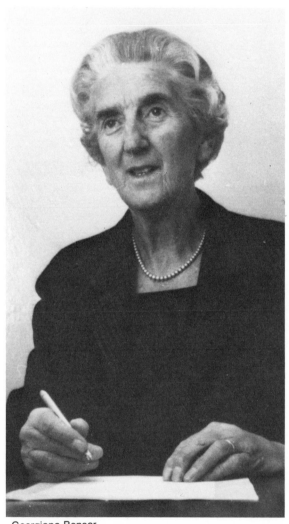

Georgiana Bonser

Harold Burrows. **Biological Actions of Sex Hormones.** Cambridge: Cambridge Univ. Press, 1945.

H. Burrows and E. S. Horning. **Oestrogens and Neoplasia.** Springfield, Ill.: C. C. Thomas, 1952.

L. Foulds. **Neoplastic Development.** London: Academic Press, 1969.

R. W. Raven (ed). **Cancer.** 6 vols. London: Butterworth & Co., 1957-59.

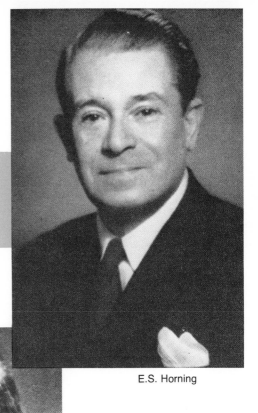

E.S. Horning

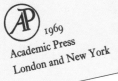

NEOPLASTIC DEVELOPMENT

LESLIE FOULDS

London

VOLUME 1

1969
Academic Press
London and New York

Leslie Foulds

THE BRITISH JOURNAL OF
CANCER

(The official journal of the British Empire Cancer Campaign)

EDITOR
R. W. Scarff

ASSISTANT EDITOR
F. R. Selbie

ADVISORY EDITORS

S. P. Bedson
Sir Stanford Cade
E. C. Dodds
Malcolm Donaldson
C. E. Dukes
L. H. Gray
W. E. Gye
A. Haddow

The Lord Horder
J. P. Lockhart-Mummery
J. McIntosh
W. D. Newcomb
Sir Heneage Ogilvie
M. J. Stewart
Percy Stocks
B. W. Windeyer

DIRECTOR
F. L. Hopwood

VOLUME ONE
1947

LONDON
H. K. LEWIS & CO. LTD.
136 GOWER STREET, W.C. 1

IX-B.

Cancer Biology

IX-B-3. Nutrition and cancer: Tannenbaum and Silverstone.

The role of nutrition in the genesis and growth of cancer has been a matter of speculation for many years. Since neoplasms are derived from, and dependent upon the host, the nutritional state must influence neoplasms; the questions, however, are the extent of such influences and whether specific dietary components can be incriminated.

During the decade, 1940 to 1950, Albert Tannenbaum conducted a series of careful experiments at the Michael Reese Hospital in Chicago, on nutrition in relation to cancer in mice. Caloric restriction, by one-third of the ad libitum, led to a reduction in the appearance of many spontaneous and induced tumors, especially of the breast. The growth of established tumors was also affected, but less impressively than their genesis. No specific material, macro- or micronutrient (vitamin or mineral) was identified as of particular importance. Clinical and statistical findings suggest that some tumors in man are partly dependent on the nutritional state, but this does not appear to be a practical means of arresting the development or growth of tumors.

Related but distinctly different aspects of nutrition and cancer are the introduction of carcinogens into foodstuffs, and the modification of the metabolism of certain carcinogens by dietary constituents. Example of the former is aflatoxin in the diet of tropical populations that is probably associated with the occurrence of hepatoma. Example of the latter is the protective effect of riboflavin in hepatomagenesis in rats ingesting azo dyes in the diet.

The review of nutrition and cancer by Tannenbaum and Silverstone is a landmark in the field. Albert Tannenbaum, born in Chicago in 1901, obtained his MD degree in 1930 at Rush Medical College and spent his career in cancer research at Michael Reese Hospital in Chicago. His associate, Herbert Silverstone (1913-1956) was a native of Philadelphia and obtained his doctorate in biochemistry at the University of Chicago in 1949.

Albert Tannenbaum and Herbert Silverstone. Nutrition in relation to cancer. **Adv. Cancer Res.** 1: 451-501, 1953.

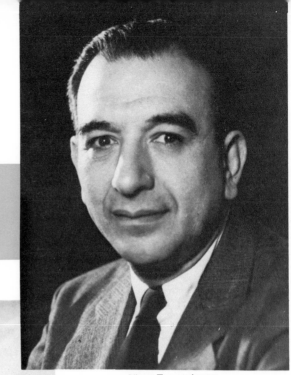

Albert Tannenbaum

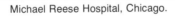

Michael Reese Hospital, Chicago.

Herbert Silverstone

315

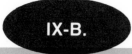

IX-B.

Cancer Biology

IX-B-4. Germ-free animals: Reyniers.

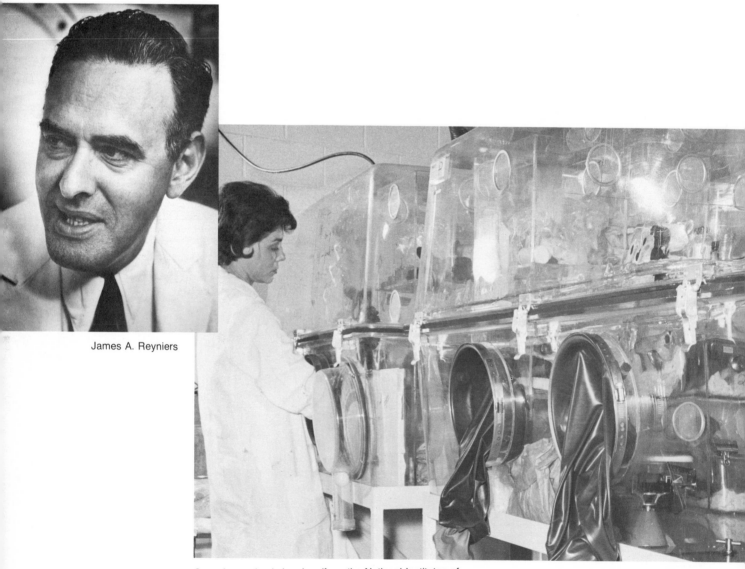

James A. Reyniers

Germ-free animal chamber (from the National Institutes of Health).

The development of conditions under which germ-free animals can be maintained over their life spans has given rise to the science of gnotobiology. Germfree animals reveal the role of bacteria in the organismal ecology, and provide information on the role of the non-stimulated immune system on physiologic and pathologic responses.

James Arthur Reyniers (1908-1967) was born in Indiana, and obtained his education at Notre Dame University in South Bend, Indiana. He remained with the University while developing the instrumentation for rearing and studying germ-free animals, and established the Lobund Institute (Laboratory of Biology, University of Notre Dame) for the purpose.

Facilities and equipment for the study of germ-free animals spread to many biological centers in Europe, Japan and the United States. The applications included experimental oncology, on the effect of the germ-free state on transplantation and induction of tumors. In general, the effects were not striking, indicating that bacteria play but a small role in the neoplastic processes. A more subtle bacterial participation was indicated by the lack of carcinogenic activity of cycasin when fed to bacteria-free animals. For absorption, cycasin has to be split into an aglycone by bacterial flora in the intestine.

J. A. Reyniers. Design and operation of apparatus for rearing germfree animals. **Ann. N. Y. Acad. Sci.** 78: 47-79, 1959.

T. D. Luckey. **Germfree Life and Gnotobiology.** New York: Academic Press, 1963.

M. Pollard, T. Matsuzawa and J. C. Salomon. Induction of neoplasms in germfree rodents by 3-methylcholanthrene. **J. Natl. Cancer Inst.** 33: 93-97, 1964.

G. L. Laqueur, E. G. McDaniel and H. Matsumoto. Tumor induction in germ-free rats with methylazoxymethanol (MAM) and synthetic MAM acetate. **J. Natl. Cancer Inst.** 39: 355-71, 1967.

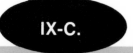

IX-C.

Cancer Genetics

IX-C-1. Animal genetics: Jackson Laboratory.

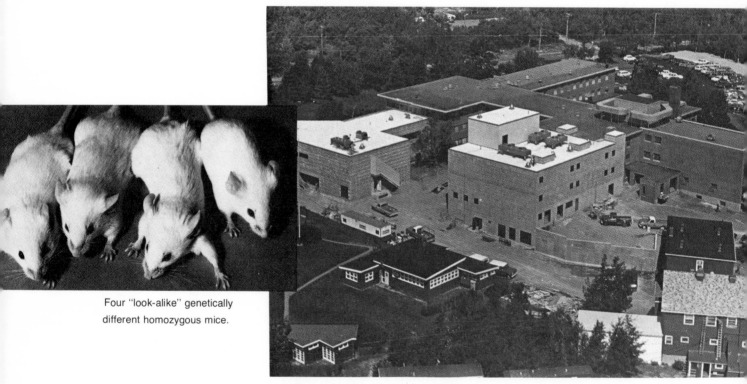

Four "look-alike" genetically different homozygous mice.

Jackson Laboratory, Bar Harbor, Maine.

The laboratory mouse, the fancy-bred descendant of the common house mouse (**Mus musculus**), is an excellent emblem for cancer research. Over 30 million mice were used in biomedical research in 1971 in the U. S. alone. Cancer research used a large proportion, especially of the genetically inbred strains that have been developed since the early years of this century.

The Jackson Laboratory of Bar Harbor, Maine, (formerly the Roscoe B. Jackson Memorial Laboratory) is the origin of many mouse strains, and is the largest research laboratory devoted to mammalian genetics in the world. Founded in 1929 by Clarence Cook Little, the laboratory was named after a Hudson motorcar magnate who summered at Bar Harbor. In addition to being an outstanding center for cancer research, the laboratory is also engaged in important programs of teaching and of production of many inbred and mutant strains of mice.

Predictability of cancer incidence and types among inbred strains of mice is

demonstrated in the pictured four white female albino "look alikes," studied by staff members of the Jackson Laboratory. Left to right, the first mouse (A/HeJ) will almost certainly develop mammary tumor. The second mouse (AKR/J) will surely die at an early age with lymphatic leukemia. The third mouse (BALB/cJ) probably will not develop mammary cancer unless she has been suckled by a foster mother. If she develops lung tumors, they will appear later in life than those of A/He mice. The fourth mouse (SJL/J) will almost certainly die with a form of reticulum-cell sarcoma similar to Hodgkin's disease. These female mice were all born at approximately the same time in the same mouse room at the Jackson Laboratory.

The director of the Jackson Laboratory from 1956 to his retirement was Earl Leroy Green, born in Pennsylvania, 1913, a doctor of genetics who graduated from Brown University and taught at Ohio State University from 1941 to 1956. Among the senior staff were two life-time members who were elected to the National Academy of Science: George Davis Snell (born in Massachusetts in 1903 and a doctor of science in genetics from Harvard), and Elizabeth Shull Russell (born in Michigan in 1913 who received her doctorate from Columbia University in New York).

The aerial view of the Jackson Laboratory was taken in August 1972. It shows the main laboratory complex with two wings under construction on the left, the summer college student quarters in the center, and the Morrell Park Laboratory facility for raising mice at the right.

C. E. Keeler. **The Laboratory Mouse.** Cambridge, Mass.: Harvard Univ. Press, 1931.
Staff of the Jackson Laboratory. **Biology of the Laboratory Mouse.** ed. 2. New York: McGraw-Hill, 1966.

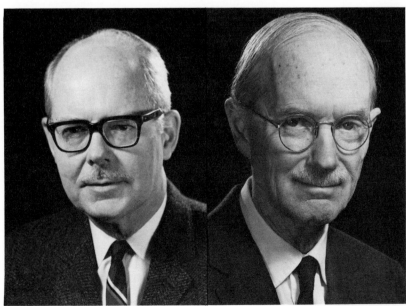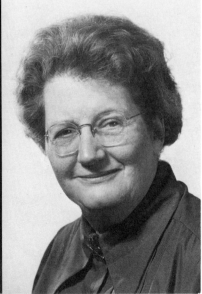

Earl L. Green   George D. Snell   Elizabeth S. Russell

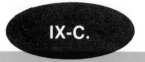

Cancer Genetics

IX-C-2. Human genetics: Macklin and Lynch.

The genetic make-up of an organism is involved in every physiological and pathological process. A role for heredity in cancer, therefore, is inescapable; the question requires specification to what degree there is genetic control for what individual types of neoplasms.

Studies of heredity in cancer of man are difficult because we are dealing with heterozygous populations, as was true of studies on mice before inbred strains were developed. Twins present a potentially valuable material for cancer genetics.

Madge T. Macklin (1893-1962) was an early investigator of the genetics of human cancer, and provided a study of twins.

Familial aggregation of cancers gained attention by the famous studies initiated by A. S. Warthin in 1913, and continued by Henry T. Lynch (1928-   ). This field of inquiry remains in need of better methodology, especially in distinguishing genetic from environmental familial factors.

There are, however, several neoplastic and preneoplastic disorders that provide evidence of Mendelian inheritance. One has been defined as an autosomal recessive inheritance: xeroderma pigmentosum, the precancerous skin lesion of extreme sensitivity to cancerous changes upon exposure to sunlight. The remaining half-dozen conditions are inherited as autosomal dominants: (1) retinoblastoma, the rare cancer of the eye; (2) familial multiple polyposis of the colon, which uniformly terminates as cancer; (3) multiple nevoid basal cell carcinoma syndrome; (4) Gardner's syndrome of colonic polyps, osteomas, fibromas and epidermal cysts; (5) polyendocrine adenomatosis; and (6) multiple neurofibromatosis of Recklinghausen. A conference on parental influence in relation to the incidence of human cancer was held at the Jackson Laboratory, Bar Harbor, Maine, in 1944. It brought together many of the workers in the field.

The subject of heredity in human cancer has been reviewed by Clemmesen, Lynch, and Fraumeni.

M. T. Macklin. Analysis of tumors in monozygous and dizygous twins; with report of 15 unpublished cases. **J. Heredity** 31: 277-90, 1940.

M. T. Macklin. Inheritance of cancer of the stomach and large intestine in man. **J. Natl. Cancer Inst.** 24: 551-71, 1960.

H. T. Lynch. **Hereditary Factors in Carcinoma. Recent Results in Cancer Research,** vol. 12. New York: Springer-Verlag, 1967.

J. Clemmesen. The status of genetical studies in human cancer. **Brit. J. Cancer** 3: 474-84, 1949.

J. F. Fraumeni, Jr. Genetic Factors. In **Cancer Medicine.** (eds. J. Holland and E. Frei III). Philadelphia: Lea and Febiger, 1973. p. 7-15.

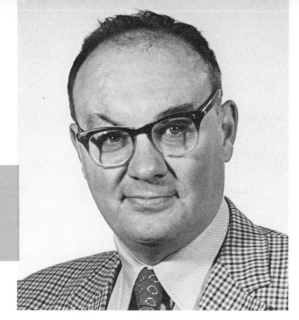

Henry T. Lynch

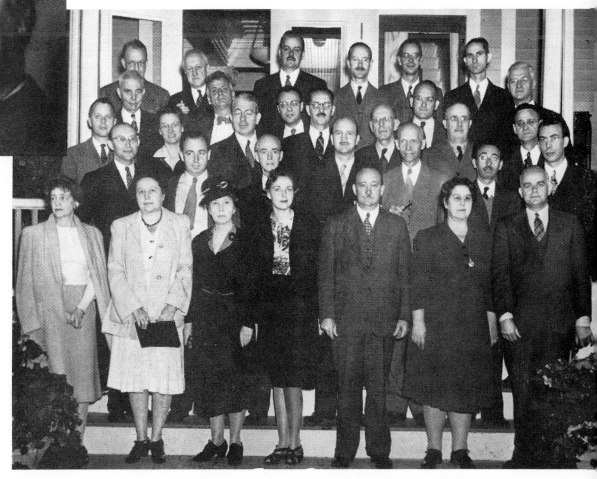

Madge Thurlow Macklin

First row: Dr. M.W.S. Schram, Elizabeth Fekete, Dr. C.J. Lynch, Dr. Margaret Kelsall, Dr. L.C. Strong, Dr. Madge Macklin, Dr. L.H.Snyder.
Second row: Dr. F. Blank, Mr. Robert Cook, Mr. J.J. O'Neill, Dr. R.G. Meader, Dr. L.J. Cole, Dr. Sigismund Peller, Dr. W.R. Bryan.

Third row: Dr. G.W. Woolley, Dr. K.P. Hummel, Dr. Herbert Lombard, Dr. C.P. Oliver, Dr. William Cramer, Dr. R.R. Spencer, Dr. H.B. Andervont.
Fourth row: Mr. Howard Blakeslee, Dr. F. Duran-Reynals, Dr. M.L. Levin, Dr. A.M. Cloudman, Dr. Douglas Murphy.
Fifth row: Dr. L.J. Evans, Dr. Waldemar Kaempffert, Dr. C.C. Little, Dr. G.D. Snell, Dr. W.L. Russell, Dr. W.E. Heston.

IX-C.

Cancer Genetics

IX-C-3. Golden hamsters: Aharoni and Adler.

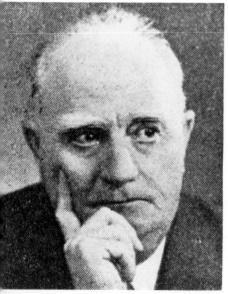

I. Aharoni

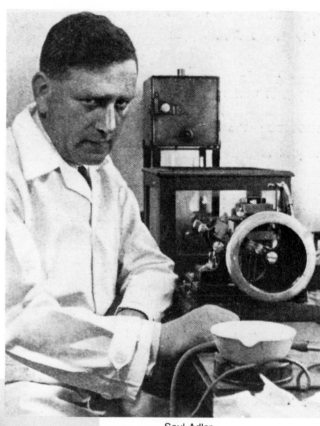

Saul Adler

Golden hamsters

The Israeli zoologist Israel Aharoni in 1930 captured for Professor Saul Adler at the University of Jerusalem one male and two female littermates of **Mesocricetus auratus**. From these three animals H. ben Menahem in Adler's laboratory quickly established that this species breeds readily in captivity. Thus the Syrian golden hamster, **Mesocricetus auratus**, replaced the hard-to-obtain Chinese hamster, **Cricetus griseus**, which Adler had to import from the Orient for his studies on Kala Azar. Since then Syrian hamsters have been used in laboratory research throughout the world at the rate of some 800,000 per year in the United States alone. Many inbred strains have been developed and much knowledge has been gained on the physiology and pathology of this species.

Syrian hamsters gained special significance in cancer research with the discovery of their ability to accept heterotransplants, especially of human neoplastic tissue, in the cheek pouch. Since 1941 they have been used extensively in carcinogenesis research. Marked differences in susceptibility have been noted for certain forms of viral and chemical carcinogenesis among various inbred strains.

Israel Aharoni was born in Lithuania in 1882 and died in Israel in 1946. He studied zoology and semitic languages at University of Prague, Czechoslovakia, and later on became lecturer in zoology at the Hebrew University of Jerusalem. He was a pioneer in the study of the fauna of Israel and its neighboring countries, especially Syria and Turkey. Aharoni discovered many species of animals hitherto unknown, and succeeded in raising the golden hamster that became one of the important experimental animals for medical research.

Saul Adler was born in Russia in 1895 and died in Israel in 1966. He graduated from the University of Leeds, England, School of Medicine and studied tropical diseases in Liverpool. During World War I he served as physician and pathologist in the British army in Iraq. In 1924 he became professor at the Hebrew University of Jerusalem, Israel, and head of the Institute of Parasitology at the University. His activities focused on the etiology, pathology and means of transfer of pathologic parasites in humans and animals and on chemotherapy of tropical diseases.

S. Adler. Origin of the golden hamster Cricetus auratus as a laboratory animal. **Nature** 162: 256-7, 1948.

R. A. Hoffman (ed). **The Golden Hamster, Its Biology and Use in Medical Research.** Ames, Iowa: Iowa State Univ. Press, 1968.

F. Homburger (ed). Pathology of the Syrian Hamster. **Prog. Exp. Tumor Res.** 16: 1-621, 1972.

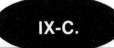

Cancer Genetics

IX-C-4. Genes and tissues: Heston and Kirschbaum.

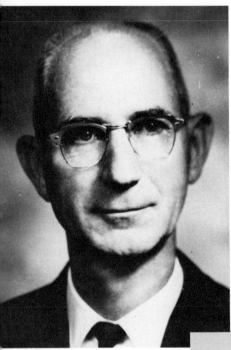

Walter E. Heston

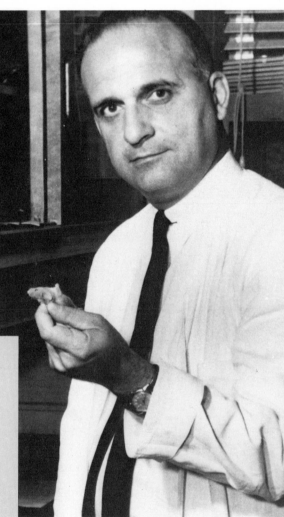

Arthur J. Kirschbaum

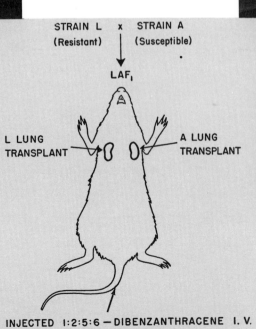

STRAIN L x STRAIN A
(Resistant)   (Susceptible)

LAF_1

L LUNG
TRANSPLANT

A LUNG
TRANSPLANT

INJECTED 1:2:5:6 — DIBENZANTHRACENE I. V.

Plan of experiment demonstrating tissue
level of carcinogenic transformation.

Two independent reports of 1951 determined that gene action controlling the development of pulmonary tumors in mice is localized in the lung tissue and is not manifested through some general systemic mechanism.

Joyce R. Shapiro and Arthur J. Kirschbaum, at the University of Minnesota obtained F_1 mice from a cross between Bagg albino, a pulmonary-tumor-susceptible strain, and dba, a pulmonary-tumor-resistant strain. Transplants of lungs from one-day-old mice from either parent strains into the subcutaneous tissue of the ear were shown to survive in these hybrids. In mice implanted with lung tissue from Bagg albino, and then injected intraperitoneally with urethane, pulmonary tumors were produced in 12 of 17 transplants. When the transplanted lung was derived from dba mice, only one pulmonary tumor was produced in 17 transplants.

Walter E. Heston and Thelma B. Dunn, of the National Cancer Institute, transplanted lungs of a resistant strain (C_{57} leaden or L) subcutaneously in one axilla, and lungs of a susceptible strain (A) in the other axilla of LAF_1 mice, who were then injected intravenously with 1,2,5,6-dibenzanthracene. Pulmonary tumors developed in 40% of the transplants from strain A donors and in 4% of transplants from strain L. This experiment is outlined in the figure.

Arthur J. Kirschbaum (1910-1958) was educated at New York University and the University of Minnesota, receiving both Ph.D. in anatomy and M.D. degrees. His interest in cancer research began at Yale, as a research fellow, and continued at Minnesota, Illinois and Baylor College of Medicine in Houston, Texas. His contributions were to mouse genetics, leukemia and other murine neoplasms.

Walter E. Heston was born in Iowa in 1909, and received his Ph.D. from Michigan State University in 1936. One of the earlier research fellows of the National Cancer Institute, first at the Jackson Laboratory at Bar Harbor, Maine, and then in Bethesda, Maryland, he became chief of the Laboratory of Biology in 1961. His contributions have been primarily to genetics of cancer and abnormal development, using the pulmonary and mammary tumors in mice as his primary material.

The interesting technique introduced by Kirschbaum and by Heston has often been applied to a multitude of questions the answers to which are obtained by observing neoplastic transformation in tissues of different genotypes growing in a common host or in tissue of one genotype growing in a host of a tolerant but different genotype. It can tie together the areas of genetics and immunology with chemical and viral carcinogenesis in experimental oncology.

Joyce R. Shapiro and Arthur J. Kirschbaum. Intrinsic tissue response to induction of pulmonary tumors. **Cancer Res.** 11: 644-7, 1951.

Walter E. Heston and Thelma B. Dunn. Tumor development in susceptible strain A and resistant strain L lung transplants in LA F_1 hosts. **J. Natl. Cancer Inst.** 11: 1057-71, 1951.

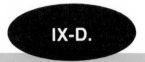

IX-D.

Oncogenic Viruses

IX-D-1. Virus isolation: Stanley.

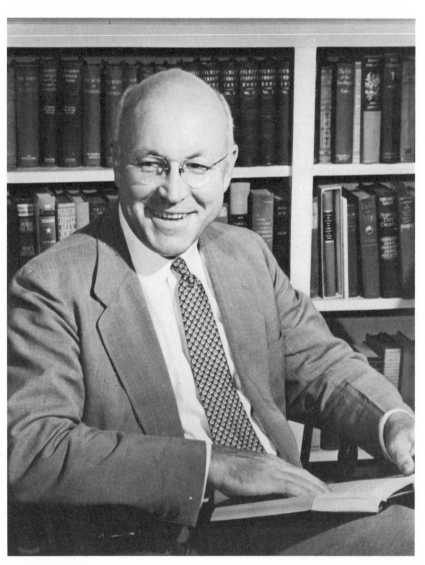

Wendell M. Stanley

W. M. Stanley. Isolation of a crystalline protein possessing the properties of tobacco-mosaic virus. **Science** 81: 644-5, 1935.

W. M. Stanley. The virus etiology of cancer. In **Proc. Third Natl. Cancer Conf.** Philadelphia: J. B. Lippincott, 1957. (p. 42-51).

W. M. Stanley and Evans G. Valens. **Viruses and the Nature of Life.** New York: E. P. Dutton and Co., 1965.

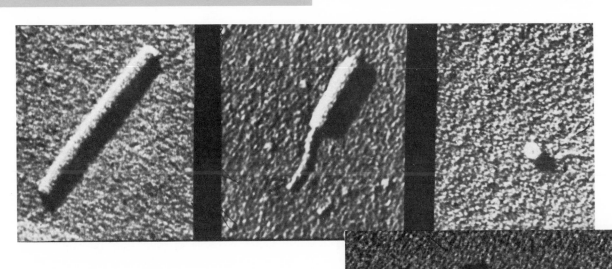

Wendell Meredith Stanley (1905-1971) was born in Indiana and obtained his doctorate in chemistry at the University of Illinois in 1929. He joined the Rockefeller Institute, and worked at its Princeton, New Jersey facilities. There, in 1935, from a ton of infected tobacco leaves, he isolated in crystalline form the tobacco mosaic virus. For this work, he shared the Nobel Prize in Chemistry for 1946.

In 1947 Stanley moved to the University of California at Berkeley and there established the Virus Laboratory, housed in a building now named after him. He became interested in cancer, and began to espouse the view of its possible viral etiology. His influence and leadership were important in the development of virus research in oncology, although he himself did not become directly involved. He was selected president of the Tenth International Congress of the International Union Against Cancer.

Tobacco mosaic virus particles, seen through an electron microscope at a magnification of × 230,000 (from W.M. Stanley and E.G. Valens, Viruses and the Nature of Life, 1965; reproduced by permission).

IX-D.

Oncogenic Viruses

IX-D-2. Avian oncogenic viruses: Beard and Bryan.

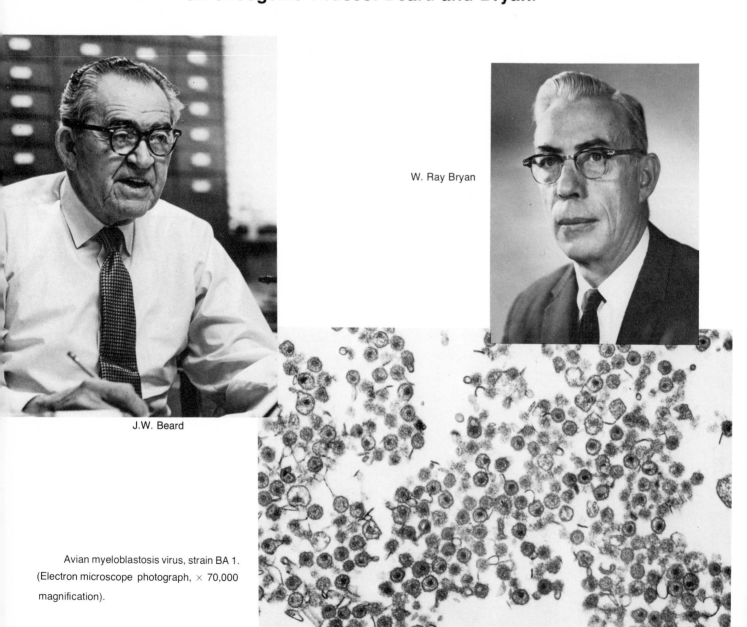

J.W. Beard

W. Ray Bryan

Avian myeloblastosis virus, strain BA 1.
(Electron microscope photograph, × 70,000
magnification).

Joseph W. Beard (1901-   ) and W. Ray Bryan (1905-1976) played pioneering roles in the science of tumor virology, contributing more than 40 years to teaching and research on the role of viruses in various animal cancers. They made major contributions in the area of avian cancer viruses.

Beard was one of the first scientists to study the role of host susceptibility in the induction of cancer by viruses. Working with Peyton Rous, Richard Shope, and associates in New York in the 1930s, he helped demonstrate that a usually benign rabbit tumor caused by a virus sometimes becomes cancerous. Later, he and Rous purified the causative virus. In the 1940s, by applying the differential centrifugation methods of Albert Claude, Beard and his associates purified the influenza and mumps viruses of humans and a similar virus which causes Newcastle disease in chickens. Since 1949, his work has been devoted primarily to the avian tumor viruses, particularly two leukemia viruses of the chicken, avian myeloblastosis, and erythroblastosis.

Bryan laid much of the groundwork for today's quantitative research on cancer viruses by applying statistical techniques to the study of viruses in animal cancers. As early as the 1930s, while a National Cancer Institute Research Fellow working at Duke University under Beard, Bryan studied the relationship between amount of Shope virus inoculated and the development of rabbit papillomas. In the early 1940s at the National Cancer Institute, he also analyzed the effects of cancer-causing chemicals on mice and helped show that the mouse breast cancer "agent" was, in fact, a filterable virus.

Bryan turned to the study of Rous sarcoma virus, a solid tumor virus of the chicken, in the 1950s. By applying statistical methods, he demonstrated correlations between the amount of virus inoculated into a chicken, the time to appearance of a tumor, and the amount of virus recoverable from that tumor. On occasion, very small amounts of virus would induce tumors from which no virus was recoverable, establishing the concept that absence of demonstrable virus in tumor tissue extracts does not prove that a tumor is not of viral origin.

The quantitative methods and principles of virus dose and tumor response established by these two leaders of animal cancer virology has enabled others to confirm and extend their studies of leukemias and solid tumors in mammals. Today, viruses of RNA type studied by Beard and Bryan in avian cancers are known to cause many kinds of cancers in mammals and are increasingly suspect of having a role in human cancers.

W. R. Bryan. Biological studies on the Rous sarcoma virus. **J. Natl. Cancer Inst.** 16: 285-335, 1955, and 843-63, 1956.
J. W. Beard. The fallacy of the concept of virus "masking." A review. **Cancer Res.** 16: 279-91, 1956.

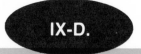

Oncogenic Viruses

IX-D-3. Vertical transmission: Gross.

Ludwik Gross

Vertical transmission of leukemia in mice.

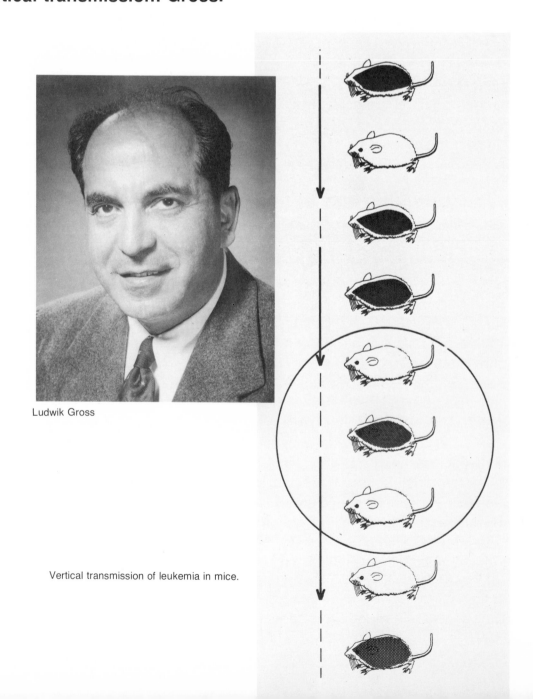

ONCOGENIC VIRUSES

SECOND EDITION
COMPLETELY REVISED AND ENLARGED

by

LUDWIK GROSS, M.D., F.A.C.P.

*Chief, Cancer Research Unit
Veterans Administration Hospital
Bronx, New York*

PERGAMON PRESS

OXFORD · LONDON · EDINBURGH · NEW YORK
TORONTO · SYDNEY · PARIS · BRAUNSCHWEIG

Gross, *Oncogenic Viruses*, 1970. Title page.

Ludwik Gross (born in 1904 in Krakow, Poland) in 1951 reported his discovery of the transmission of mouse leukemia by cell-free extracts inoculated into newborn mice, and the vertical transmission of the leukemic virus by passage of filtrates prepared from leukemic mouse organs. He had proposed as early as 1944 the concept of transmission of pathogenic agents from one generation to another, as in the passage of rickettsia through eggs in ticks.

In 1958 Gross reported the isolation of a transmissible, leukemogenic virus from radiation-induced leukemia in mice. He also isolated from leukemic mouse tissues an oncogenic virus causing parotid gland tumors and other neoplasms following inoculation into newborn mice, in parallel with similar studies by Stewart and Eddy.

Gross began cancer research during his postgraduate clinical years at the Pasteur Institute in Paris, from 1932 to 1939. He served in the Medical Corps of the United States Army, and since 1946 has been chief of the Cancer Research Unit of the Veterans Administration Hospital, Bronx, New York. He has been consultant and recipient of many honors for his research, including the WHO United Nations prize in 1962. He is the author of the now classical monograph, **Oncogenic Viruses**, first published in 1961 and in a second edition in 1970.

L. Gross. Spontaneous leukemia developing in C3H mice following inoculation, in infancy, with AK-leukemic extracts, or AK-embryos. **Proc. Soc. Exp. Biol. and Med.** 76: 27-32. 1951.

L. Gross. A filterable agent, recovered from AK leukemic extracts, causing salivary gland carcinomas in C3H mice. **Proc. Soc. Exp. Biol. and Med.** 83: 414-21, 1953.

L. Gross. **Oncogenic Viruses,** ed. 2. New York: Pergamon Press, 1970.

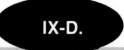

IX-D.

Oncogenic Viruses

IX-D-4. Polyoma virus: Stewart and Eddy.

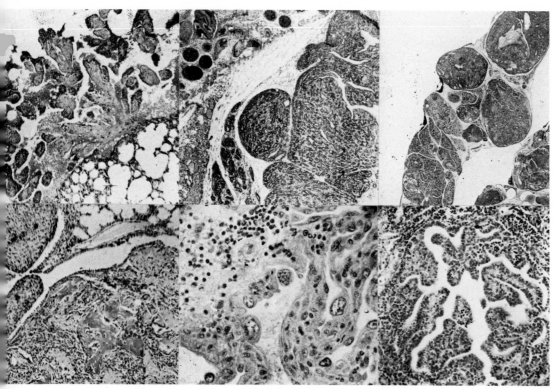

Some tumors induced by the Polyoma virus, left to right, upper: mesothelioma; hair follicle and mammary cancer; parotid tumor. lower: metastatic osteogenic sarcoma; endothelial tumor; proliferative lesion of kidney tubules.

The identification of the polyoma virus by Sarah E. Stewart and Bernice E. Eddy of the National Institutes of Health, is a milestone in viral carcinogenesis.

Studies initiated by Ludwik Gross between 1951 and 1953, and carried along similar but separate lines by Stewart, resulted in simultaneous publications on the production of salivary (parotid) tumors in newborn C3H mice inoculated with cell-free extract of leukemic tissues from AKR strain mice. Subsequent reports by Stewart further delineated neoplasms in hybrid mice, inoculated shortly after birth with cell-free extracts or filtrates prepared from leukemic mouse tumors, specifically of parotid and adrenal gland origins.

Ensuing investigations, published in 1957 by Stewart, Eddy, and their coworkers, showed that minced mouse parotid tumors cultivated on monkey kid-

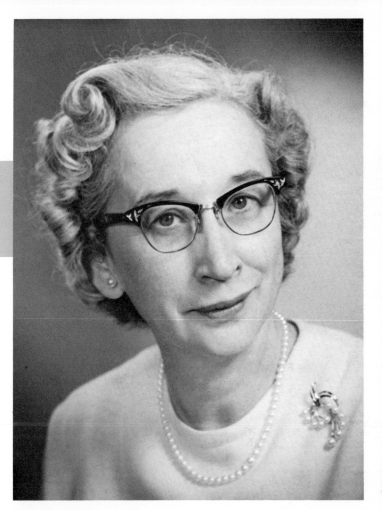

Sarah E. Stewart

ney cells **in vitro** and on chick chorioallantoic membranes resulted in propagation of a virus.

The oncogenic versatility of this agent in hamsters, rabbits, rats, guinea pigs, and other rodents later led to its being named "polyoma" and to its full characterization under a wide spectrum of experimental conditions. In work reported during this era, purified DNA isolated from the polyoma virus was found to be infective.

Sarah Elizabeth Stewart was born in 1906 in Mexico. She obtained a Ph.D. in bacteriology from the University of Chicago in 1939 and an M.D. from Georgetown University School of Medicine, Washington, D.C., in 1949. Her professional career was at the National Institutes of Health.

Bernice Elaine Eddy was born in 1903 in West Virginia, and obtained her doctorate in bacteriology from the University of Cincinnati, Ohio, in 1927. She performed bacteriological studies on leprosy for the U.S. Public Health Service and was assigned to the National Institutes of Health in 1937.

S. E. Stewart. Leukemia in mice produced by a filterable agent present in AKR leukemic tissues, with notes on a sarcoma produced by the same agent. **Anat. Rec.** 117: 532, 1953.

S. E. Stewart. Neoplasms in mice inoculated with cell-free extracts of filtrates of leukemic mouse tissue. I. Neoplasms of the parotid and adrenal glands. **J. Natl. Cancer Inst.** 15: 1391-1415, 1955.

S. E. Stewart, B. E. Eddy, and N. G. Borgese. Neoplasms in mice inoculated with a tumor agent carried in tissue culture. **J. Natl. Cancer Inst.** 20: 1223-43, 1958.

B. E. Eddy et al. Tumors induced in hamsters by injection of Rhesus monkey kidney cell extracts. **Proc. Soc. Exp. Biol. Med.** 107: 191-7, 1961.

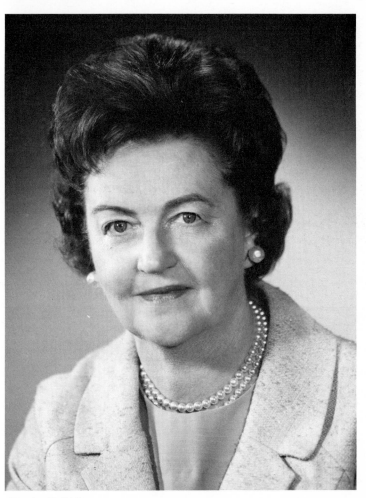

Bernice E. Eddy

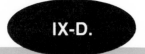

Oncogenic Viruses

IX-D-5. Human adenovirus tumors: Trentin.

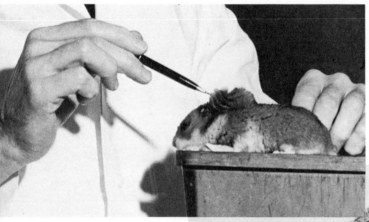

Hamster injected with human adenovirus type 12 during first week of life; a sarcoma arose at the site of injection within 2 months.

Intranuclear crystalline array of human adenovirus type 12 particles growing in HeLa cell culture.

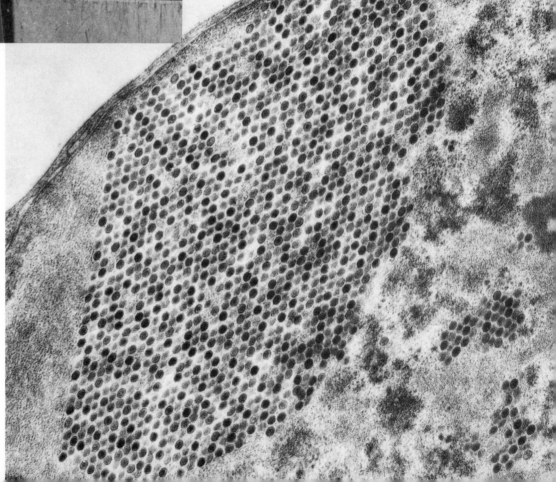

In 1962, John J. Trentin, Yoshiro Yabe and Grant Taylor reported that "in hamsters injected intrapulmonarily with tissue culture fluid of human type 12 adenovirus within 24 hours after birth there was a very high incidence of malignant tumors at the site of injection in from 1 to 3 months. The tumor-inducing activity was not lost by filtration . . ." No tumors were obtained with adenovirus types 2, 3, 7, 7a, 9, 10, 11 and 14, nor with appropriate control materials, and the possibility of contamination with polyoma virus and simian virus 40 was excluded by a variety of tests.

This was the first demonstration of oncogenic activity of a human virus. Subsequent work failed to establish that adenoviruses were associated with cancer in man, indicating that the oncogenic property is not manifested in the natural host.

John J. Trentin (born in 1918 in New Jersey), received his doctorate in endocrinology at the University of Missouri in 1947. He joined the faculty of Baylor College of Medicine in Houston in 1954, and since 1960 has been Professor of Experimental Biology.

John J. Trentin, Yoshiro Yabe and Grant Taylor. The quest for human cancer viruses. **Science** 137: 835-41, 1962.

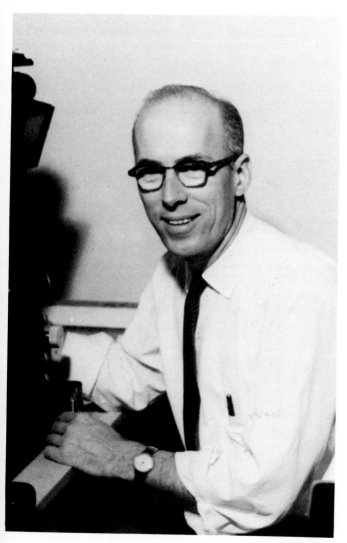

John J. Trentin (1962)

IX-D.

Oncogenic Viruses

IX-D-6. Oncologic virology comes of age.

The publication of a special journal, **Virology**, can be used as a marker in the development of virology as a scientific discipline. The first number of the first volume, of May, 1955, started with an article by Francis O. Holmes, appropriately on tobacco mosaic virus. The first article on oncogenic virus, by Harry Rubin, was printed in the last issue of the volume; appropriately, it concerned Rous chicken sarcoma.

A historic gathering of virologists and proponents of the viral etiology of cancer occurred at the M. D. Anderson Institute in Houston, Texas, as participants in a symposium on fundamental research in 1957.

Oncologic virology expanded rapidly as the scientific community recognized its research opportunities. The availability of effective vaccines against poliomyelitis turned the attention of many virologists who had worked on poliomyelitis toward problems of neoplasia. By 1960 specifically designated funds for viral oncology to the National Cancer Institute led to the development of a program centered around a task force on virus research.

The First Twenty Years of the University of Texas M. D. Anderson Hospital and Tumor Institute. Houston, Texas: M. D. Anderson Institute, 1964.

Eleventh Annual Symposium on Fundamental Cancer Research. **Texas Rep. Biol. Med.** 15: 431-826, 1957.

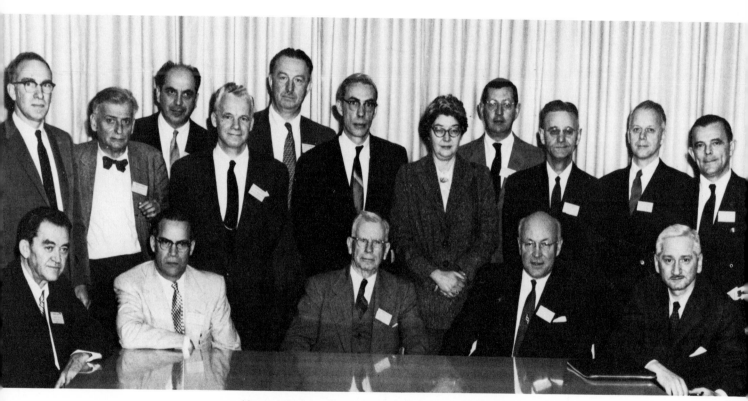

Many of the proponents of the theory on the viral etiology of cancer met at a 1957 symposium at the M. D. Anderson Hospital in Houston. **Seated,** left to right: J.W. Beard, John Bittner, Ernest Goodpasture, W.M. Stanley, and A.B. Sabin. **Standing:** B.R. Burmester, Francisco Duran-Reynals, Ludwik Gross, J.T. Syverton, George Gey, W.R. Bryan, Alice E. Moore, E.A. Evans, Howard Adervont, George Woolley, and Leon Dmochowski.
(Copyright, M.D. Anderson Institute, reproduced by permission).

IX-E.

Chemical Carcinogens

IX-E-1. Acetaminofluorene: Wilson, DeEds and Cox.

Robert H. Wilson (1903-   ) and Floyd DeEds (1894-   ), both of the U. S. Western Regional Agriculture Laboratory, and Alvin J. Cox, Jr. (1907-   ) of the Department of Pathology, Stanford University School of Medicine at San Francisco, uncovered in 1941 the carcinogenic effect of 2-acetaminofluorene (N-2-fluorenylacetamide; 2-FAA). In 1940, 2-FAA received a U. S. patent for use as an insecticide. The studies of the Wilson group revealed that the compound had no demonstrable acute toxicity for rats. Among the chronic toxic effects in rats fed continuously with food containing 2-FAA were malignant epithelial proliferations of bladder, renal, pelvic, hepatic, pancreatic, and lung tissues. Subsequent studies on 2-FAA have provided valuable insights into the mechanisms of action of chemical carcinogens. It is one of the "indirect" carcinogens requiring metabolic conversion in the liver to the N-hydroxy derivative.

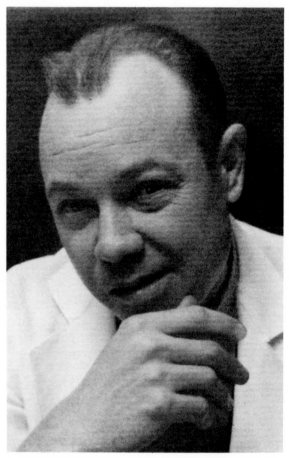

Robert H. Wilson

R. H. Wilson, F. DeEds and A. J. Cox, Jr. Toxicity and carcinogenic activity of 2-acetaminofluorene. **Cancer Res.** 1: 595-608, 1941.

E. K. Weisburger and J. H. Weisburger. Chemistry, carcinogenicity and metabolism of 2-fluorenamine and related compounds. **Adv. Cancer Res.** 5: 331-431, 1958.

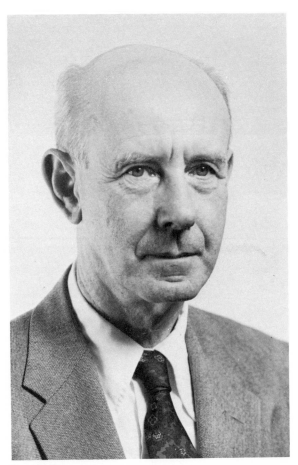

Floyd DeEds

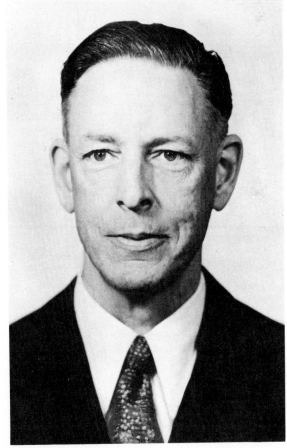

Alvin J. Cox

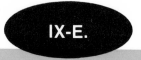

IX-E.

Chemical Carcinogens

IX-E-2. Urethane: Nettleship and Henshaw.

Anderson Nettleship (1910-   ) and Paul S. Henshaw (1902-   ), assisted by Henry L. Meyer, in 1943, issued from the National Cancer Institute a report on the carcinogenic activity of urethane (ethyl carbamate) in mice. This finding was unanticipated in the original experiment; it emerged as an accidental discovery based upon alert observation. Mulitple pulmonary tumors were detected in 26 of 29 mice anesthetized through intraperitoneal injections of urethane, preliminary to skin exposures to X-irradiation. Strain C3H mice used in these experiments have a low incidence of spontaneous lung tumors. The possibilities of carcinogenesis by direct radiation or through scattered radiation were subsequently eliminated. Direct tests defined urethane as the carcinogenic factor. Subsequent long-term tests on mice and rats showed that urethane induces hepatomas and other tumors as well as those in the lung.

The biochemical and physiologic action of urethane carcinogenesis has not been elucidated. Experimentation with analogues has not revealed chemical intermediates that exceed the carcinogenic capacities of urethane itself. Urethane was the first carcinogen to have been demonstrated to be active transplacentally on the fetus. For several years urethane was used as a chemotherapeutic agent in leukemia and multiple myeloma, but there are no reports of carcinogenic hazards to man.

A. Nettleship and Paul S. Henshaw. Induction of pulmonary tumors in mice with ethyl carbamate (urethane). **J. Natl. Cancer Inst.** 4: 309-19, 1943.

Sidney S. Mirvish. The carcinogenic action and metabolism of urethan and N-hydroxyurethan. **Adv. Cancer Res.** 11: 1-42, 1968.

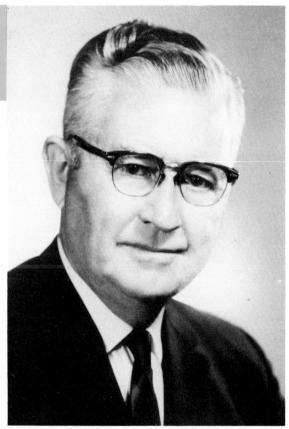

Paul S. Henshaw

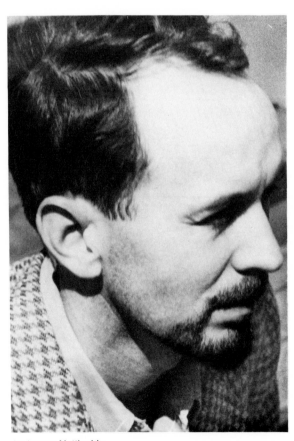

Anderson Nettleship

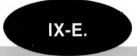

Chemical Carcinogens

IX-E-3. Nitrosamines: Magee and Barnes.

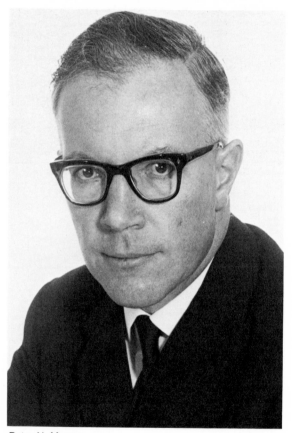

Peter N. Magee

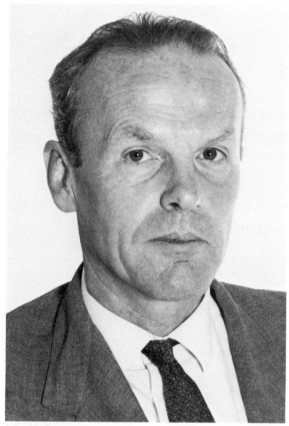

John M. Barnes

DIMETHYLNITROSAMINE

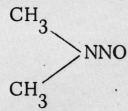

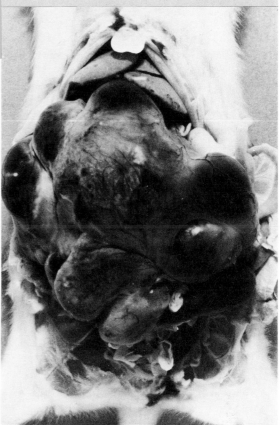

Kidney tumor in a rat 9 months after a single dose of dimethylnitrosamine, 125 μg, administered during the first 24 hours of life.

Peter N. Magee (1921-   ) and John M. Barnes (1913-   ), at the Medical Research Council (M.R.C.) Unit for Research in Toxicology (Carshalton, Surrey, England) in 1956 reported evidence for liver carcinogenesis by dimethylnitrosamine (DMN). Previous investigations (1954) by Magee and Barnes disclosed that DMN is severely toxic. Doses of 25 mg/kg, administered orally or parenterally, produced extensive liver damage in rats.

In the carcinogenesis experiments, albino rats were fed a normal diet containing 50 ppm DMN, which induced a very high incidence of liver tumors, many with metastatic spread. Subsequently, a number of different N-nitroso compounds have been reported by other workers to induce tumors in many organs of a wide range of animal species. DMN and other nitrosamines have proved to be very valuable agents for the study of experimental carcinogenesis.

P. N. Magee and J. M. Barnes. The production of malignant primary hepatic tumors in the rat by feeding dimethylnitrosamine. **Brit. J. Cancer** 10: 114-22, 1956.

P. N. Magee and J. M. Barnes. Carcinogenic nitroso compounds. **Adv. Cancer Res.** 10: 163-246, 1967.

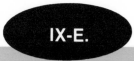

IX-E.

Chemical Carcinogens

IX-E-4. Nitroso analogues: Druckrey.

Hermann Druckrey (1904-) received his education in Giessen, Heidelberg, and Leipzig. In 1942, he became professor of pharmacology and toxicology at the University of Berlin, and by 1965, he became Director of Forschergruppe Praeventivmedizn, a foundation of Deutsche Forschungsgemeinschaft, Freiburg.

Druckrey has devoted his career to research in cancer biochemistry, chemotherapy, and carcinogenesis. His systematic studies on the relationships between chemical structure, dose, time, route of administration, and the condition of the host have been especially fruitful with N-nitroso compounds, hydrazo-, azo-, and azoxylalkanes, and triazenes. He and his co-workers recorded their important findings in a long series of papers during the 1960's in **Naturwissenschaften** and in **Zeitschrift für Krebsforschung.**

Nitrosamine carcinogenesis gained significance when it was shown that such compounds occur in foods and in cigarette smoke, and that they were formed in food in the presence of nitrites. These compounds are among candidates as environmental carcinogens in human cancer, especially of the gastrointestinal tract.

H. Druckrey, R. Preussman, S. Ivankovic, and D. Schmähl. Organotrope carcinogene Wirkungen bei 65 verschiedenen N-Nitroso-Verbindungen an BD-Ratten. **Z. Krebsforsch.** 69: 103-201, 1967.

Editorial. Nitrites, nitrosamines and cancer. **Lancet** 1: 1071-2, 1968.

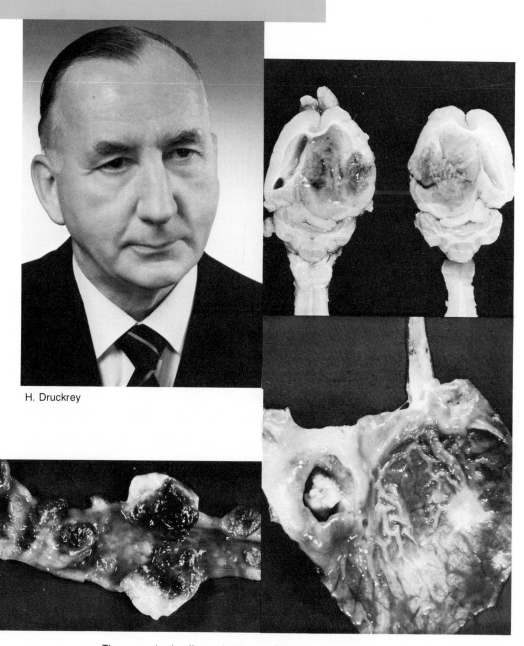

H. Druckrey

Three neoplastic effects of nitroso compounds: Upper, brain glioma in a rat following a single transplacental dose of ethylnitrosourea; center, gastric carcinoma in a guinea pig fed methylnitrosourathan; Lower, multiple adenocarcinomas of the colon in a rat given subcutaneous injections of azoxymethane.

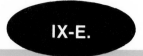

IX-E.

Chemical Carcinogens

IX-E-5. Cocarcinogenesis: Shear and Berenblum.

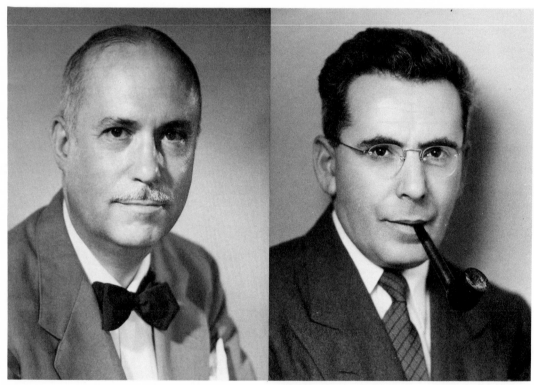

M.J. Shear   I. Berenblum

Murray Jacob Shear, of the National Cancer Institute, reported in 1938 that a basic fraction of creosote oil enhanced the production of mouse skin tumors by 3:4-benzpyrene. He considered this fraction to be the source of a "co-carcinogen." Subsequent investigations by Shear and his associates uncovered cocarcinogenic action of several fractions with other carcinogens.

Shear was born in 1899 in Brooklyn, New York, and received his doctorate in biochemistry from Columbia University in 1925. He joined the Office of Cancer Investigations at Harvard in 1931, and continued in cancer research until his retirement. He tested polycyclic hydrocarbons synthesized by L. F. Fieser and isolated a polysaccharide from **Serratea marcescens** of Coley's toxin that had antitumor effects.

Isaac Berenblum (1903-), of the Weizmann Institute of Science (Rehovot, Israel) and formerly of the Dunn School of Pathology (Oxford University, England), in 1941 reported the cocarcinogenic properties of croton oil resin. If a mouse receives a single skin painting of a carcinogen such as 20-methylcholanthrene, only a few papillomas are produced. Later repeated paintings of the site, however, will induce skin carcinomas in almost all animals. Croton oil itself is not carcinogenic. This work suggested a multistage mechanism underlying the effect of croton oil in the development of epidermal neoplasms. The two-stage hypothesis of cocarcinogenic action was extended by quantitative studies.

Berenblum devoted his life to cancer research and his contributions extended into many phases of biology and pathology of experimental cancer.

M. J. Shear. Studies in carcinogenesis. V. Methyl derivatives of 1:2-benzanthracene. **Am. J. Cancer** 33: 499-537, 1938.

R. D. Sall and M. J. Shear. Studies in carcinogenesis. XII. Effect of the basic fraction of creosote oil on the production of tumors in mice by chemical carcinogens. **J. Natl. Cancer Inst.** 1: 45-55, 1940.

I. Berenblum. The mechanism of carcinogenesis: A study of the significance of carcinogenic action and related phenomena. **Cancer Res.** 1: 807-14, 1941.

I. Berenblum and P. Shubik. A new quantitative approach to the study of the stages of chemical carcinogenesis in the mouse's skin. **Brit. J. Cancer** 1: 383-91, 1947.

IX-E.

Chemical Carcinogens

IX-E-6. Chemical carcinogen index: Hartwell and Shubik.

In 1941, there appeared from the National Cancer Institute the multilithed **Survey of Compounds Which Have Been Tested for Carcinogenic Activity**, by Jonathan L. Hartwell. This compilation of 696 compounds indicated 169 as active. The Survey was expanded for a second edition in 1951, which appeared in 1963 (Washington, D.C., Government Printing Office, Public Health Service Publication No. 149, 1951). In it, Hartwell tabulated data on 1329 compounds, of which 322 were reported as having carcinogenic activity.

The third and fourth editions, listed as Supplement 1 and 2, were prepared by Philippe Shubik and Hartwell, and were printed in 1957 and 1969. Three subsequent updates were prepared for the National Cancer Institute under contracts, and appeared as volumes "1961-1967," "1970-1971," under the same title and printer, retaining the identification of P.H.S. Publication 149. The

later volume contains 1667 pages. These Surveys are an important resource for investigators and other workers concerned with chemical carcinogens.

Jonathan L. Hartwell was born in Boston in 1906 and obtained his doctorate in chemistry from Harvard in 1935. He was with the National Cancer Institute from 1938 until his retirement in 1975. He is shown holding the 1969 volume.

Philippe Shubik was born in London in 1921 and received his doctorate in medicine from Oxford in 1949. He was Professor of Oncology at the Chicago Medical School, 1960-1968, Director of the Eppley Institute and Eppley Professor of Oncology and Pathology, of the College of Medicine of the University of Nebraska, Omaha.

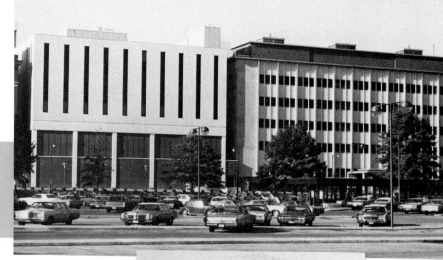

Eppley Institute, Omaha, Nebraska.

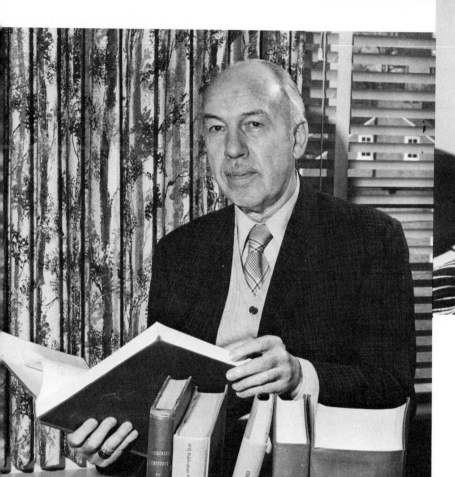

J.L. Hartwell

Philippe Shubik

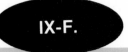

Natural Carcinogenic Products

IX-F-1. Aflatoxin: Lancaster, Halver and Wogan.

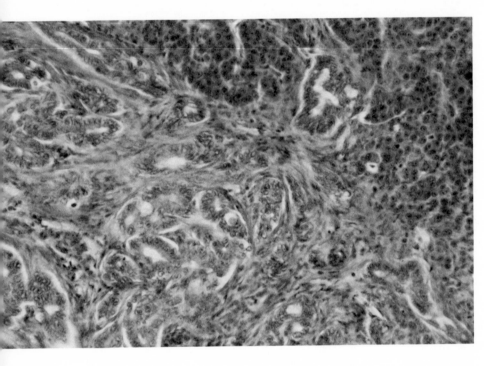

A hepatoma induced with aflatoxin in a trout.

Aflatoxin is a historical landmark in chemical carcinogenesis. It is a potent environmental carcinogen from "natural" sources rather than from industrial contaminants or synthetic chemistry.

In 1961, there occurred two epizootic outbreaks. In England, thousands of turkey poults, ducklings and chicks died of hepatic necrosis. In the northwestern United States, rainbow trout, the favorite game fish of the region, died with hepatomas. Initially, there was no evident relationship between these outbreaks.

The fowl epidemic of hepatotoxicity was traced quickly to food sources, then to peanut meal, and finally to the contamination of the food by a common fungus, **Aspergillus flavus**. M. C. Lancaster, F. P. Jenkins, and J. McL. Philp, of the Unilever Laboratories in England, fed rats with food containing the toxic material and, in 6 months, 9 of 11 survivors developed hepatomas.

Two teams of chemists, one in England and the other in the United States, isolated and identified the active chemi-

experiments were arranged. Hepato-magenic fish diets were sent to Gerald N. Wogan at the Massachusetts Institute of Technology, Cambridge, Massachusetts, for analysis for aflatoxin, and aflatoxin was likewise sent to Halver for feeding to trout. Crystalline aflatoxin B_1 prepared by Wogan produced hepatomas in rainbow trout, and there was an almost perfect

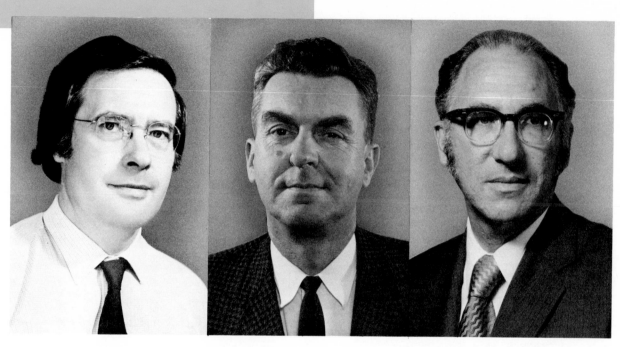

M.C. Lancaster   John E. Halver   Gerald N. Wogan

cals, the aflatoxins (**A. flavus toxins**). These compounds, on a molecular-weight basis, are among the most active hepatocarcinogens in the rat; they produce sarcomas at the site of subcutaneous injection and have other carcinogenic effects.

Hepatomas in trout also were rapidly related to food sources. Fractionation of fish diets for the carcinogen was initiated by John E. Halver at the Western Fish Nutrition Laboratory of the United States Department of Interior at Cook, Washington. Isolation of aflatoxin from **A. flavus** contamination of poultry food kept under warm, humid conditions pointed to the possibility of a similar etiology of trout hepatomas.

To test this relationship, concurrent

relationship between the appearance of hepatomas in trout and the aflatoxin content in the food.

Epidemiological investigations in Africa and in Thailand show correlations between the prevalence of hepatoma in man and the aflatoxin levels in the food. Aflatoxicosis thus may be an important environmental carcinogenic hazard for man.

H. F. Kraybill and M. B. Shimkin. Carcinogenesis related to foods contaminated by processing and fungal metabolites. **Adv. Cancer Res.** 8: 191-248, 1964.

M. C. Lancaster, F. P. Jenkins and J. McL. Philp. Toxicity associated with certain samples of groundnuts. **Nature** 192: 1095-96, 1961.

J. E. Halver and I. A. Mitchell, eds. **Trout Hepatoma, Research Conference Paper No. 70,** United States Department of the Interior, Fish and Wildlife Service, Washington, D.C. 1967.

G. N. Wogan, ed. **Mycotoxins in Foodstuffs.** Cambridge, Mass.: MIT Press, 1965.

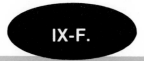

IX-F.

Natural Carcinogenic Products

IX-F-2. Cycasin: Laqueur and Matsumoto.

Observations, from 1950 to 1953, of an unusually high incidence of amyotrophic lateral sclerosis and other neurological disorders endemic to Guam were subsequently (1963) correlated with the ingestion of cycad nut meal. This discovery was accomplished by epidemiological investigations, especially those of Leonard T. Kurland and Marjorie G. Whiting. The cycad (**Cycas circinalis**) is a plant indigenous to the Mariana Islands, and cycad varieties occur widely from the Japanese Archipelago to the subcontinent of India. The plant is of local economic importance as a source of foodstuffs, fiber, and medicinal products. The studies of Kurland and Whiting suggested the possibility of the existence of a neurotoxic agent in the nut meal and edible starch extracted from cycad roots, stems, and leaves.

In 1963 Gert L. Laqueur (born 1912, Strasbourg, France), Chief, Laboratory of Experimental Pathology at the National Institute of Arthritis and Metabolic Diseases, and his associates uncovered carcinogenic activity in the cycad. Crude nut meal from **C. circinalis** fed to rats failed to elicit neurological symptoms but induced cancers of the liver, kidney, and intestinal tract. This work indicated that a glycoside isolated from cycads, and known as cycasin, might yield in its metabolic breakdown a compound with a carcinogenic potential similar to that of dimethylnitrosamine (DMN). This inference was supported by comparable pathological alterations in rats fed toxic cycad nut meal and those reported for rats treated with DMN. Collateral investigations revealed that cycasin was ineffective as a hepatotoxin and a hepatocarcinogen when administered to germfree rats.

A later report by Laqueur and his co-workers showed that a metabolic degra-

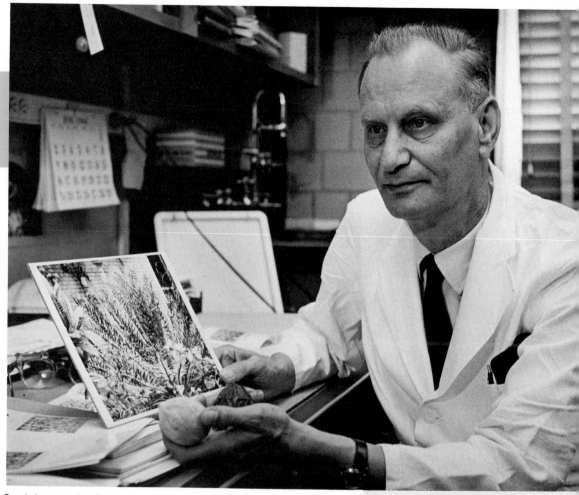

Gert L. Laqueur, holding picture of *Cycas circinalis* and its nut.

dation via β-glucosidase of bacterial origin in the intestinal tracts of rats released the aglycone, a potent carcinogen. The aglycone of cycasin, methylazomethanol (MAM) and the synthetic aglycone acetate ester produced tumors in germfree animals, thus establishing MAM as the proximate carcinogen. The chemical work was done by Hiromu Matsumoto (born 1920, Honolulu, Hawaii) and his group at the Department of Agricultural Chemistry, University of Hawaii.

G. L. Laqueur, O. Mickelsen, M. Whiting, and L. T. Kurland. Carcinogenic properties of nuts from *Cycas circinalis* L. indigenous to Guam. **J. Natl. Cancer Inst.** 31: 919-51, 1963.

G. L. Laqueur, E. G. McDaniel, and H. Matsumoto. Tumor induction in germfree rats with methylazoxymethanol (MAM) and synthetic MAM acetate. **J. Natl. Cancer Inst.** 39: 335-71, 1967.

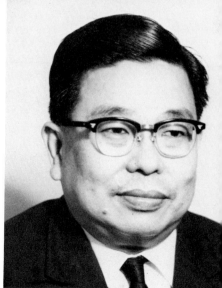

H. Matsumoto

IX-F.

Natural Carcinogenic Products

IX-F-3. Bracken fern: Pamukcu and Price.

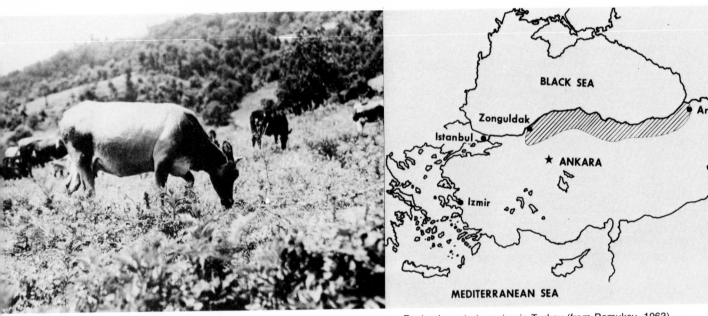

Typical wooded mountainous area of endemic disease occurrence of enzootic hematuria in cattle.

Bovine hematuria region in Turkey (from Pamukcu, 1963)

Enzootic hematuria of cattle occurs in most countries of the world. The disease is usually confined to small, well-defined areas and occurs in cattle raised in mountainous, wooded wastelands. A. M. Pamukcu demonstrated that the serious problem of enzootic hematuria in cattle and water buffalo along the Black Sea area of Turkey was a manifestation of carcinoma of the urinary bladder.

Initial epidemiological studies convinced Pamukcu that an environmental factor was involved, it being the common fern of the mountain forests (**Pteris aquilina**). Collaborative investigations between Pamukcu and J. M. Price extended the field studies. Cattle from non-disease areas around Ankara were fed bracken fern from mountainous farms where the problem existed. Bladder cancer was induced in virtually all cattle that survived for more than 3 years on a feeding regimen patterned after the field observations. The induced bladder cancers were indistinguishable from the disease seen under natural conditions.

Bracken fern feeding also produces intestinal and urinary cancers in rats and leukemia and pulmonary tumors in mice.

A. M. Pamukcu was born in 1912 in Turkey. He received a D.V.M. degree from the University of Ankara, Turkey, in

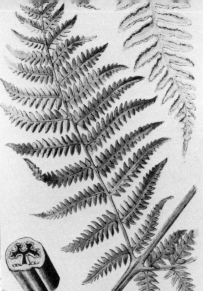

Bracken fern

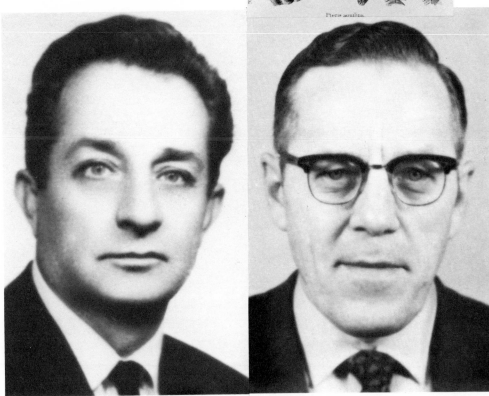

A.M. Pamukcu

James M. Price

1938, and Ph.D. in Animal Pathology from Michigan State University, East Lansing, in 1948. In 1957 he became professor at the University of Ankara and in 1959 was made chairman of the Department of Pathology, Faculty of Veterinary Medicine, at the University.

James M. Price was born in 1921 in Wisconsin. He received a Ph.D. in physiology, and an M.D. degree from the University of Wisconsin, where he joined the faculty. In 1957 he obtained the first American Cancer Society-sponsored

Lifetime Professorship in Cancer Research and in 1967 joined Abbott Laboratories as Director of Experimental Therapy.

A. M. Pamukcu, S. K. Göksoy and J. M. Price. Urinary bladder neoplasms induced by feeding bracken fern (*Pteris aquilina*) to cows. **Cancer Res.** 27: 917-24, 1967.

A. M. Pamukcu, E. Ertürk, J. M. Price and G. T. Brown. Lymphatic leukemia and pulmonary tumors in female Swiss mice fed bracken fern (*Pteris aquilina*). **Cancer Res.** 32: 1442-5, 1972.

A. M. Pamukcu. Epidemiologic studies on urinary bladder tumors in Turkish cattle. **Ann. N.Y. Acad. Sci.** 108: 938-47, 1963.

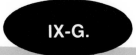

Hormones

IX-G-1. Steroid hormones: Allen and Gardner.

Edgar Allen (1892-1943) was an internationally known authority on the physiology of sex and reproduction and was one of the best-known anatomists of his era. He demonstrated, in 1923, that the ovarian follicle was a source of a hormone, which was extracted and purified in collaboration with E. A. Doisy. Allen was born in Colorado and obtained his doctorate in anatomy from Brown University at Providence, Rhode Island, in 1921. He was with the School of Medicine of Washington University in St. Louis, Missouri from 1919 to 1933, and then became professor of anatomy at Yale University in New Haven, Connecticut.

William Ullman Gardner (1907-   ), an associate of Allen, succeeded him as professor of anatomy at Yale University. Gardner has made many contributions to our knowledge of the role of steroid hormones in neoplasia, of the role of heredity to hormonal and neoplastic responses, and of hormonal imbalance in tumorigenesis. His influence extends through his students, many of whom made their initial discoveries under his guidance. Gardner was born in Minnesota and obtained his Ph.D. from the University of Missouri in 1933.

The interest in steroid hormone carcinogenesis, of course, involved many cancer research workers in the United States and Europe.

E. Allen and W. U. Gardner. Cancer of cervix of the uterus in hybrid mice following long-continued administration of estrogen. **Cancer Res.** 1: 359-66, 1941.

W. U. Gardner. Studies on steroid hormones in experimental carcinogenesis. **Recent Prog. Hormone Res.** 1: 217-59, 1947.

W. U. Gardner. Hormonal imbalances in tumorigenesis. **Cancer Res.** 8: 397-411, 1948.

M. B. Shimkin. Hormones and neoplasia. In, R. W. Raven (ed), **Cancer**, Vol. 1, p. 161-213. London: Butterworth, 1957.

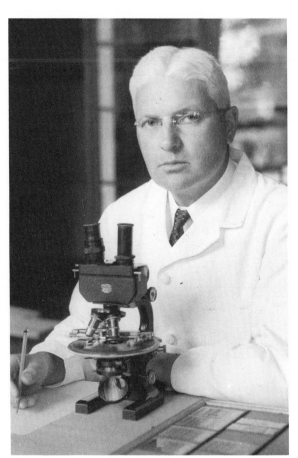

Edgar Allen

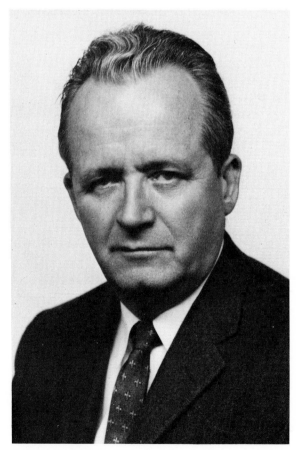

William U. Gardner

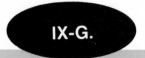

Hormones

IX-G-2. Pituitary hormones: Evans and Li.

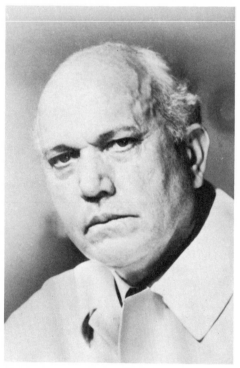

H.M. Evans

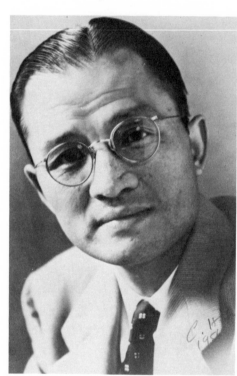

C.H. Li

The understanding of the role of the anterior pituitary gland secretions in normal and abnormal growth has been advanced by the work of H. M. Evans and C. H. Li, both of the University of California at Berkeley and San Francisco.

Herbert M. Evans (1882-1971), born in Modesto, California, was educated at the University of California and Johns Hopkins University, graduating with an M.D. in 1908. In 1915, Evans became affiliated with the Department of Anatomy at the University of California, where he engaged in teaching and in research on reproduction physiology, hormones, and vitamins until his final retirement in 1966. With J. A. Long, he described the estrous cycle in the rat in 1921, produced gigantism in rats with anterior pituitary fractions in 1922, and separated the growth-promoting substance in 1939.

Choh Hao Li (1913-), a native of China, graduated from the University of Nanking in 1933. He received a doctorate in chemistry from the University of California, Berkeley, in 1938. His whole career has been spent at the University of California where, since 1950, he has been professor of biochemistry, professor of experimental endocrinology, and director of the Hormone Research Laboratory. Since 1938, he has devoted his research to the biochemical aspects of the pituitary hormones, initially collaborating with Evans in the studies. Through the efforts of Li and his associates, as well as those at other laboratories, all of the 10 adenohypophyseal hormones have now been isolated, and the primary structure of 9 has been elucidated. The list includes interstitial cell-stimulating hormone, 1940; lactogenic hormone, 1942; bovine growth hormone, 1944; adrenocorticotropic hormone, 1953; β-melantropin, 1956; follicle-stimulating hormone, 1964; and β-lipotropin, 1965. Human growth hormone was isolated and purified in 1956 and its structure determined in 1966. In 1970, Li and D. Yamashiro succeeded in synthesizing a protein with human growth hormone activities. The work on the chemical biology of pituitary hormones was summarized by Li in 1972.

Herbert M. Evans. The function of the anterior hypophysis. **Harvey Lectures** 19: 212-35, 1923-24.

C. H. Li and D. Yamashiro. The synthesis of a protein possessing growth-promoting and lactogenic activities. **J. Am. Chem. Soc.** 92: 7608-9, 1970.

C. H. Li and L. Gráf. Human pituitary growth hormone: isolation and properties of two biologically active fragments from plasmin digests. **Proc. Nat. Acad. Sci.** (USA) 71: 1197-1201, 1974.

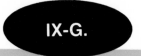

Hormones

IX-G-3. Hormonal imbalance: Biskind and Biskind.

M. S. Biskind and G. R. Biskind in 1944 reported the development of granulosa cell tumors of the ovary in female rats that were castrated and had one ovary transplanted into the spleen.

This interesting physiological method of inducing tumors of the endocrine tissues dependent upon anterior pituitary stimulation was based upon the following facts. Castrated rats with an ovary transplanted to the spleen remain anestrous, due to inactivation in the liver of estrogen thus secreted into the portal circulation. The resultant low levels of estrogen in the general circulation induce the production of increased levels of pituitary gonadotropic hormones, stimulating the ovary in the spleen.

In the original experiment, all of nine rats by 12 months following the operation had ovarian masses in the spleen that on histologic examination were tumors of the granulosa cell type. Subsequently, it was found that the transplanted ovary first formed masses of corpora lutea. These transformed into a luteoma, and then the granulosa cell tumor arose in the luteoma. Later research showed that testicular interstitial cell tumors were induced by similar splenic transplants in male rats. Retention of one ovary or testis in normal position, or the supply of exogenous steroid hormones, prevented the neoplastic formation.

Morton Sidney Biskind, born in Cleveland, Ohio, in 1906, a medical graduate of Western Reserve University in 1930, was a research endocrinologist at the Beth Israel Hospital in New York. His career has been in pharmacology, endocrinology and nutrition and tumor research. Since 1950 he has been in the private practice of medicine in Westport, Connecticut.

Gerson R. Biskind, born in Cleveland, Ohio, in 1908, is a cousin of M. S. Biskind. He is a graduate of the University of California Medical School, in 1932, and after training in pathology at the University of California Hospital and at Mt. Zion Hospital in San Francisco has conducted research, teaching and service in pathology at these institutions.

M. S. Biskind and G. R. Biskind. Development of tumors in the rat ovary after transplantation into the spleen. **Proc. Soc. Exp. Biol. and Med.** 55: 176-79, 1944.

G. R. Biskind, D. E. Bernstein and S. M. Gospe. The effect of exogenous gonadotropins on the development of experimental ovarian tumors in rats. **Cancer Res.** 13: 216-20, 1953.

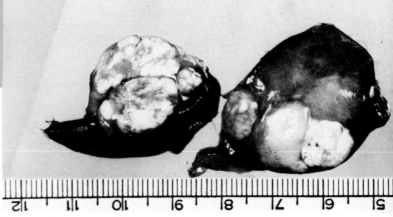

Cross section of a tumor in the spleen in a rat, 625 days following transplant of an ovary into the spleen and removal of the other ovary, showing nodules of granulosa cells in a luteoma.

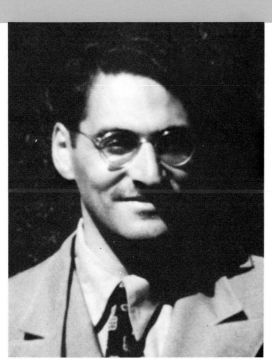

M.S. Biskind

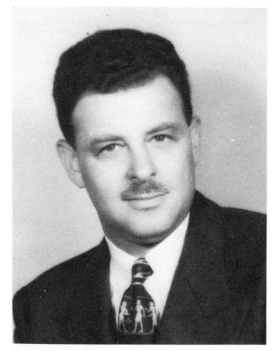

G.R. Biskind

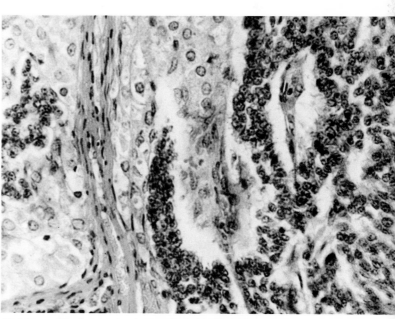

Histology of the tumor, showing small, dark cells of the granulosa cell tumor on the right, and the larger luteoma cells on the left.

IX-G.

Hormones

IX-G-4. Role of pituitary in carcinogenesis: Mühlbock.

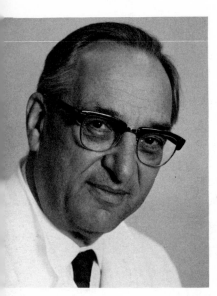

Otto Mühlbock

Otto Mühlbock (1906-   ) was educated at the University of Berlin, obtaining a Ph.D. in chemistry in 1927 and an M.D. in 1933. He specialized in gynecology and endocrinology, as assistant to Ernest Laqueur in Amsterdam from 1935 to 1940. After the war he joined the staff of the Antoni van Leeuwenhoek Huis (The Netherlands Cancer Institute) in Amsterdam.

Mühlbock's scientific contributions have centered around the problem of hormones as carcinogenic agents. Work on ovarian tumors (with R. van Nie), hypophyseal tumors (with H. G. Kwa), and especially mammary tumors in mice served as models. Mühlbock, in collaboration with L. M. Boot and G. Röpcke, developed a system to induce mammary tumors in mice with isografts of pituitaries, thus demonstrating that these tumors can develop in the absence of an active virus. For comparative studies, he and W. van Ebbenhorst Tengbergen developed a number of inbred strains of mice of European origin. Mühlbock and P. Bentvelzen found that one of these, the GR strain, proved to be of special interest because of the mammary tumor virus (MTV) variant which is transmitted not only by milk but also by the genome. With A. Dux he demonstrated that the genetic resistance against MTV, located in the mammary gland, is associated with a diminished replication of the virus. This resistance was shown to be related to a certain allele of the **H-2** locus.

The Netherlands Cancer Institute, Amsterdam.

The Netherlands Cancer Institute was founded with the help of private funds in 1913 on the premise that the only way to conquer cancer is for clinical observation and basic research to be closely combined. Named after the 17th Century Dutch scientist Antoni van Leeuwenhoek, it was begun as a research clinic with a limited number of beds, with the selection of cancer patients made in accordance with the research interests of the clinicians; for many years the emphasis was on research on mammary cancer. The Institute is managed by a committee that handles the administrative and financial affairs of its 390 clinical and laboratory workers. Having outgrown its original housing in Amsterdam, in a Napoleonic military hospital, it was moved to new facilities on the outskirts of Amsterdam.

Antoni van Leeuwenhoek Hospital, Amsterdam.

O. Mühlbock and L. M. Boot. Induction of mammary cancer in mice without the mammary tumor agent by isografts of hypophyses. **Cancer Res.** 19: 402-12, 1959.

IX-G.

Hormones

IX-G-5. Diethylstilbestrol cancer in man: Herbst et al.

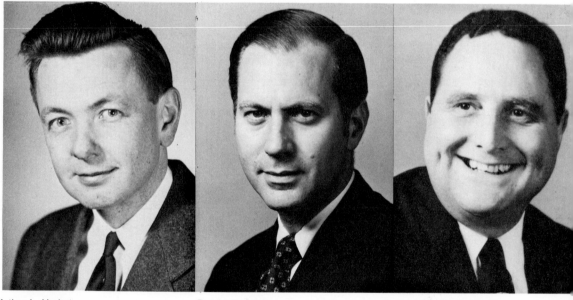

Arthur L. Herbst   Robert E. Scully   David C. Poskanzer

The multiple carcinogenic properties of estrogens are easily demonstrable in experimental animals. In man, however, data on carcinogenic effects of estrogens were uncertain until 2 reports were released from a group of investigators in Boston, on the association of adenocarcinoma of the vagina with maternal diethylstilbestrol therapy.

·   Arthur L. Herbst (born 1931 in New York City), associate professor of obstetrics and gynecology, and Robert E. Scully (born 1921 in Pittsfield, Mass.), professor of pathology, reported 7 cases of adenocarcinoma of the vagina in adolescent girls.

This clustering of a rare tumor in an unusual age group during a period of 4

Poskanzer (born 1929 in Albany, N. Y.), associate professor of neurology, was the epidemiologist for the project. Herbst, Ulfelder, and Poskanzer published a definitive report in 1971. In 7 of 8 cases, there was a history of diethylstilbestrol administration to the mother during pregnancy. Of 32 matched control women, none had received diethylstilbestrol during pregnancy. The therapy for these patients was administered between 1946 and 1951.

Thus, the orally potent, nonsteroidal estrogen, diethylstilbestrol, given during pregnancy, exerted an effect on the fetus that became clinically evident 14 to 22 years later. Although the initial studies suggest a small risk to the exposed offspring, it is possible that the full story at older ages and among males may change these estimates. The effect of dose and other specific factors also require more study. Herbst and his colleagues are continuing their studies in this area and have established a Registry to study the epidemiological, pathological, and therapeutic details of cases of these cancers that are occurring throughout the world. Over 100 such cases have been reported to them to 1974.

The data already are unequivocal that diethylstilbestrol is carcinogenic for man during the gestational period and that its use during pregnancy, therapeutically or in food sources, should not be tolerated.

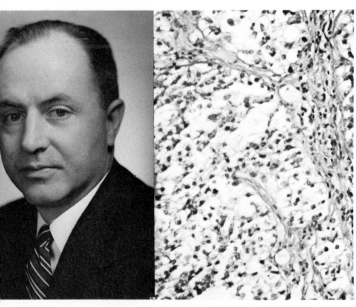

Howard Ulfelder   Photomicrograph of an adenocarcinoma
of the vagina (Case 6
of Herbst and Scully, 1970).

years led to the design of a classical retrospective, case-control epidemiological study. The undertaking of a study was suggested by Howard Ulfelder (born 1911 in Mexico City), professor of gynecology, after the mother of one of his patients with vaginal adenocarcinoma indicated that she had taken diethylstilbestrol during her pregnancy. David C.

A. L. Herbst and R. E. Scully. Adenocarcinoma of the vagina in adolescence. **Cancer** 25: 745-57, 1970.

A. L. Herbst, H. Ulfelder and D. C. Poskanzer. Adenocarcinoma of the vagina: association of maternal stilbestrol therapy with tumor appearance in young women. **New England J. Med.** 284: 878-81, 1971.

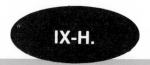

IX-H.

Biochemistry of Cancer

IX-H-1. Biochemistry of cancer: Greenstein.

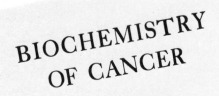

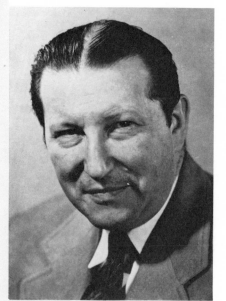

Jesse P. Greenstein

Greenstein, Biochemistry of Cancer, 1947. Title page.

Biochemistry, as a pursuit of professional stature, was added to the oncological sciences by Otto Warburg by 1930. Forays into the chemistry of cancer before that time have been criticized as blunders committed by poor oncology and bad chemistry. A compilation of the work was made by Stern and Wilheim in 1943.

Jesse P. Greenstein (1905-1959), on the basis of 20 years of intensive work, attempted to analyze and synthesize oncologic biochemistry in his important monograph, **Biochemistry of Cancer**, which appeared in 1947 and in a revised and enlarged edition in 1954. Working primarily with transplantable tumors in rodents, and analyzing the enzymes of the tissues, Greenstein concluded that tumors as a biochemical class converged toward each other rather than having the diversity of normal tissues.

Greenstein was born in New York City, and obtained his doctorate in biochemistry from Brown University in 1930. He held various teaching posts during the great economic depression, and finally stabilized himself and his family in 1939 as one of the earlier Research Fellows of the newly-created National Cancer Institute. A prodigious worker and writer, he rose to the position of Chief of the Laboratory of Biochemistry in 1946. Author of some 300 papers on enzymology, nucleoproteins and aminoacid resolution, he initiated the **Advances in Cancer Research** annual with Alexander Haddow and was honored by many prizes and membership in the National Academy of Sciences (USA).

Otto Warburg. **The Metabolism of Tumors.** London: Constable and Co., 1930.

Kurt Stern and Robert Willheim. **Biochemistry of Malignant Tumors.** Brooklyn, N.Y.: Reference Press. 1943.

J. P. Greenstein. **Biochemistry of Cancer.** Ed. 2. New York: Academic Press, 1954.

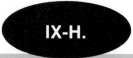

IX-H.

Biochemistry of Cancer

IX-H-2. Metabolism of carcinogens: Millers and Weisburgers.

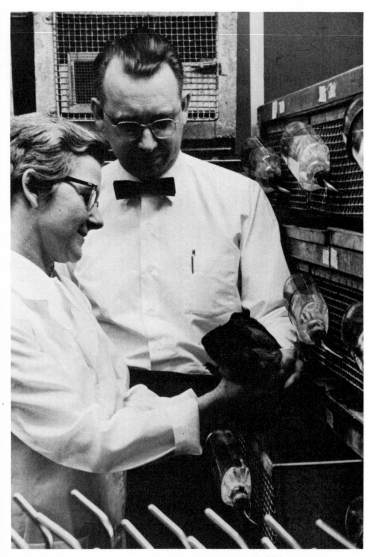

James and Elizabeth Miller

James Alexander Miller and his wife, Elizabeth Cavert Miller, were among the pioneer investigators of the metabolism of carcinogenic chemicals, especially in the aminoazo dyes. These chemicals produce hepatomas of the liver in rats and in mice, but are inactive at the site of application, indicating that they require metabolic conversion to a carcinogen. The Millers established that a key activation reaction is hydroxylation on the nitrogen to form the corresponding hydroxylamine derivatives.

James Miller was born in 1915 in Pennsylvania and obtained his doctorate in biochemistry from the University of Wisconsin in 1943. His wife, Elizabeth, was born in 1920 in Minnesota and obtained her doctorate at Wisconsin in 1945. Their careers were at the McArdle Laboratory for Cancer Research at the University of Wisconsin, Madison.

John Hans Weisburger and Elizabeth K. Weisburger were prominent contributors to the chemistry and metabolism of carcinogenic compounds, using the fluorenamines as their primary material. Their studies also established the concept of indirect carcinogenesis and the role of the host's metabolic mechanisms in the reactions.

John Weisburger was born in Germany in 1921, and obtained his doctorate in organic chemistry at the University of Cincinnati in 1949. Elizabeth Weisburger was born in Pennsylvania in 1924 and obtained her doctorate at Cincinnati in 1947. They worked at the National Cancer Institute, Bethesda, Maryland, 1949 to 1972, when John Weisburger became vice-president for research at the American Health Foundation in New York City.

J. A. Miller and E. C. Miller. The carcinogenic aminoazo dyes. **Adv. Cancer Res.** 1: 339-96, 1953.

J. A. Miller and E. C. Miller. Chemical carcinogenesis: mechanisms and approaches to its control. **J. Natl. Cancer Inst.** 47: v-xiv, 1971.

E. K. Weisburger and J. H. Weisburger. Chemistry, carcinogenicity, and metabolism of 2-fluorenamine and related compounds. **Adv. Cancer Res.** 5: 331-431, 1958.

J. H. Weisburger and E. K. Weisburger. Biochemical formation and pharmacological, toxicological, and pathological properties of hydroxylamines and hydroxamic acids. **Pharmacol. Rev.** 25: 1-66, 1973.

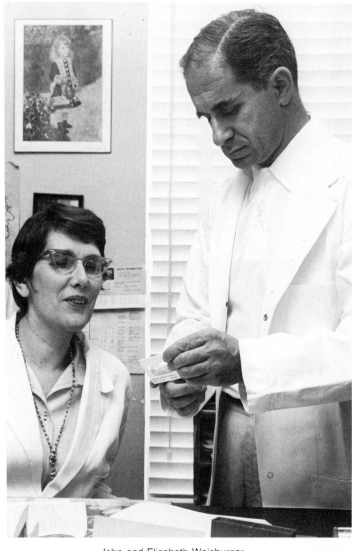

John and Elizabeth Weisburger

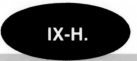

IX-H.

Biochemistry of Cancer

IX-H-3. Endocrine influences in carcinogenesis: Bielschowsky and Cantarow.

Endocrine factors in hepatocarcinogenesis in rats fed 2-acetylaminofluorene were discovered almost simultaneously by two groups of workers, F. Bielschowsky and Marianne Bielschowsky in New Zealand, and A. Cantarow and K. Paschkis in Philadelphia.

F. D. Bielschowsky (1902-1965), after medical service on the European Continent, migrated to Sheffield, England where, influenced by Dr. Georgiana Bonser, he turned his interests to cancer research, and began to study the involvement of endocrines in the action of the carcinogen 2-acetylaminofluorene. In 1949 he assumed the directorship of the Cancer Research Laboratory of the University of Otago in Dunedin, New Zealand, where Griesbach and Purves assisted in extending his approaches to include goitrogens and modifiers of carcinogen response. By elegant experimentation, applying parabiotic and endocrine-modified animal systems, he developed the now classic concept of pituitary-thyroid and pituitary-gonad-adrenal relationships.

Contemporary with these studies, a group at the Jefferson Medical College in Philadelphia developed similar, yet quite independent approaches in the area of endocrine influences in carcinogenesis. Abraham Cantarow (1901-   ) and Karl E. Paschkis (1896-1961), were also concerned with the mechanisms of endocrine influences in cancer induced by 2-acetylaminofluorene. They likewise utilized goitrogenic chemicals to study pituitary-thyroid relationships, and later, developed into the gamut of endocrine factors controlling the growth of tumors at various sites. They formulated the principle that normally functioning hyperplastic tissue does not cancerize as readily as non-functioning or abnormally functioning hyperplastic tissue. Also from their laboratory came the fundamental biochemical observation on differences in incorporation of uracil between hepatoma and normal liver which stimulated interest in the metabolism of pyrimidine nucleotides in cancer and led Charles Heidelberger to the development of 5-fluorouracil in cancer chemotherapy.

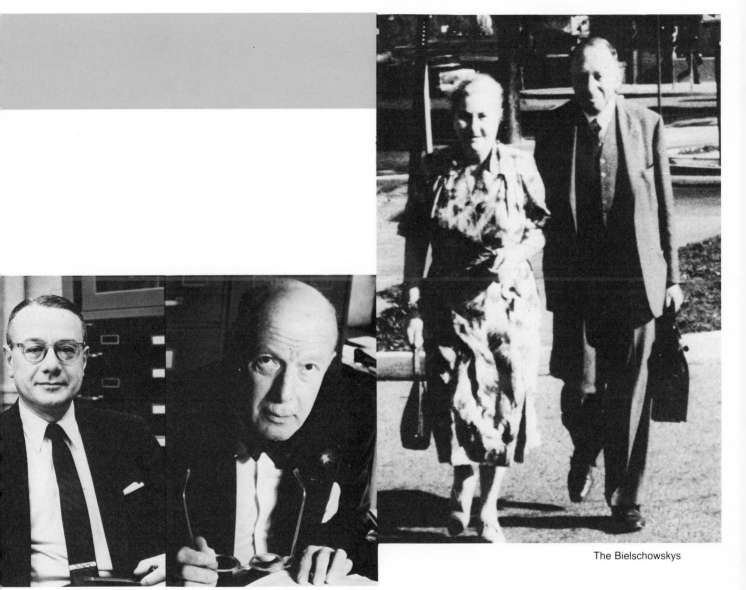

A. Cantarow

Karl E. Paschkis

The Bielschowskys

F. Bielschowsky. Neoplasia and internal environment. **Brit. J. Cancer** 9: 80-116, 1955.

A. Cantarow, K. E. Paschkis, J. Stasney and M. S. Rothenberg. The influence of sex hormones upon the hepatic lesions produced by 2-acetaminofluorene. **Cancer Res.** 6: 610-16, 1946.

R. J. Rutman, A. Cantarow and K. E. Paschkis. Studies in 2-acetylaminofluorene carcinogenesis: III. The utilization of uracil-2C^{14} by preneoplastic rat liver and rat hepatoma. **Cancer Res.** 14: 119-23, 1954.

IX-H.

Biochemistry of Cancer

IX-H-4. Biochemistry of hepatomas: Morris et al.

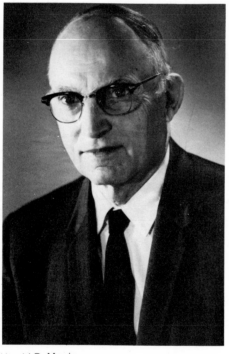

Harold P. Morris

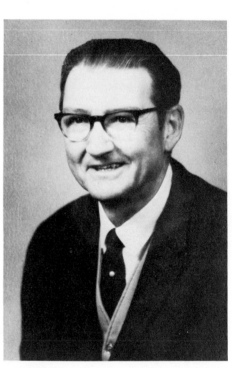

Van R. Potter

The discovery of the hepatomagenic activity of the azo dyes in rats, made by Yoshida in the mid-1930s, provided biochemists with a favorite material for studies in carcinogenesis. Livers are easily identified and removed, and fetal, adult and regenerating liver tissue can be compared with liver tissue following exposure to carcinogens.

The biochemical oncologic investiga-

tions were greatly facilitated by the patient work of Harold P. Morris, who was using a variety of chemical carcinogens at a variety of dose levels, and by careful transplantation selection, derived a large series of hepatomas with specific, producible characteristics of growth and other behavior. These tumors include the "minimal deviation" hepatomas, which despite their malignant biological behavior demonstrate few biochemical changes presumably associated with neoplastic growth.

The Morris hepatomas have been sent around the world to more than 150 interested biochemists. A collaborative

Indiana, in 1900. He obtained his doctorate in biochemistry and nutrition from the University of Minnesota in 1930. After serving with the Department of Agriculture and the Food and Drug Administration, Morris joined the staff of the National Cancer Institute in 1938, conducting research in biochemistry and nutrition in experimental oncology. In 1968, upon retirement from the National Cancer Institute, he became Research Professor of Biochemistry at the College of Medicine, Howard University, Washington, D.C.

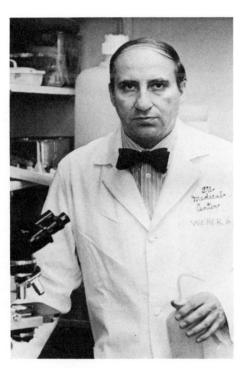

George Weber

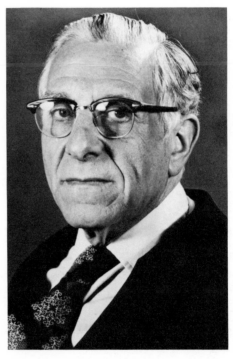

Sidney Weinhouse

group of research workers in the United States and Japan recorded their findings in a monograph. Among the many workers in the United States who have used the materials and participated in hepatoma research have been Van R. Potter of Wisconsin, George Weber of Indiana, and Sidney Weinhouse of Philadelphia.

Harold P. Morris was born in Salem,

Harold P. Morris and Billie P. Wagner. Induction and transplantation of rat hepatomas with different growth rate (including "minimal deviation" hepatomas). In Harris Busch, ed., **Methods in Cancer Research**, Vol. 4: 125-52. New York: Academic Press, 1968.

Biological and Biochemical Evaluations of Malignancy in Experimental Hepatomas. Gann Monograph 1, July 1966. Tokyo, Japan: Japanese Cancer Association, 1966.

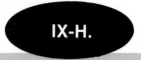

Biochemistry of Cancer

IX-H-5. Fetal antigens: Zilber and Abelev.

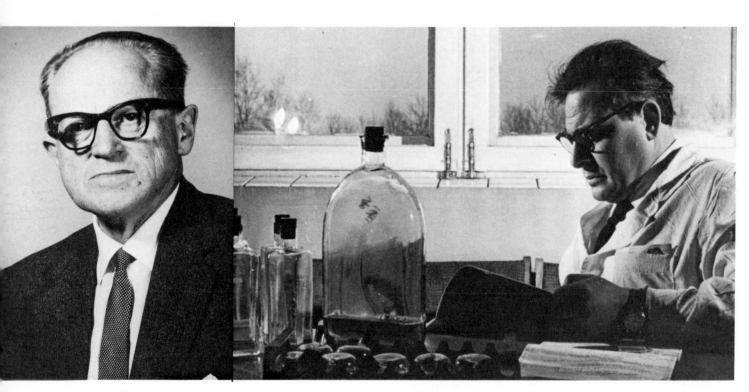

L.A. Zilber   G.I. Abelev

Lev Alexandrovich Zilber (1894-1966), doctor of medical sciences and member of the U.S.S.R. Academy of Medical Sciences, was the founder of the Russian school of viral oncology. A graduate of Moscow State University in 1919, his earlier experimental work was on autoserotherapy of typhus (1921), hereditary transformation of serotypes in **Proteus vulgaris** (1922-1923), and the replication of viruses in unnatural hosts, as vaccinia virus in yeast (1932-1934). He and his coworkers identified the tick-borne, summer-spring encephalitis of the Far East regions of the U.S.S.R. He began work on the virological aspects of cancer in 1944, heading the Department of Immunology and Virology of Tumors in the Gamaleya Institute of Epidemiology and Microbiology, Moscow.

Zilber and his associates described specific tumor antigens and the induction of tumors in mammals by Rous sarcoma virus.

The Selected Works of L. A. Zilber, edited by N. N. Blokhin (Meditsina, Leningrad, 1971), lists 11 monographs and over 260 articles published by Zilber.

G. I. Abelev (1928-   ) doctor of biological sciences and professor of biochemistry, graduated from Moscow State University in 1950. He was an assistant of Zilber, whom he succeeded as departmental chairman at the Gamaleya Institute in 1966. Abelev and his colleagues devoted their attention to tumor-specific antigens and demonstrated striking immunological individuality in mouse hepatomas.

The most important contribution from Abelev's groups was the 1963 discovery of embryo-specific α-globulin (α-fetoprotein, or AFP) in experimental hepatomas. This led to the development of an immuno-diagnostic test for hepatocellular carcinoma and teratocarcinoma in man.

L. A. Zilber. Specific tumor antigens. **Adv. Cancer Res.** 5: 291-329, 1958.

L. A. Zilber. Pathogenicity and oncogenicity of Rous sarcoma virus for mammals. **Prog. Exp. Tumor Res.** 7: 1-48, 1965.

G. I. Abelev. Antigenic structure of chemically-induced hepatomas. **Prog. Exp. Tumor Res.** 7: 104-157, 1965.

G. I. Abelev. Alpha-fetoprotein in oncogenesis and its association with malignant tumors. **Adv. Cancer Res.** 14: 295-358, 1971.

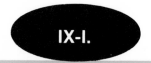

Tumor Immunology

IX-I-1. Cellular immunology: Burnet and Medawar.

Optimism regarding the solution of the cancer problem rests to a great extent on the application to oncology of scientific advances in immunology and virology. In turn, oncology is making contributions to immunology and virology.

The founders of modern immunology are F.M. Burnet and P. B. Medawar, who shared in the 1960 Nobel Prize in Physiology or Medicine "for their discovery of acquired immunological tolerance." Both have received many honors and have been knighted.

Frank Macfarlane Burnet was born in 1899 in Australia. He completed his medical course at Melbourne University, graduating M.B., B.S., in 1922 and M.D. in 1923.

His first research work on the agglutinin reactions in typhoid fever was begun in the Walter and Eliza Hall Institute of the Melbourne Hospital in 1923 and, except for periods overseas, all his professional career was in the Hall Institute, of which he was director from 1944 to 1965. In 1926-1927 he worked at the Lister In-

stitute, London, and in 1932-1933 he was at the National Institute for Medical Research, Hampstead, England.

Burnet's work has covered several fields but, until 1957, was primarily concerned with viral and rickettsial disease with special interest in influenza virus. He has had a continuing interest in immunology since his early work on staphylococcal toxin and antitoxin and is well known for his formulation of the clonal selection theory of antibody production.

Peter Brian Medawar was born in 1915, in Rio de Janeiro, Brazil, son of a naturalized British subject. He studied zoology at Oxford University and after graduation began his research at the School of Pathology at Oxford. In 1944 he became a University Lecturer in zoology at Oxford, but he left three years later to assume the post of Mason Professor of Zoology at the University of Birmingham. He continued his earlier work at Oxford on the mechanism of skin graft reactions in Birmingham with studies of ac-

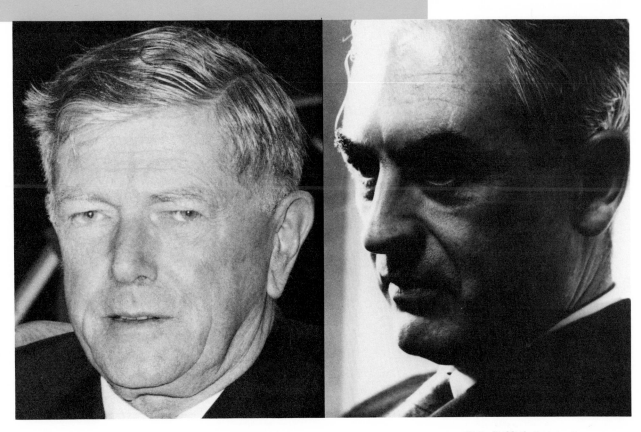

Frank Macfarlane Burnet   Peter B. Medawar

quired tolerance to skin grafts in cattle. In 1951 Medawar went to University College, London, as the Jodrell Professor of Zoology. In 1962 Medawar was appointed to his position as the director of the National Institute for Medical Research, Mill Hill, London.

The key references to the contributions of Burnet and Medawar are in their Nobel lectures.

Nobel Lectures. Physiology or Medicine 1942-1962. p. 681-715. New York: Elsevier Publishing Co., 1964.
F. M. Burnet. Immunological surveillance in neoplasia. **Transplant. Rev.** 7: 3-25, 1971.

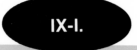

IX-I.

Tumor Immunology

IX-I-2. Tumor antigens: Klein and Prehn.

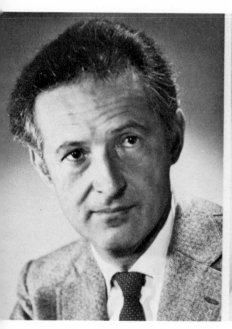

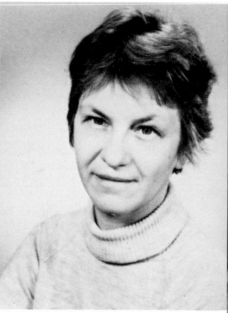

George and Eva Klein

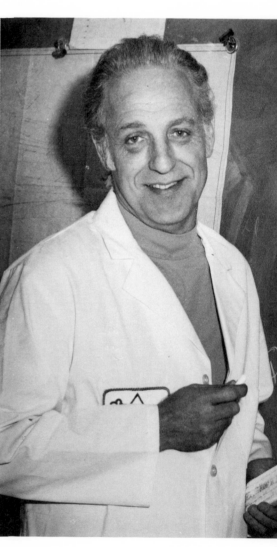

Richmond T. Prehn

Tumor-specific transplantation antigens are defined as cellular components capable of inducing host-rejection responses in autochthonous and syngeneic hosts. Evidence for this type of tumor immunity can be traced to several workers, but its clear demonstration is attributed to E. J. Foley in 1953. However, in the development of the field, much subsequent work was performed by George Klein, Eva Klein and their coworkers at the Karolinska Institutet in Stockholm, Sweden and by Richmond T. Prehn in the United States. The potentials of the work include the possible identification of specific tumor antigens, and the enhancement of effects in therapy.

George Klein was born in 1925, in Sweden, and obtained his doctorate at the Karolinska Institutet in Stockholm. He is professor of tumor biology at the Institutet.

Richmond Talbot Prehn was born in 1922 in New York City, and graduated with an M.D. degree in 1947 from the Long Island Medical College. He was with the National Cancer Institute, 1948-1956, with Washington University in Seattle until 1966, and then at the Institute for Cancer Research in Philadelphia, Pennsylvania. In 1976 he became Director of the Jackson Laboratory in Bar Harbor, Maine.

E. J. Foley. Antigenic properties of methylcholanthrene-induced tumors in mice of the strain of origin. **Cancer Res.** 13: 835-37, 1953.

G. Klein, H. O. Sjögren, E. Klein and K. E. Hellström. Demonstration of resistance against methylcholanthrene-induced sarcomas in the primary autochthonous host. **Cancer Res.** 20: 1561-72, 1960.

R. T. Prehn. Tumor-specific immunity to transplanted dibenz (a, h)-anthracene-induced sarcomas. **Cancer Res.** 20: 1614-17, 1960.

G. Klein. Tumor-specific transplantation antigens. **Cancer Res.** 28: 625-35, 1968.

IX-I.

Tumor Immunology

IX-I-3. Marek's disease vaccine: Biggs and Burmester.

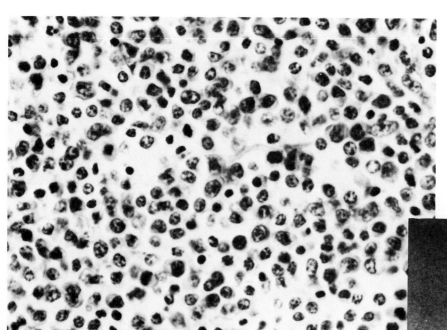

Marek's Disease histology

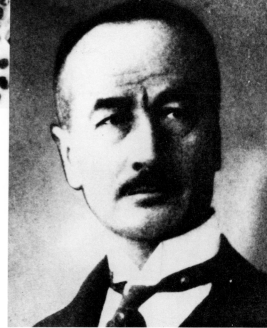

J. Marek

Marek's disease is a lymphoproliferative disease of the domestic chicken, which was first described by Joseph Marek (1868-1952) of Hungary in 1907. It is important to the poultry industry.

The infectious nature of Marek's disease was recognized from field experience. In 1967 the causative agent was shown to be a herpesvirus. Two years later pathogenic Marek's disease virus had been attenuated by growth in cultured cells and attenuated virus was shown experimentally to be an effective vaccine. In 1970 field trials established this as a safe and effective vaccine when used under commercial conditions. Soon after, a naturally apathogenic field Marek's disease virus and a herpesvirus from turkeys antigenically related to Marek's disease virus were also shown to be effective and safe vaccines. For various practical and commercial reasons, the herpesvirus of turkeys became the more widely used vaccine.

Two groups of investigators were primarily involved in these advances. Houghton Poultry Research Station at Huntingdon, England, introduced the earlier attenuated chicken virus vaccine. The Station was directed by Peter M. Biggs. Biggs was born in 1926, in Petersfield, Hampshire, and received his education in veterinary science at the Royal College of Veterinary Surgeons in London, and a doctorate at the University of Bristol in 1958. He was with the Houghton Poultry Research Station since 1959, and its director since 1974. Important contributions to the investigations were made by A. E. Churchill, who conducted the field trials of the vaccine, and L. N. Payne and R. C. Chubb.

Investigators at the Regional Poultry Research Laboratory of the U. S. Department of Agriculture at East Lansing, Michigan, conducted parallel studies and introduced the turkey virus vaccine. The Laboratory is directed by Ben Roy Burmester. Burmester was born in Petaluma, California, in 1910, and educated at the University of California, receiving a Ph.D. in 1936, and at Michigan State University, receiving a DVM in 1951. In 1940 he joined the Regional Poultry Research Laboratory at East Lansing and became its director in 1964. Important contributions to the investigations of Marek's disease were made by R. L. Witter, K. Nazerian, and H. G. Purchase.

J. Marek. Kakasokban (Polyneuritis in roosters). **Allatorvosi lapok, Budapest** 30: 315-18, 1907. (Translated in Deutsche **Tierärtl. Wchnschr.** 15: 417-21, 1907.)

K. Nazerian. Marek's disease, a neoplastic disease of chickens caused by a herpesvirus. **Adv. Cancer Res.** 17: 279-315, 1973.

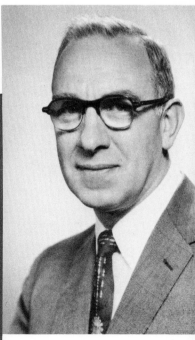

B.R. Burmester

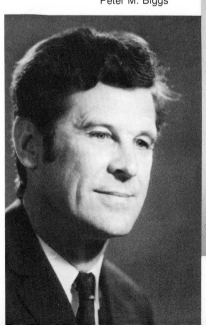

Peter M. Biggs

IX-I.

Tumor Immunology

IX-I-4. Tumor immunology comes of age.

On October 20, 1975, there was held a ceremony in New York City, under the auspices of the Cancer Research Institute of New York, honoring 15 scientists for their pioneer contributions to the field of cancer immunology. The recognitions were as follows:

Ludwig Gross (Veterans Administration Hospital, Bronx, N.Y.), Edward J. Foley (Schering Corporation, Bloomfield, N.J.), Richmond T. Prehn (University of Pennsylvania, Philadelphia, Pa.). For finding evidence that cancer cells have specific antigens that can elicit a cancer-destructive immune response.

Hans O. Sjögren (University of Lund, Lund, Sweden). For demonstrating that tumor viruses can impart antigens to the surface of cells they render cancerous, and so render them immunologically foreign.

Garri I. Abelev (Gamaleya Institute of Epidemiology and Microbiology, Moscow, U.S.S.R.). For the discovery that antigens that are normally evident only in the embryo may reappear in cancer (fetoproteins).

Robert J. Huebner (National Cancer Institute, Bethesda, Md.). For the recognition that viral antigens may persist in animal cancers from which the causative virus itself can no longer be recovered (T-antigens).

Donald L. Morton (School of Medicine, University of California, Los Angeles, Calif.). For studies on immunological tolerance, and clinical observations which relate immune capacity of cancer patients to their prognosis.

Edmund Klein (Roswell Park Memorial Institute, Buffalo, N.Y.). For the first reproducibly effective immunological therapy for a form of human cancer.

Robert A. Good (Sloan-Kettering Institute for Cancer Research, New York, N.Y.). For research on the immune deficiencies of cancer patients and the increased incidence of certain tumors in immunologically deficient patients.

Werner and Gertrud Henle (Children's Hospital, Philadelphia, Pa.). For immunological research which elucidated the relation of the Epstein-Barr herpes virus to Burkitt's lymphoma, and to the self-limiting proliferative disease, infectious mononucleosis.

George and Eva Klein (Karolinska Institutet, Stockholm, Sweden). For discoveries of tumor-specific antigens in the mouse, to the most comprehensive immunological analysis of a human cancer, Burkitt's lymphoma.

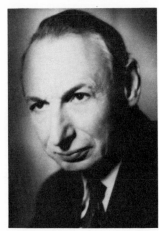

Peter A. Gorer

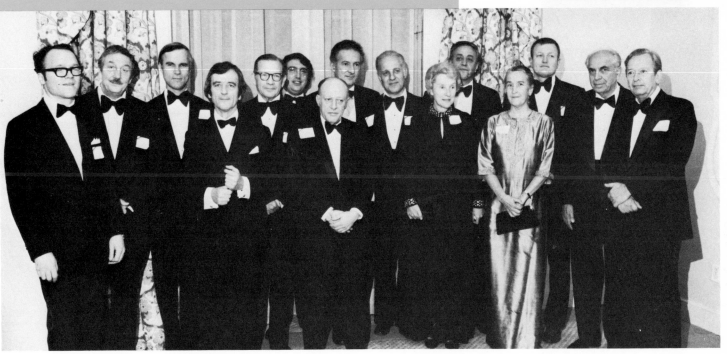

Tumor immunologists. Award ceremony, 1975.

Edward A. Boyse and Lloyd J. Old (Sloan-Kettering Institute for Cancer Research, New York, N.Y.). For studies on the antigenic composition of normal and malignant cells, and the way in which this is governed by cellular and viral genes.

In addition, a posthumous award was given to Peter A. Gorer (1907-61), of England for his basic work on the immunogenetic analysis of the mouse. A special William B. Coley Memorial Award was presented to Helen C. Nauts, executive director of the Cancer Research Institute of New York.

The photograph of the occasion includes, from left to right: Drs. Hans O. Sjögren, Robert J. Huebner, Lloyd J. Old,

Edward A. Boyse, Edward J. Foley, Peter A. Gorer, Jr. (for his father), Edmund Klein, George Klein, Richmond T. Prehn, Gertrud Henle, Robert A. Good, Helen C. Nauts, Donald L. Morton, Ludwik Gross and Werner Henle.

Not present were Garri Abelev and Eva Klein.

The photograph of Peter Gorer is reproduced by permission from Jan Klein, **Biology of the Mouse Histocompatability-2 Complex**, New York: Springer-Verlag, 1975. Gorer's contributions are memorialized by Peter B. Medawar, in the **Biographical Memoirs of Fellows of the Royal Society**, 7:95-109, 1961.

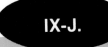

Diagnosis of Cancer

IX-J-1. Vaginal cytology: Papanicolaou and Traut.

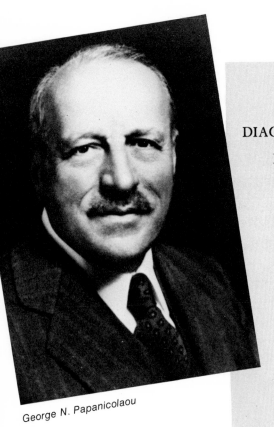

George N. Papanicolaou

DIAGNOSIS OF UTERINE CANCER

BY THE VAGINAL SMEAR

GEORGE N. PAPANICOLAOU, M.D., Ph.D.
Department of Anatomy, Cornell University Medical College

AND

HERBERT F. TRAUT, M.D.
*Department of Obstetrics and Gynecology, Cornell
University Medical College and the New York Hospital*

NEW YORK: THE COMMONWEALTH FUND
1943

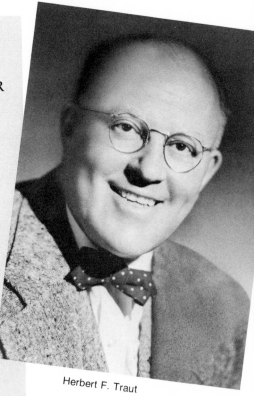

Herbert F. Traut

Papanicolaou and Traut, *Diagnosis of Uterine Cancer by the
Vaginal Smear,* 1943. Title page.

The clinical diagnosis of cancer is based upon histologic criteria developed by pathologists during the 19th Century. Such criteria are obtained from the examination under a microscope of a relevant piece of tissue, or exudated cells, from the suspected lesion.

Long before the techniques of imbedding, cutting and staining tissues became commonplace in the pathology laboratory, observations were made on individual cancer cells. The return to cytologic diagnosis of cancer was made by G. N. Papanicolaou and H. F. Traut in the 1940s, with the publication of their correlative studies on the use of the method for cancer of the uterine cervix.

George Nicholas Papanicolaou (1883-1962), born and educated in Greece, pursued his scientific career at Cornell Medical College, New York. He studied the cellular aspects of the vaginal content of animals and humans, and thereby correlated cytologic changes with physiologic states. Papanicolaou, by 1928, suggested the relevance of his method to the diagnosis of uterine cancer. An identical suggestion was made also in 1928 by Aurel A. Babes, of the Faculty of Medicine of Bucharest, as indicated by Douglass.

Herbert Frederick Traut (1894-1963) was the clinical collaborator of Papanicolaou. Traut was on the faculty of Cornell Medical College, and later became professor and head of the Department of Obstetrics and Gynecology at the University of California Medical School in San Francisco. The combined efforts of Papanicolaou and Traut established the efficacy and simplicity of the method in the diagnosis of preclinical uterine cancer, and introduced the "Pap smear" as a clinical and public health measure. Since the procedure does recognize an important cancer before it is invasive, its full application would significantly reduce mortality from cervical cancer.

G. N. Papanicolaou and H. F. Traut. **Diagnosis of Uterine Cancer by the Vaginal Smear.** New York: Commonwealth Fund, 1943.

G. N. Papanicolaou. New cancer diagnosis. **Third Race Betterment Conf. Proc.** pp. 528-34. Battle Creek, Mich.: Race Betterment Fdn., 1928. (Reproduced in **CA** 23: 171-79, 1973.)

L. E. Douglass. A further comment on the contributions of Aurel Babes to cytology and pathology. **Acta Cytologica** 11: 217-24, 1967.

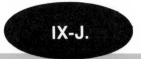

IX-J.

Diagnosis of Cancer

IX-J-2. Breast cancer detection: Gershon-Cohen and Shapiro.

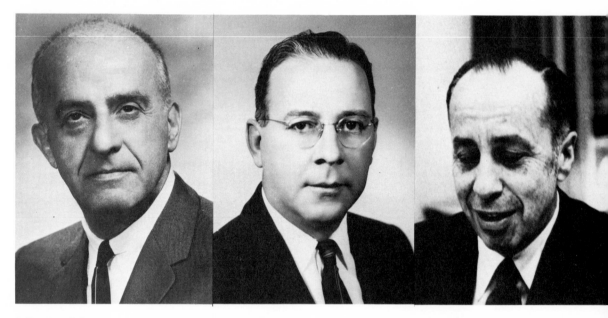

J. Gershon-Cohen   Robert L. Egan   Sam Shapiro

Soft-tissue X-ray mammography for breast cancer diagnosis was revived in the United States by Jacob Gershon-Cohen (1898-1970) of Philadelphia and Robert L. Egan (1920-   ) while he was at the M. D. Anderson Hospital in Houston. A systematic application of X-ray mammography as a **screening** method for breast cancer, in combination with clinical palpation of the breast, was undertaken by three investigators at the Health Insurance Plan of Greater New York, under contract with the National Cancer Institute. The question was whether periodic screening results in lower breast cancer mortality.

Mammography and clinical examination were performed in 31,000 women, 40-64 years old, selected and invited for screening, of whom two-thirds accepted; comparison was with 31,000 women in a matched control group. After five years of

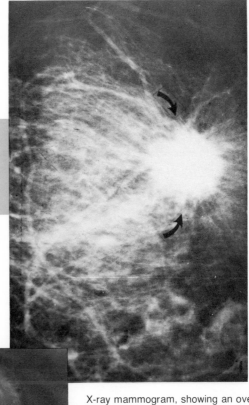
X-ray mammogram, showing an overt cancer.

Philip Strax   Louis Venet

follow-up, there was a significant reduction in mortality from breast cancer in the study group women: 40% versus 63%. Reduced mortality was concentrated among women 50 years of age or older.

The study was a model of a systematic, designed field evaluation of a screening procedure for cancer.

Sam Shapiro, B.S., born in New York City in 1914, was vice-president and director of the Department of Research and Statistics of the Health Insurance Plan of Greater New York. Philip Strax, M.D., was the chief radiologist and Louis Venet, M.D. was the supervising surgeon of the study.

J. Gershon-Cohen, M. B. Hermel and S. M. Berger. Detection of breast cancer by periodic X-ray examinations. A five-year survey. **J. Am. Med. Assn.** 176: 1114-16, 1961.

R. L. Egan. Experience with mammography in a tumor institution. **Radiology** 75: 894-900, 1960.

S. Shapiro, P. Strax and L. Venet. Periodic breast cancer screening in reducing mortality from breast cancer. **J. Am. Med. Assn.** 215: 1777-85, 1971.

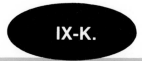

Cancer Surgery

IX-K-1. Supraradical procedures: Pack and Brunschwig.

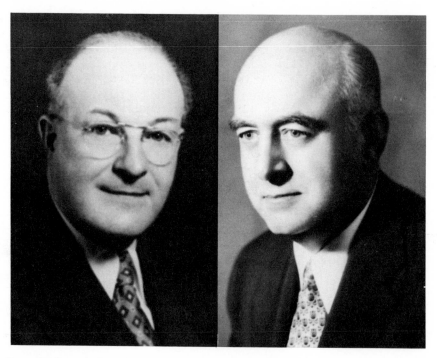

Alexander Brunschwig   George T. Pack

By the last quarter of the 20th Century, surgery and radiotherapy remained the curative methods of cancer therapy for all but a small proportion of patients. The primary treatment of over 60% of all patients with cancer was by surgery.

Surgery for cancer reached its apogee after World War II, with better control of shock, blood replacement and antibiotics making possible incursions and excisions of ever greater extent.

Two American surgeons are selected as examples of cancer surgery during this period. Both were connected with the Memorial Hospital for Cancer and Allied Diseases in New York for much of their professional life.

George Thomas Pack (1898-1969) was a proponent and practitioner of radical operations for cancer. His views are gathered in the massive volumes he edited from 1940 to 1964. A native of Ohio, Pack graduated from Yale University School of Medicine in 1922.

Alexander Brunschwig (1901-1969) also developed extensive resections, including pelvic exenteration for advanced carcinoma of the cervix. Brunschwig was

agement of colostomy following resection of rectal cancer, speech restoration following removal of laryngeal cancer, and muscular and psychological rehabilitation following radical mastectomy were among the more frequent, important procedures.

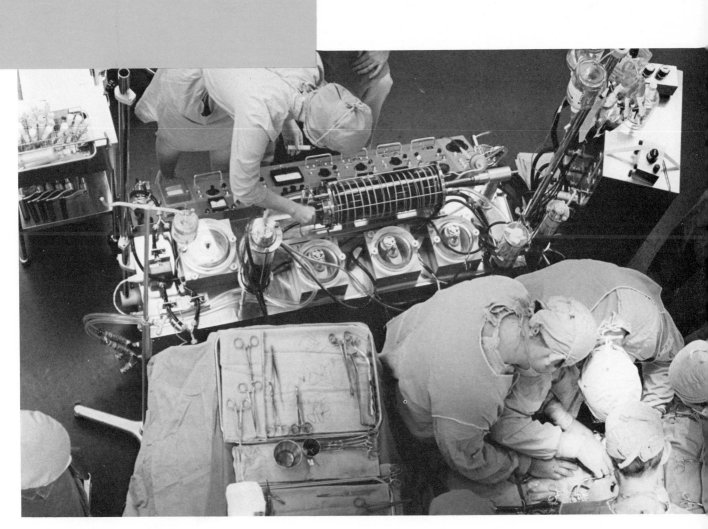

Surgery at the Clinical Center, National Institutes of Health, 1972.

born in Texas, and obtained his M.D. degree from Rush Medical College of the University of Chicago in 1927. Perhaps the limit of the surgical approach was reached in hemicorporectomy.

As the number of successfully treated patients rose, problems of rehabilitation became of increasing importance. Programs were developed in the use of devices and retraining of salvaged cancer patients, such as those of Dietz at the Memorial Hospital. The care and man-

George T. Pack and Irving M. Ariel (eds). **Treatment of Cancer and Allied Diseases.** Ed. 2, 9 vols. New York: Paul B. Hoeber, 1958-1964.

Alexander Brunschwig and William Daniel. The surgical treatment of cancer of the cervix uteri. **Am. J. Obst. and Gyn.** 75: 875-81, 1958.

T. R. Miller, A. R. MacKenzie and H. T. Randall. Translumbar amputation for advanced cancer: indications and physiologic alterations in four cases. **Ann. Surg.** 164: 514-21, 1966.

J. Herbert Dietz, Jr. Rehabilitation of the cancer patient. **Med. Clin. N. A.** 53: 607-24, 1969.

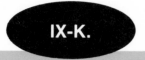

IX-K.

Cancer Surgery

IX-K-2. Challenge to radical surgery: McWhirter and Crile.

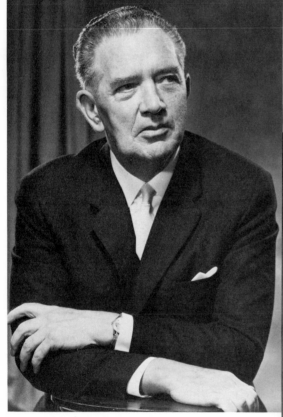

Robert McWhirter

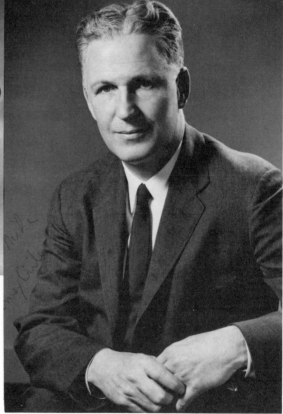

George Crile, Jr.

Mastectomy for breast cancer, one of the oldest surgical procedures for cancer, typifies the surgical approach to malignant disease. The removal of the breast en bloc with its lymphatic drainage and its muscle attachments, as developed by William S. Halsted in 1894, was the acknowledged technique for over a half-century. Procedures were developed to extend the operation, especially to include the internal mammary chain of lymphatics for cancers arising medial to the nipple. Statistical support for the more extensive (supraradical) operations, in comparison with the results of more limited resections, however, were hard to marshal.

Robert McWhirter, (1904-   ), graduate of Glasgow University in 1927 and radiotherapist of Edinburgh, conducted an actual clinical trial of breast cancer. In 1948 he reported that the results of simple mastectomy plus radiotherapy were equal to those of radical mastectomy. His paper aroused wide reappraisal of breast cancer treatment, and even wider arguments.

George Crile, Jr. (1907-   ), graduate of Harvard in 1933, was surgeon at the Crile Clinic, Cleveland, Ohio. In 1955 he published a plea for a more conservative approach to cancer, in his book, **Cancer and Common Sense**. These views were in opposition to the surgical precepts of the period, and a rebuttal was quickly forthcoming in a popular magazine. Nevertheless, the apogee of radical surgery was passed, and with the advent of chemotherapy, new directions of combined treatment became evident.

Robert McWhirter. Value of simple mastectomy and radiotherapy in treatment of cancer of the breast. **Brit. J. Radiol.** 21: 599-610, 1948.

George Crile, Jr. **Cancer and Common Sense.** New York: Viking Press, 1955.

Life. 31 Oct. 1955, p. 129.

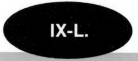

IX-L.

Radiotherapy

The history of radiotherapy is a topic unto itself. It includes the development of radiation sources of increasing power and versatility, the use of more exact dosimetry and exploitation of time-dose relationships, and the application of radiobiologic data, such as cell-replication cycles, to clinical problems of cancer. Franz Buschke edited an informative collection of essays on these topics.

Radiotherapy is the primary modality for approximately 20% of patients with cancer, excluding most cancers of the gastro-intestinal tract. In another 25% of patients radiation is used in conjunction with surgery, post-operatively or for recurrence. Primary surgical and radiological approaches are combined with chemotherapy with increasing frequency.

The trend in radiotherapy during the mid-century was toward larger doses and fields, more exact direction of the beams, and reexamination of the role of X-irradiation in cancers previously considered radio-resistant. Gilbert H. Fletcher (1911-   ), of the M. D. Anderson Hospital and Cancer Institute in Houston, Texas, exemplified the period.

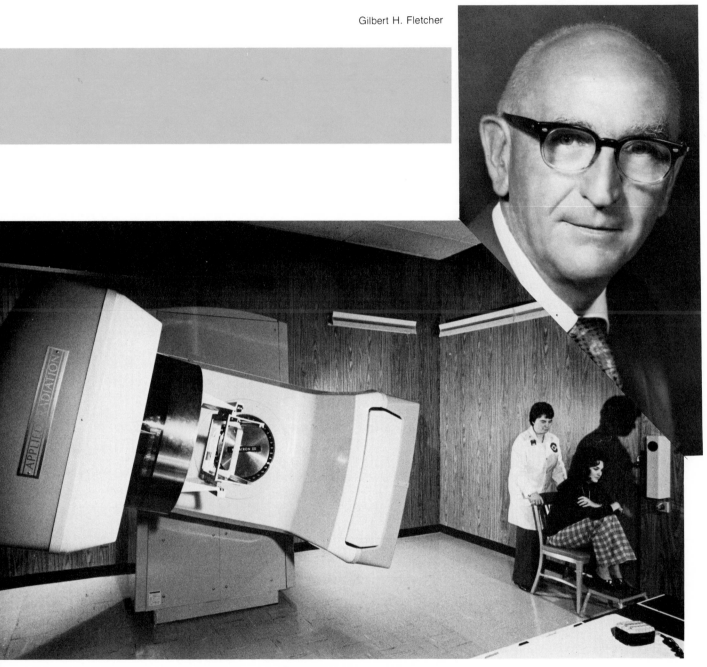

Gilbert H. Fletcher

Radiation therapy: 12 MEV linear accelerator (from the Clinical Center, National Institutes of Health).

James T. Case. History of radiation therapy. In, F. Buschke, ed., **Progress in Radiation Therapy,** vol. 1. New York: Grune & Stratton, 1958. (p. 13-41).

E. Dale Trout. History of radiation sources for cancer therapy. In, F. Buschke, ed., **Progress in Radiation Therapy**, vol. 1. New York: Grune & Stratton, 1958. (p. 42-61).

IX-L.

Radiotherapy

IX-L-1. International studies: Heyman and Denoix.

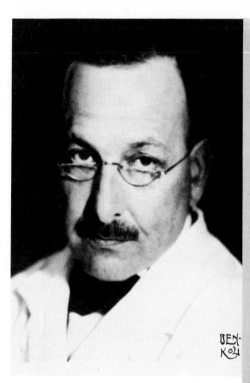

J. Heyman

ANNUAL REPORT ON THE RESULTS OF
RADIOTHERAPY IN CARCINOMA OF
THE UTERINE CERVIX

Seventh Volume

STATEMENTS OF
RESULTS OBTAINED IN 1945 AND
PREVIOUS YEARS
(collated in 1951)

SPONSORED BY

American Cancer Society
British Empire Cancer Campaign, London
Cancerföreningen, Stockholm
Donner Foundation, Philadelphia
Landsforeningen mot Kreft, Oslo
World Health Organization

Editorial Committee

DR. J. HEYMAN (EDITOR)
Stockholm

DR. M. DONALDSON   DR. JOE V. MEIGS
London   Boston

Editorial office: STOCKHOLM 60, SWEDEN

In 1928, the Health Organization of the League of Nations initiated a study comparing results being achieved in the radiotherapy of cancer of the uterine cervix. The task of obtaining and analyzing the data was entrusted to James Heyman (1882-1956) of Stockholm, A. Lacassagne of Paris, and F. Voltz of Munich.

The first report appeared in 1937, and the seventh in 1952. By then 65 institutions in 14 European and American countries pooled data on 70,178 cases, of whom 93.2% were submitted to treatment. The 5-year overall survival without clinical evidence of disease was 32.6%, a gradual steady improvement from 26.3% reported in the second report of 1938.

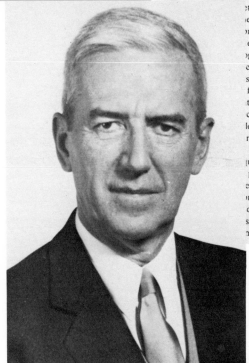

Pierre Denoix

Denoix, Hamperl and Harmer,
Le Système TNM, 1973.

This long-term international cooperative project developed important criteria for clinical staging and reporting of cancer, allowing more uniform comparisons of data from different clinics and different therapeutic approaches.

Another step toward comparable clinical data was the development of the TNM System espoused by Pierre Denoix of France and developed between 1943 and 1967 under the International Union Against Cancer and the World Health Organization. This system includes the size and extent of the primary tumor (T), the involvement or non-involvement of the regional lymph nodes (N), and the presence or absence of metastases (M).

Comparison of end-results with various therapeutic approaches was facilitated by the use of the TNM System. Its acceptance overlaps the more general use of formal clinical trials in which patients are not only staged as uniformly as possible but assigned to treatment groups by randomization.

J. Heyman (ed). **Annual Report on the Results of Radiotherapy in Carcinoma of the Uterine Cervix.** Vol. 7. Stockholm: P. A. Norstedt & Söner, 1952.

P. Denoix. **Clefs pour la Cancérologie.** Paris: Seghers, 1974.

International Union Against Cancer. Committee on Professional Education. **Clinical Oncology. A Manual for Students and Doctors.** New York: Springer-Verlag, 1973.

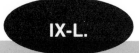

IX-L.

Radiotherapy

IX-L-2. Treatment of Hodgkin's disease: Peters and Kaplan.

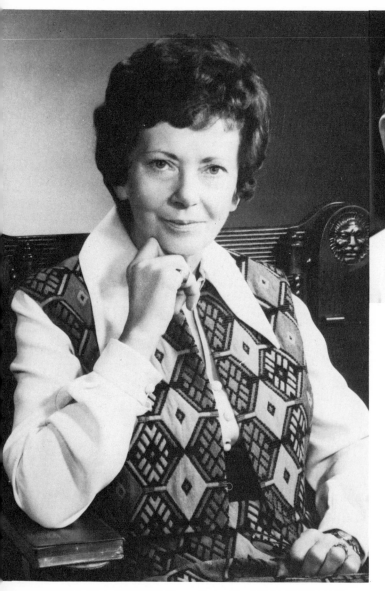

M. Vera Peters

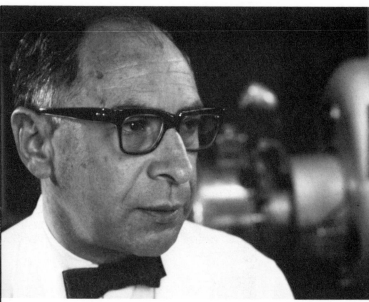

Henry Kaplan

A modern application of radiotherapy was to Hodgkin's disease. Over 30 years ago, René Gilbert and Nándor Ratkoczy in Europe advocated intensive radiotherapy for Hodgkin's based on the concept that generalized disease evolves from a localized stage. Since then, improved radiation sources allowed more aggressive, systematized radiotherapy. A new histopathologic classification devised by R. J. Lukes, more detailed clinical staging schemes, lymphangiography, and chemotherapy encouraged further progress.

M. Vera Peters of Toronto and Henry S. Kaplan spearheaded improved radiotherapy of Hodgkin's disease during the two decades, 1950-70.

M. Vera Peters (born 1911 in Toronto) graduated from the University of Toronto Medical School in 1934. Soon thereafter she became associated with the Ontario Institute of Radiotherapy at the Toronto General Hospital, which later evolved into the Ontario Cancer Institute incorporating Princess Margaret Hospital. Her analysis of survival experiences in Hodgkin's disease at Toronto in 1950 was an important impetus to more aggressive radiotherapy. The crude 5-year survival rate at the Ontario Cancer Institute has risen gradually from 35% to 70%. Further changes in therapeutic approach resulted in the division of patients with Hodgkin's disease into several major clinicopathological types.

Henry Seymour Kaplan (born 1918 in Chicago) graduated from Rush Medical College in 1940, trained in radiology at thd University of Minnesota, and from 1948-1972 was professor and chairman of the Department of Radiology at Stanford University School of Medicine, Palo Alto, California. His contributions include basic studies in radiobiology and on the role of radiation and viruses in rodent leukemia. Kaplan accelerated the use of radical radiation of regionally localized Hodgkin's disease, and achieved over 70% five-year survival.

M. Vera Peters. A study of survivals in Hodgkin's disease treated radiologically. **Am. J. Roentgenol.** 63: 299-311, 1950.

M. Vera Peters, T. C. Brown and D. F. Rideout. Prognostic influences in radiation therapy according to pattern of disease. **J. Am. Med. Assn.** 223: 53-9. 1973.

H. S. Kaplan. The radical radiotherapy of regionally localized Hodgkin's disease. **Radiology** 78: 553-61, 1962.

Henry Kaplan. **Hodgkin's Disease.** Cambridge, Mass.: Harvard Univ. Press, 1972.

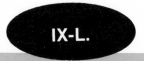

IX-L.

Radiotherapy

IX-L-3. Cancer management at mid-century: Ackerman and del Regato.

"**Cancer, Diagnosis, Treatment and Prognosis**," by L. V. Ackerman and J. A. del Regato was one of the best single-volume textbooks on cancer that reflected the clinical approaches to neoplastic diseases at mid-twentieth century. It went through four editions since 1947, appearing in revised editions in 1954, 1962, and 1970.

The textbook, with del Regato as senior author, also appeared in a Spanish translation of the first edition in 1951 and in a Polish translation of the second edition in 1967.

Lauren V. Ackerman was born in 1905 in New York, and graduated in 1932 from the University of Rochester, New York, with a doctorate in medicine. He was pathologist at the Ellis Fischel State Cancer Hospital in Missouri from 1940 to 1948, when he joined the faculty of Washington University at St. Louis as professor of pathology and surgical pathology until he moved to the State University of New York at Stony Brook in 1973.

Juan A. del Regato was born in 1909 in Cuba, and received his doctorate in medicine at the University of Paris in 1937; he trained in radiotherapy under Regaud, Coutard, and Lacassagne. In 1938 he came to the United States, where he served as a radiotherapist at Ellis Fischel Cancer Hospital from 1943 to 1948. From 1949 until 1973, he was director of the Penrose Cancer Hospital in Colorado Springs, Colorado, and professor of radiobiology at the University of Colorado, when he moved to the University of South Florida College of Medicine, Tampa.

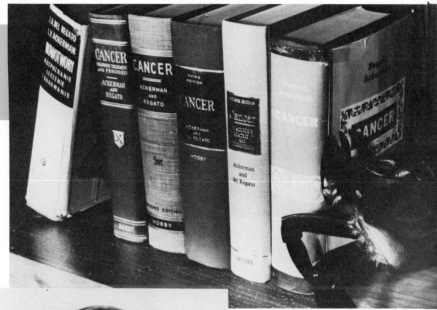

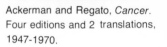

Ackerman and Regato, *Cancer*.
Four editions and 2 translations,
1947-1970.

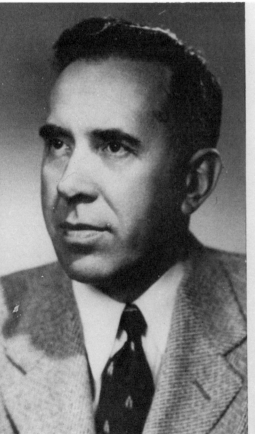

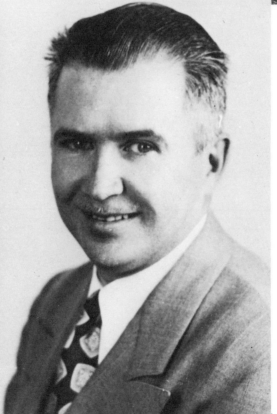

Lauren V. Ackerman   Juan A. del Regato

IX-M.

Cancer Chemotherapy

IX-M-1. Hormonal treatment of prostatic cancer: Huggins.

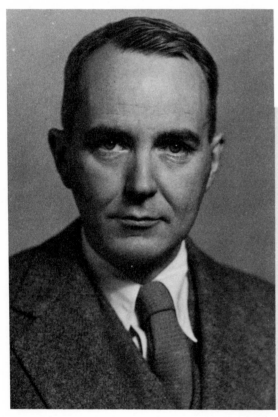

Charles Huggins

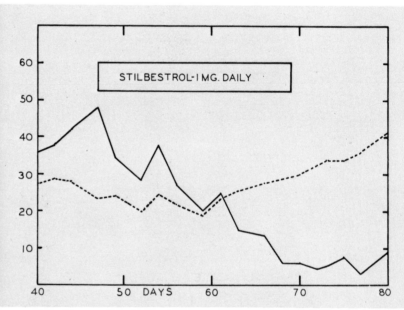

STILBESTROL-I MG. DAILY

Effect of 1 mg diethylstilbestrol daily on serum phosphatases in metastatic carcinoma of the prostate. Solid line, acid phosphatase; dashed line, alkaline phosphatase; the ordinate, units per 100 ml of serum; abscissa, time in days.

Charles Brenton Huggins was born in 1901 in Halifax, Nova Scotia. He was educated at Acadia University in Nova Scotia, received his M.D. from Harvard Medical School, and trained in surgery at the University of Michigan. In 1927 he began his career as a urologist at the University of Chicago, where later he headed the Ben May Laboratory for Cancer Research until his retirement in 1969.

In 1941 Huggins and his students showed that patients with disseminated prostatic cancer were dramatically improved by castration. The alleviation of bone pain was associated with reduction in the levels of acid phosphatase. Subsequent observations showed that the synthetic estrogen, diethylstilbestrol, caused effects similar to those of castration. The use of estrogens in prostatic cancer initiated the modern era of cancer chemotherapy.

Huggins investigated the field of endocrine relations in cancer in the laboratory as well as the clinic. He developed the technique of production of mammary tumors in rats with single doses of 7,12-dimethylbenz(a)anthracene, and the role of adrenalectomy in advanced breast cancer in women.

His contribution of hormonal control in prostatic cancer led to a Nobel Prize in physiology or medicine for 1966, which he shared with Peyton Rous.

Elwood V. Jensen, who succeeded Huggins at the Ben May Laboratory, has extended the studies by showing that hormone responsiveness of neoplasms is related to intracellular estrogen-receptor sites.

C. B. Huggins, R. E. Stevens, Jr. and C. V. Hodges. Studies on prostatic cancer. II. The effect of castration on advanced carcinoma of the prostate gland. **Arch. Surg.** 43: 209-23, 1941.

Charles Huggins and C. V. Hodges. "Studies on prostatic cancer, I. The effect of castration, of estrogen and of androgen injection on serum phosphatase in metastatic carcinoma of the prostate." **Cancer Res.** 1: 293-7, 1941.

Charles Huggins. "Endocrine-induced regression of cancers." **Science** 156: 1050-54, 1967.

E. V. Jensen and E. R. DeSombre. "Mechanism of action of the female sex hormones." **Ann. Rev. Biochem.** 41: 203-30, 1972.

IX-M.

Cancer Chemotherapy

IX-M-2. Nitrogen mustard: Gilman and Goodman.

Cancer chemotherapy by alkylating agents was discovered under the cloak of war-time secrecy, and the full story was published in 1963.

Alfred Gilman recalled that work on chemical warfare agents started at Yale University under contract with the Office of Scientific Research and Development (OSRD) in 1943. Nitrogen mustards, especially the bis and tris β-chlorethyl amines were studied thoroughly by chemists and pharmacologists, especially Louis S. Goodman, Alfred Gilman and Frederick S. Philips. The remarkable sensitivity of normal lymphoid tissue to the cytotoxic action of the nitrogen mustards led to a test by Thomas Dougherty on one mouse with a transplanted lymphoma, with encouraging results that led to a more extensive investigation. A therapeutic trial in man was organized by Gustav D. Lindskog, with the first patient being an X-ray resistant patient with lymphosarcoma. A dose of 0.1 mg per kilogram of bis β-chlorethylamine daily for 10 days was selected. "The response of the first patient was as dramatic as that of the first mouse." Five additional patients were treated at Yale, and the studies shifted to Chicago under Leon O. Jacobson and to the Memorial Hospital in New York under David A. Karnofsky. Reports of their findings were published in 1946, when secrecy restrictions were lifted.

Elaboration of analogues of nitrogen mustard and related compounds led to the eventual clinical use of a wide variety of such drugs. Of particular interest were Busulfan (Myleran), an alkyl alkanesulfonate discovered by G. M. Timmis in England, Cyclophosphamide (Cytoxan), introduced by G. Domagk of Germany, Chlorambucil (Leukeran), and l-Phenylalanine mustard (Melphalan).

Alfred Gilman was born in 1908 in Connecticut, and graduated from Yale with a Ph.D. in pharmacology in 1931. Louis Stanford Goodman was born in 1906 in Oregon and obtained an M.D. degree at the University of Oregon in 1932. Both are chairmen of departments of pharmacology, at Albert Einstein College of Medicine in New York and at University of Utah School of Medicine, respectively. They collaborated in the writing of the influential **Pharmacological Basis of Therapeutics**, first issued in 1941 and in a fifth edition in 1975.

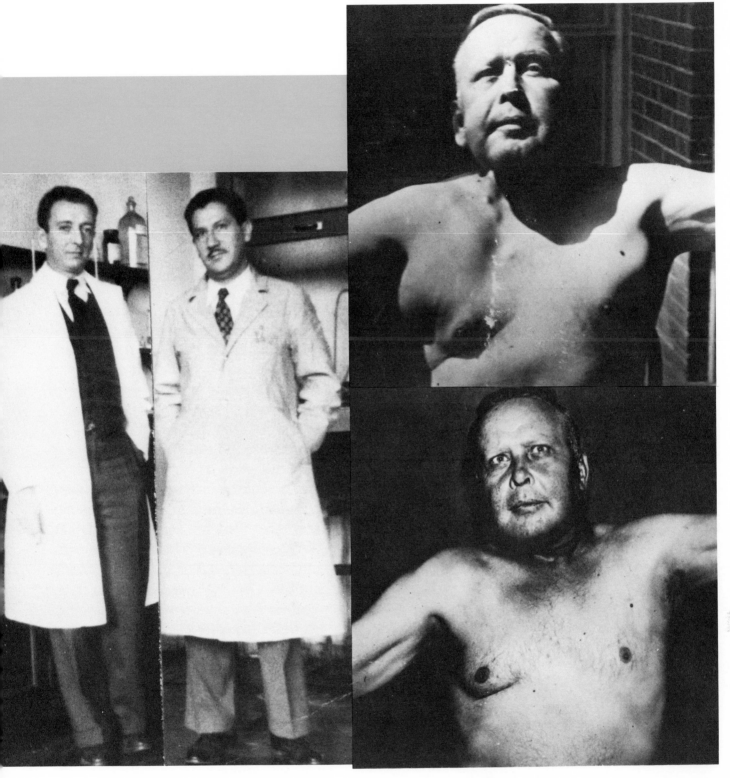

Alfred Gilman and Louis Goodman, circa 1942.

First patient with lymphosarcoma treated with nitrogen mustard, photographed before and after therapy. Note reduction in lymph nodes and facial edema.

Alfred Gilman. The initial clinical trial of nitrogen mustard. **Am. J. Surg.** 105: 574-8, 1963.

L. S. Goodman, M. M. Wintrobe, W. Dameshek, M. J. Goodman, A. Gilman and M. T. McLennan. Nitrogen mustard therapy. **J. Am. Med. Assn.** 132: 126-32, 1946.

L. S. Goodman and A. Gilman. **The Pharmacological Basis of Therapeutics.** New York: Macmillan, 1941.

IX-M.

Cancer Chemotherapy

IX-M-3. Cancer chemotherapy program: Rhoads, Stock and Sugiura.

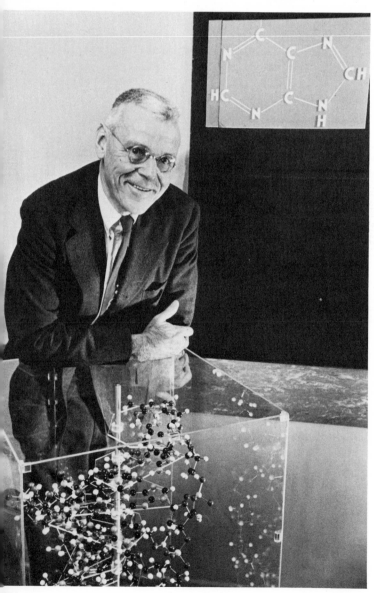

C.P. Rhoads

An important pioneer program in experimental cancer chemotherapy was initiated by Cornelius Packard Rhoads (1898-1959) in New York during the 1940s.

Rhoads was born in Springfield, Massachusetts, completed his medical education at Harvard School of Medicine in 1924, and following training in pathology, joined the research staff of the Rockefeller Institute for Medical Research in New York. In 1940 he succeeded James Ewing as Director of the Memorial Hospital for Cancer and Allied Diseases in New York City. During World War II he served in the United States Army Chemical Warfare Service. Under the cloak of wartime secrecy, nitrogen mustard was shown to have therapeutic effects in patients with leukemia and lymphoma. This led to the exploration for therapeutic effects of many analogues of nitrogen mustard and subsequent synthesis of many other alkylating chemicals.

Following the war, the Sloan-Kettering Institute for Cancer Research was organized, and the Memorial Hospital expanded. Rhoads was the Director until his sudden death in 1959. Cancer

K. Sugiura. Reminiscence and experience in experimental chemotherapy of cancer. **Med. Clin. N. Am.** 55: 667-82, 1971.

C. C. Stock. Cornelius Packard Rhoads, 1898-1959. [Obituary.] **Cancer Res.** 20: 409-11, 1960.

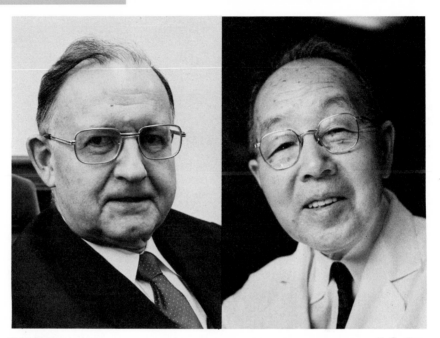

C.C. Stock   K. Sugiura

chemotherapy was emphasized in the research program. Among the key personnel brought together by Rhoads were Joseph H. Burchenal, the late David A. Karnofsky, Frederick S. Philips, C. Chester Stock, and K. Sugiura.

The experimental cancer chemotherapy program was organized at the Sloan-Kettering Institute by C. Chester Stock (1910-   ) as Chief of the Division of Experimental Chemotherapy. In addition, he subsequently became the director of the subsidiary Donald S. Walker Laboratory in Rye, New York.

Kanematsu Sugiura (1890-   ) became head of the Tumor Spectrum Section of the chemotherapy program, with responsibility in the bioassay procedures. A native of Japan, Sugiura was brought to the United States in 1905, and his subsequent education and career developed in New York, in close association with many of the cancer research programs that evolved in the city. Sugiura's contributions to experimental cancer chemotherapy extend back to 1912 and are recorded in his many publications. Sugiura has published a charming account of his reminiscences and experiences in the experimental chemotherapy of cancer.

Cancer Chemotherapy

IX-M-4. Antifolates: Farber and SubbaRow.

Sidney Farber (1903-1973) and his associates of the Children's Cancer Research Foundation in Boston in 1947 produced the first temporary remissions of acute leukemia in children by the use of folic acid antagonists. This initiated the fertile area of research on the antineoplastic activity of antimetabolites.

Sidney Farber was born in Buffalo, New York, to a family of distinguished scholars. He graduated from the University of Buffalo in 1923, and from Harvard Medical School in 1927, where he spent his entire professional life. Farber was an international authority in pediatric pathology, with special interest in pediatric oncology. He was an influential and respected advisor to many national and international medical organizations in cancer. A large, gracious man, his spirit was indomitable. The Children's Cancer Research Foundation was renamed the Sidney Farber Cancer Center after his death.

Yellapragada SubbaRow (1896-1948), onetime member of the Department of Biological Chemistry of the Harvard Medical School, was, after 1942, research director of Lederle Laboratories. The chemists in Lederle Laboratories synthesized and made available to the Farber clinical group a series of folic acid (pteroylglutamic acid) analogues, among which were found the first effective antileukemic agents.

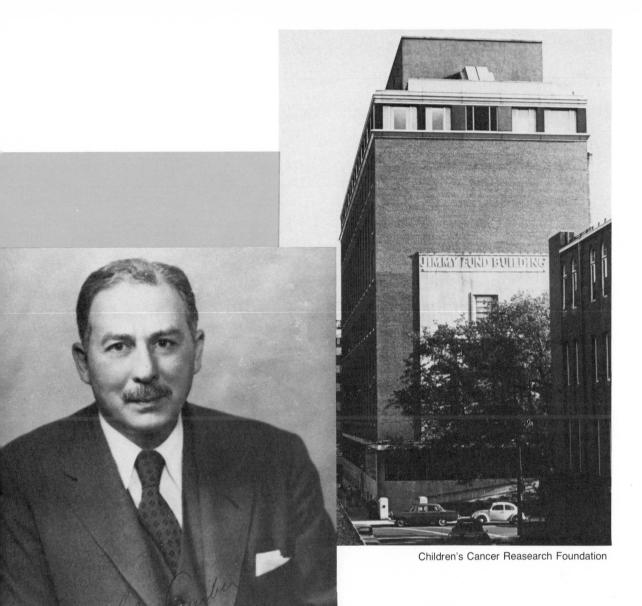

Children's Cancer Reasearch Foundation

Sidney Farber

Y. SubbaRow

S. Farber, L. K. Diamond, R. D. Mercer, R. F. Sylvester, and James A. Wolff. Temporary remissions in acute leukemia in children produced by folic acid antagonist, 4-aminopteroylglutamic acid (aminopterin). **New Engl. J. Med.** 238: 787-93, 1948.

S. Farber, R. Toch, E. M. Sears and D. Pinkel. Advances in chemotherapy of cancer in man. **Adv. Cancer Res.** 4: 1-71, 1956.

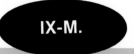

IX-M.

Cancer Chemotherapy

IX-M-5. Choriocarcinoma in women: Hertz and Li.

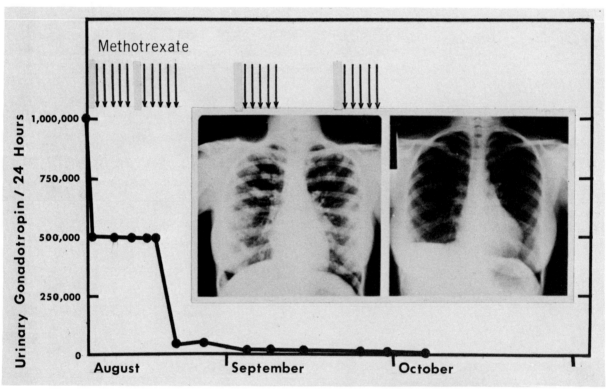

Course of a patient with disseminated choriocarcinoma treated with intermittent courses of Methotrexate.

The most impressive results of cancer chemotherapy were obtained with the antifolic, Methotrexate, in women with disseminated choriocarcinoma.

Roy Hertz, born in 1909, in Cleveland, Ohio, while chief of the Endocrinology Branch of the National Cancer Institute, Bethesda, Maryland, was instrumental in introducing and developing the therapy. The first observations, however, were

M. C. Li, R. Hertz and D. B. Spencer. Effect of Methotrexate therapy upon choriocarcinoma and chorioadenoma. **Proc. Soc. Exp. Biol. & Med.** 93: 361-66, 1956.

R. Hertz, J. Lewis, Jr., and M. B. Lipsett. Five years' experience with the chemotherapy of metastatic choriocarcinoma and related trophoblastic tumors in women. **Am. J. Obst. & Gyn.** 82: 631-40, 1961.

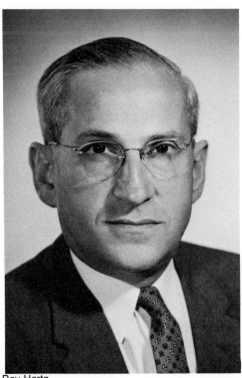

Roy Hertz

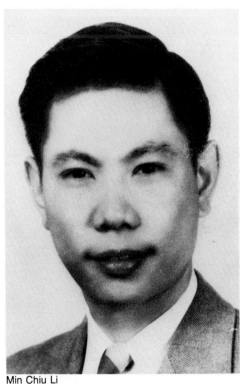

Min Chiu Li

made in collaboration with Min Chiu Li, who was born in 1919 in Canton, China.

Complete and sustained remissions of this otherwise fatal disease were achieved in over 50% of patients. Some of these cured women even experienced subsequent normal pregnancies. The results were further improved by the use of actinomycin D in Methotrexate-resistant patients.

IX-M.

Cancer Chemotherapy

IX-M-6. Purine and pyrimidine antagonists: Hitchings and Heidelberger.

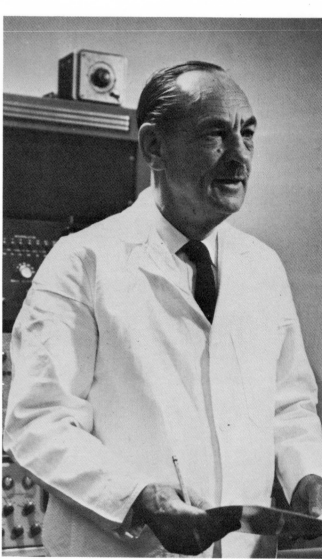

Another class of antineoplastic agents were purine and pyrimidine antagonists, particularly 6-mercaptopurine and 5-fluorouracil.

George Hubert Hitchings at the Burroughs Wellcome Company in the Research Triangle Park, North Carolina, was the chief biochemist of the group that developed 6-mercaptopurine. Hitchings was born in Washington in 1905, and received his doctorate in biochemistry from Harvard in 1933. The purine

George H. Hitchings

antagonists synthesized at Burroughs Wellcome were tested clinically primarily at the Memorial Cancer Hospital in New York, by J. H. Burchenal and his associates.

Charles Heidelberger was born in New York City in 1920, and in 1946 obtained a Ph.D. in organic chemistry at Harvard. He pioneered the use of radioactive carcinogens to study metabolic pathways at the University of California in Berkeley and joined the McArdle Laboratory for Cancer Research of the University of Wisconsin in 1948. In 1960 he was a recipient of one of the first American Cancer Society Professorships. In 1976 he transferred to the University of Southern California.

Heidelberger is best known for his invention, synthesis and applications of 5-fluorouracil (5-FU) as a cancer chemotherapeutic agent. His wide interests and participation in research on carcinogenesis, including chemical carcinogenesis **in vitro**, have been productive.

5-FU was tested clinically by the Wisconsin group headed by F. J. Ansfield and A. R. Curreri. This antipyrimidine affects "solid" tumors, particularly of the breast and the lower intestinal tract.

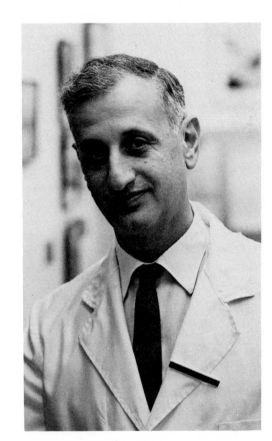

Charles Heidelberger

G. H. Hitchings and C. P. Rhoads (eds). 6-Mercaptopurine. **Ann. N. Y. Acad. Sci.** 60: 183-507, 1954.

J. H. Burchenal et al. Clinical evaluation of a new antimetabolite, 6-mercaptopurine, in the treatment of leukemia and allied diseases. **Blood** 8: 965-99, 1953.

C. Heidelberger et al. Fluorinated pyrimidines, a new class of tumour-inhibitory compounds. **Nature** 179: 663-66, 1957.

F. J. Ansfield et al. A ten-year study of 5-fluorouracil in disseminated breast cancer with clinical results and survival times. **Cancer Res.** 29: 1062-66, 1969.

IX-M.

Cancer Chemotherapy

IX-M-7. Cancer Chemotherapy National Service Center: Endicott.

On the basis of the discoveries of the alkylating agents and antimetabolites in leukemia and lymphoma, and of hormones in cancer of the breast and prostate, a national program of research in chemotherapy of cancer was initiated in 1954 by Congressional mandate. An earmarked appropriation that rose to 19 million dollars by 1956 represented almost half of the total funding of the National Cancer Institute.

Kenneth M. Endicott was selected to organize and direct the targeted chemotherapy program. The Cancer Chemotherapy National Service (CCNSC) was established with Sidney Farber as chairman of the directing committee.

The program enlisted other cancer agencies as well as pharmaceutical companies. Procurement of chemicals and bioassay was systematized, new mouse breeding centers were established to meet animal needs, and clinical trials were organized by multi-institutional groups of physicians who were treating patients with advanced cancers. Surgical groups were also organized around "adjuvant chemotherapy," in which drugs were cautiously added to standard resection procedures.

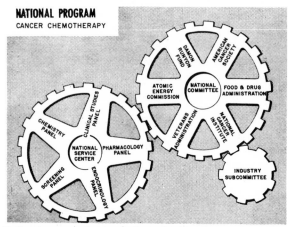

National program in cancer chemotherapy; constituent parts.

All groups designed "protocols" with appropriate controls of contratests and with biometric surveillance.

Fifteen years later thousands of compounds and crude materials had been tested in animals and several hundred in patients with cancer. Definitely successful results were achieved in a significant proportion of patients with many types of rapidly-proliferating neoplasms.

Kenneth M. Endicott was born in 1916 in Colorado, and obtained his M.D. from the University of Colorado Medical School in 1939. A pathologist by training, he became a career officer of the Public Health Service and an expert in administration. He was Director of the National Cancer Institute, 1960-69.

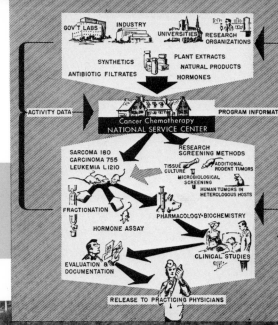

Relationships of activities of the Cancer Chemotherapy National Service Center.

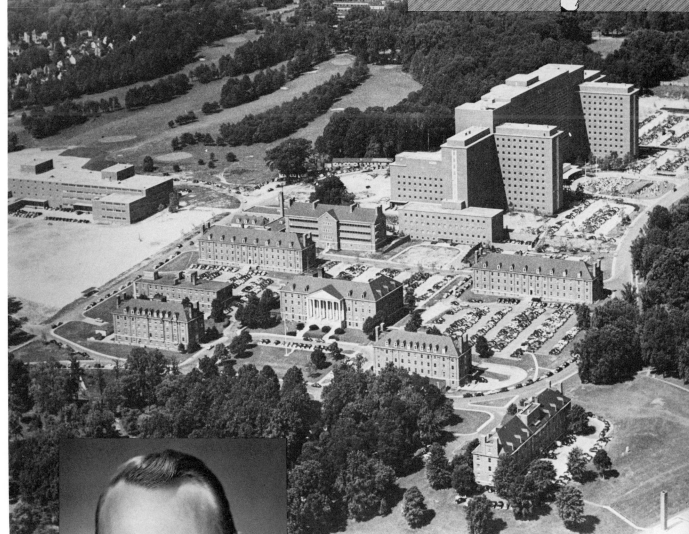

National Institutes of Health, ca 1955.

Kenneth M. Endicott

K. M. Endicott. The chemotherapy program. **J. Natl. Cancer Inst.** 19: 275-93, 1957.

M. B. Shimkin and George E. Moore. Adjuvant use of chemotherapy in the surgical treatment of cancer. **J. Am. Med. Assn.** 167: 1710-14, 1958.

C. G. Zubrod *et al.* The chemotherapy program of the National Cancer Institute. History, analysis, and plans. **Cancer Chemother. Rep.** 50: 349-540, 1966.

S. K. Carter and M. Slavik. Chemotherapy of cancer. **Ann. Rev. Pharmacol.** 14: 157-83, 1974.

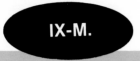

IX-M.

Cancer Chemotherapy

IX-M-8. Principles of chemotherapy: Skipper, Greenspan and Fisher.

The number of agents with clinical antineoplastic activity increased, and the investigators sought some guiding principles for their use. Two emerged: the "total kill" concept, and combinations of several agents.

Howard E. Skipper, born in 1915 in Florida, received his doctorate in nutritional biochemistry from the University of Florida in 1941. Since 1946 he has been with the Southern Research Institute in Birmingham, Alabama. The Kettering-Meyer Laboratory of the Institute, headed by Skipper, has developed over 100 compounds, including nitrosourea derivatives and imidazole triazines. The theoretical models developed by Skipper and his group, visualizing therapeutic response in terms of the target cell population, were important in guiding research, particularly on acute leukemia.

Ezra M. Greenspan, born in 1919 and on the staff of Mount Sinai School of Medicine in New York, was a pioneer in using several antineoplastic agents in combination. This lead was followed by some of the cooperative clinical groups of the national program. Significant improvement in response rates and maintenance of remissions were elicited. The effects were not limited to leukemia, but were evident in osteogenic sarcoma and in breast cancer.

Combination therapy was also extended to patients being treated surgically or radiologically. That such adjuvant therapy improved the salvage in patients with breast cancer with limited lymph node metastases was shown by a nationally organized group of surgeons chaired by Bernard Fisher. Fisher, born in 1923 in Pittsburgh, Pennsylvania, was educated in the city of his birth and was the professor of surgery at the University of Pittsburgh School of Medicine.

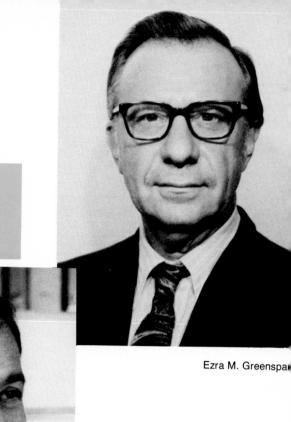

Ezra M. Greenspan

Bernard Fisher

Howard E. Skipper. Criteria associated with destruction of leukemia and solid tumors in animals. **Cancer Res.** 27: 2636-45, 1967.

E. M. Greenspan. Combination cytotoxic chemotherapy in advanced disseminated breast carcinoma. **J. Mt. Sinai Hospital** 33: 1-27, 1966.

Emil Frei III. Combination cancer chemotherapy. **Cancer Res.** 32: 2593-2607, 1972.

B. Fisher et al. I-Phenylalanine mustard (L-Pam) in the management of primary breast cancer. A report of early findings. **New Engl. J. Med.** 292: 117-22, 1975.

Howard E. Skipper

IX-M.

Cancer Chemotherapy

IX-M-9. Cancer chemotherapy comes of age.

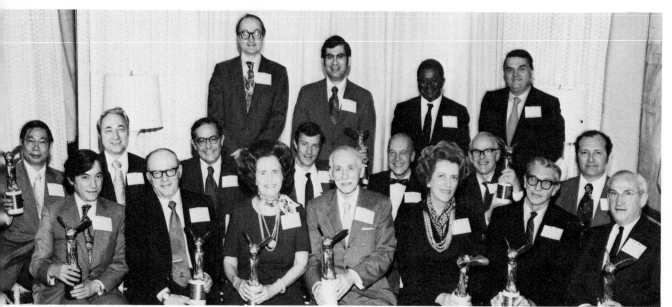

Cancer chemotherapy investigators, at Lasker awards ceremony, 1972.

The group picture of the awards ceremonies, held on November 16, 1972, in New York, shows: **Left to right, seated in first row**: Isaac Djerassi, Director of Research Hematology at Mercy Catholic Medical Center (Fitzgerald Division), Darby, Pa.; Edmund Klein, Chief of Department of Dermatology at Roswell Park Memorial Institute, Buffalo, N. Y.; Mrs. Albert D. Lasker, President of the Albert and Mary Lasker Foundation; Sidney Farber, Chairman of the Awards Jury, also President and Director of the Children's Cancer Research Foundation, Boston, Mass.; Mrs. Alice Fordyce, Vice President of the Albert and Mary Lasker

Foundation; Special Award Winner, C. Gordon Zubrod, Director of the Division of Cancer Treatment at the National Cancer Institute, Bethesda, Md.; Roy Hertz, Professor of Obstetrics and Gynecology and Director of Clinical Research at New York Medical College, Valhalla, N.Y. **Seated in second row**: Min Chiu Li, Director of Medical Research at Nassau Hospital, Mineola, N.Y.; Eugene J. Van Scott, Professor of Dermatology at the Skin and Cancer Hospital at Temple University, Philadelphia, Pa.; Paul P. Carbone, Associate Scientific Director for Medical Oncology at the National Cancer Institute and National Institutes of Health, Bethesda, Md.; John L. Ziegler, Director at Uganda Cancer Institute, Kampala, Uganda, Africa; Joseph H. Burchenal, Director of Clinical Investigation at Memorial Hospital for Cancer and Allied Diseases, New York, N.Y.; Denis Burkitt, Surgeon at Medical Research Council, London,

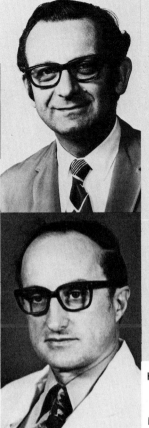

James F. Holland

Emil Frei, III

Cancer

Medicine

JAMES F. HOLLAND, M.D.
Professor and Chairman
Department of Neoplastic Diseases
Mt. Sinai School of Medicine
of the
City University of New York
Formerly Chief of Medicine A
Roswell Park Memorial Institute
Buffalo, New York

EMIL FREI, III, M.D.
Professor of Medicine
Harvard Medical School
Physician-in-Chief
Children's Cancer Research Foundation, Inc.
Boston, Massachusetts
Formerly Associate Director, Clinical Research, and
Professor of Medicine, University of Texas
M.D. Anderson Hospital and Tumor Institute
Houston, Texas

In Collaboration with 158 Contributors

LEA & FEBIGER · 1973 · PHILADELPHIA

Holland and Frei (eds), *Cancer Medicine*, 1973.

Title page.

England; Emil J. Freireich, Professor of Medicine and Chief of Research Hematology at the University of Texas, Houston, Texas. **Standing**: Emil Frei, III, Physician-in-Chief at Children's Cancer Research Foundation, Boston, Mass,; Vincent T. DeVita, Jr., Chief of Medicine Branch at National Cancer Institute, Bethesda, Md.; V. Anomah Ngu, Professor of Surgery at Centre of Health Sciences, Yaounde, United Republic of Cameroun, Africa; Donald Pinkel, Medical Director at St. Jude Children's Research Hospital, Memphis, Tenn. Absent was James F. Holland, Director, Cancer Clinical Research Center at Roswell Park Memorial Institute, Buffalo, N.Y., who was on a medical exchange visit to the Soviet Union.

The entry of meaningful chemotherapy in oncology was summarized by a 3000-page **Cancer Medicine** edited by Holland and Frei, who became directors of oncology programs at the Mt. Sinai Medical School in New York and at the Sidney Farber Cancer Center in Boston, respectively.

The 1972 Albert Lasker Medical Research Awards were extended to 17 individuals, for 7 categories of accomplishment in clinical cancer chemotherapy: (1) Use of drugs in cures of gestational choriocarcinoma (Li and Hertz). (2) Use of drugs in long-term disease-free survivors with Burkitt's tumor (Burkitt, Burchenal, Ngu, and Ziegler). (3) Use of topical chemotherapy and enhancement of host response for cures in skin cancer

(Klein). (4) Use of combination drug therapy resulting in prolonged survival, in acute lymphatic leukemia (Frei, Freireich, Holland, and Pinkel). (5) Use of combination drug therapy, resulting in prolonged survival, in Hodgkin's disease (Frei, Carbone, and DeVita). (6) Treatment of mycosis fungoides, with topical chemotherapy and enhancement of host response (Van Scott). (7) Supportive measures in treatment of toxicity, infection, and hemorrhage due to side effects of drugs (Djerassi and Freireich).

A special Award was presented to C. Gordon Zubrod of the National Cancer Institute, for his leadership in the National Cancer Institute program of chemotherapy.

[Lasker Awards]. **J. Am. Med. Assoc.** 222: 1160-73, Nov. 27, 1972.

J. F. Holland and E. Frei, III (eds). **Cancer Medicine.** Philadelphia: Lea & Febiger, 1973.

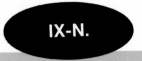

Cancer Statistics

IX-N-1. Cancer incidence: Dorn and Haenszel.

National and international comparisons of cancer mortality and incidence have been important sources of hypotheses regarding cancer causation since the turn of this century. Better diagnostic criteria, registration schemes, and designed studies on specific topics have increased the value of this type of research. Attention has been directed to the analysis of the effects of migration of human populations on the incidence of cancer and other diseases. This "experiment in nature" allows dissociation of environmental and genetic influences, and leads to further inquiries of possible causative factors.

Harold F. Dorn (1906-1963) was an outstanding practitioner of statistics, demography and cancer research. Born in New York State, he received his education at Cornell and Wisconsin Universities, with a Ph.D. in sociology in 1933. He spent most of his career in government service, at the National Institutes of Health. He conducted the 1937 and 1947 cancer incidence surveys in metropolitan areas of the United States, and extended his interests to international studies as secretary-general of the International Union Against Cancer from 1953. A third cancer survey in the United States was conducted between 1969 and 1971.

William M. Haenszel was born in 1910 in Rochester, New York, and received his education at the University of Buffalo, New York. He worked as a statistician for the New York and Connecticut Departments of Health from 1933 to 1952, when he joined the biometry group at the National Cancer Institute. His productive career encompassed many statistical considerations of cancer in the United States and around the world.

Harold F. Dorn and Sidney J. Cutler. **Morbidity from Cancer in the United States.** Public Health Monograph No. 56, Washington, D. C.: U.S. Govt. Printing Office, 1959.

William Haenszel (ed). **Epidemiological Approaches to the Study of Cancer and Other Chronic Diseases.** National Cancer Institute Monograph No. 19. Washington, D.C.: U.S. Govt. Printing Office, 1966.

Sidney J. Cutler and John L. Young (eds). **Third National Cancer Survey: Incidence Data.** National Cancer Institute Monograph No. 41. Washington, D.C: U.S. Govt. Printing Office, 1975.

L. J. Dunham and H. F. Dorn. Techniques in the geographic pathology of cancer. **Transactions, 5th Meeting, Internat. Soc. Geographic Path.** New York: Karger, 1955 (p. 472-81).

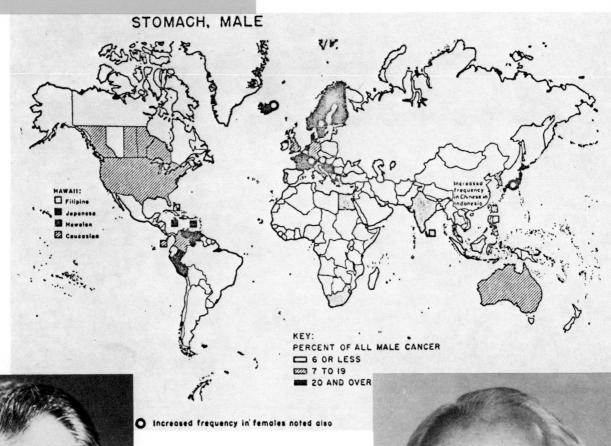

Distribution of cancer of the stomach in men, from Dunham and Dorn, 1955.

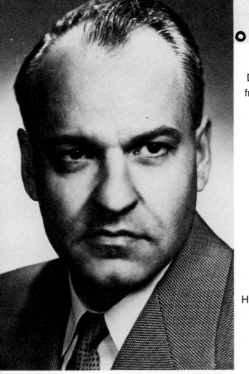

Harold F. Dorn

William Haenszel

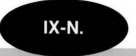

IX-N.

Cancer Statistics

IX-N-2. Connecticut Tumor Registry: Griswold and Macdonald.

The Connecticut Tumor Registry, housed in the Connecticut State Department of Health in Hartford, is the oldest continual cancer registry based upon a defined population. It gathers data on incidence, mortality, and survival for all cancers in the state, and thus provides irreplaceable material for special epidemiological studies on cancer in man.

The Division of Cancer and Other Chronic Diseases was founded in 1935 by the Connecticut General Assembly, providing for cancer studies by the Department of Health. During 1936 to 1940, the programs organized cancer mortality statistics and public information, and established tumor clinics. In 1941 the registry was begun to which all hospitals sent standard abstracts, including data going back to 1935. Case histories and life-long follow-up are maintained on all cancer patients of the total state population, which was 1.6 million in 1935. The Registry issues periodic reports, published by the Connecticut State Department of Health, Hartford.

Matthew H. Griswold (1887-1969) was chief of the Division of Cancer and Other Chronic Diseases at the inception of the Registry and served as its director until his retirement in 1959. He was succeeded by Henry Eisenberg, who served until his death in 1968. Barbara Christine headed the activity during the 1970s.

Eleanor J. Macdonald (1906-   ) was the statistician who organized the statewide Registry during its formative years. In 1948 she became Research Statistician at the M.D. Anderson Hospital for Cancer Research in Houston, Texas.

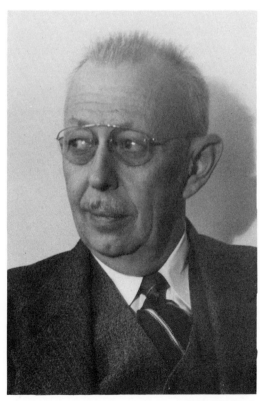

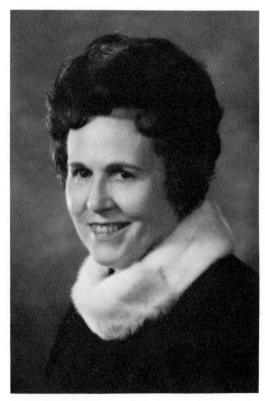

M.H. Griswold   Eleanor Macdonald

M. H. Griswold, et al. **Cancer in Connecticut 1935-1951.**
Hartford: Connecticut State Dept. Health, 1955.

IX-N.

Cancer Statistics

IX-N-3. Danish Cancer Registry: Clemmesen.

The Danish Cancer Registry (Cancer-registeret, Copenhagen), is the oldest nation-based tumor registry in the world. It forms one of the human population laboratories that record the incidence and distribution of cancer and yield material for epidemiological studies on cancer.

The Danish Tumor Registry was opened in 1942 under the joint auspices of the Danish Cancer Society, National Health Service, and the Medical Association. In 1950 it moved to the Finsen Institute. Its records include information on all cancer cases in Denmark, which had a population in 1950 of 4.3 million.

The history of epidemiological cancer statistics, the operation, gathered data, and many special studies of the Registry have been published in a four-volume work by Clemmesen.

Johannes Clemmesen was the founder and has been the director of the Danish Cancer Registry from its inception. He was born in 1908, in Copenhagen, and received his education at the University of Copenhagen. He is a specialist in clinical medicine as well as in pathology and is the chief pathologist of the Finsen Institute.

Clemmesen has made many contributions to pathology, immunology, and radiation of tumors, and to the statistical-epidemiological studies of cancer. Of particular note were his observations on the distribution of cancer by socioeconomic classes, on cancer of the breast and the uterine cervix, on smoking and lung cancer, and on leukemia. He has played a major role in international cancer studies, such as those carried out under the auspices of the World Health Organization.

Johannes Clemmesen. **Statistical Studies in the Aetiology of Malignant Neoplasms.** 4 vols. København: Munksgaard, 1965-1974.

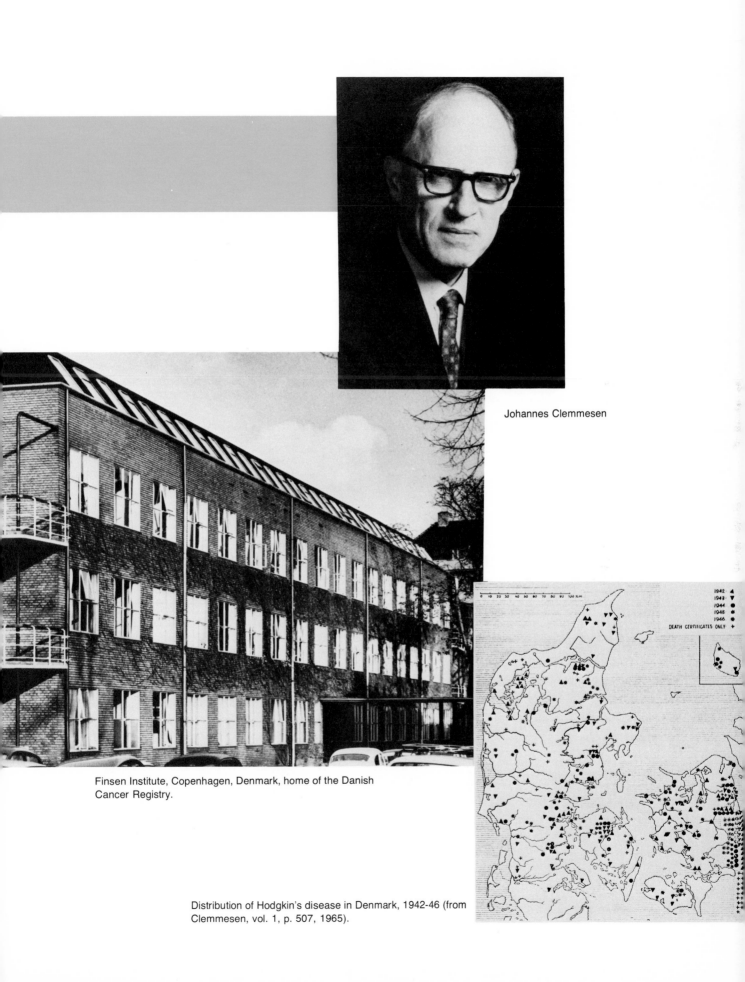

Johannes Clemmesen

Finsen Institute, Copenhagen, Denmark, home of the Danish
Cancer Registry.

Distribution of Hodgkin's disease in Denmark, 1942-46 (from
Clemmesen, vol. 1, p. 507, 1965).

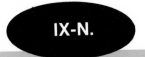

Cancer Statistics

IX-N-4. International cancer statistics: Segi and Doll.

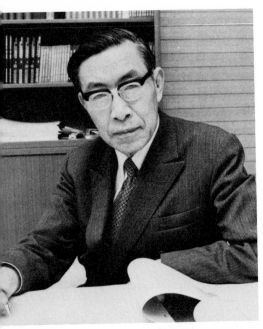

Mitsuo Segi

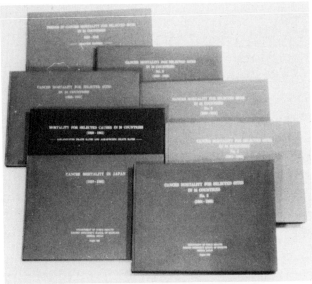

Eight publications by Segi and his coworkers on cancer mortality throughout the world, issued between 1960 and 1966.

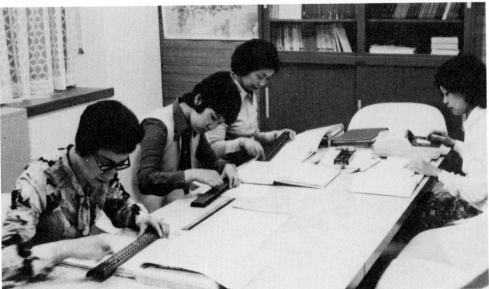

Staff at Tohoku University School of Medicine in Sendai, Japan, calculating data on cancer mortality.

Data on cancer mortality and incidence are important for epidemiology and for public health.

Mitsuo Segi and his coworkers at Tohoku University School of Medicine in Sendai, Japan, during the decade of 1960 published 5 volumes of cancer mortality statistics from 24 countries for 1950 to 1965. The data were made comparable by age adjustment and, with 3 supplemental volumes, became standard reference works on the subject throughout the world.

Mitsuo Segi was born in 1908 and is a graduate of Tokyo University School of Medicine. He was trained in obstetrics and became Director of Maternal and Child Hygiene in the Japanese Ministry of Health and Welfare in 1940. In 1950 he became Professor of Public Health at Tohoku University, retiring in 1971 from this post and becoming President of Mizuho College in Nagoya, as well as continuing as research associate at the Aichi Cancer Center Research Institute in Nagoya, and founding the Segi Institute of Cancer Epidemiology.

Richard Doll, Peter Payne and John Waterhouse analyzed for the International Union Against Cancer data on cancer incidence in the world, and issued the first report in 1966. This was the most comprehensive collation of the most comparable information on the subject available at the time.

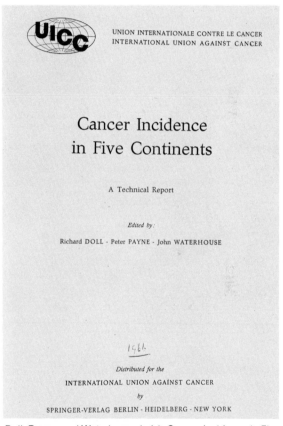

Doll, Payne, and Waterhouse (eds), *Cancer Incidence in Five Continents,* 1966. Title page.

IX-N.

Cancer Statistics

IX-N-5. End-results in cancer: Cutler.

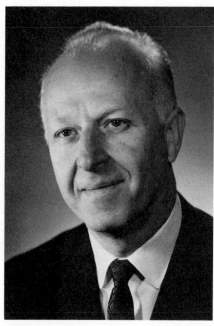

Sidney J. Cutler

The need for long-term follow-up of patients with cancer was recognized by surgeons during the 19th Century, and became a requirement in all cancer treatment centers. Systematic regional or national registries of treated patients with cancer, however, were a more recent development.

In the United States, a cancer end-results evaluation program was initiated in 1956, as part of the cancer chemotherapy endeavors. Information on 66,000 patients was collected for presentation at the Third National Cancer Conference. The responsibility for the development was placed under Sidney Cutler.

In 1959, a meeting was held of representatives of six national cancer registration programs, for the purpose of organizing a cooperative international effort in the evaluation of end-results of cancer therapy and in the investigation of epidemiological questions. The countries represented were Denmark, England and Wales, Finland, France, Norway and the United States. Their labors thus organized were reported as a symposium held in Norway in 1963.

Sidney J. Cutler was born in Russia in 1917, and graduated in statistics from Columbia University in New York in 1941, with a doctorate from the University of Pittsburgh in 1961. He was statistician with the National Cancer Institute from 1948 to 1975, when he moved to the Michigan Cancer Foundation in Detroit.

Meeting of Ad Hoc Group on International Cooperation in Evaluation of End Results, January, 1959, Bethesda, Maryland, USA.

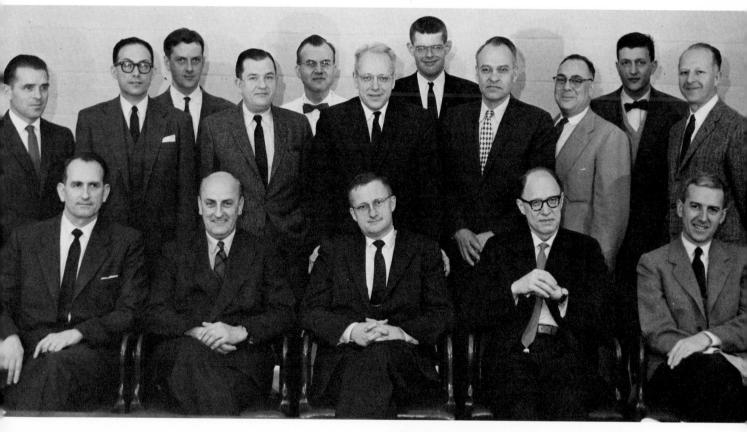

Left to right, seated: Einar Pedersen, Norway; W.P.D. Logan, England; Howard B. Latourette, U.S.A.; Johannes Clemmensen, Denmark; Pierre Denoix, France. **Standing, left to right:** George Linden, U.S.A.; Piero Mustacchi, U.S.A.; Erkki Saxén, Finland; Michael B. Shimkin, U.S.A.; Benno K. Milmore, U.S.A.; William Haenszel, U.S.A.; John C. Bailar, III, U.S.A.; Harold F. Dorn, U.S.A.; William I. Lourie, U.S.A.; Charles B. Clayman, U.S.A.; and Sidney J. Cutler, U.S.A.

Sidney J. Cutler (ed.). **International Symposium on End Results of Cancer Therapy.** National Cancer Institute Monograph 15. Washington, D. C.: U.S. Govt. Printing Off., 1964.

IX-O.

Cancer Epidemiology

IX-O-1. Ionizing radiation cancers: ABCC and Alice Stewart.

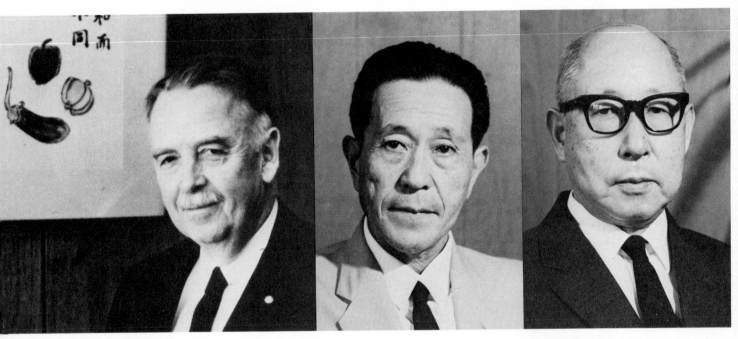

George B. Darling   Hiroshi Maki   Isamu Nagai

Following the tragedy of the atomic bomb explosions over Hiroshima and Nagasaki in 1945, an Atomic Bomb Casualty Commission (ABCC) was established to monitor the effects of the radiation exposure. Following a period of organization, the endeavor was structured along epidemiological principles under the guidance of Keith Cannon.

George B. Darling directed ABCC for the 15 years in concert with Hiroshi Maki and Isamu Nagai, Associate Directors in Hiroshima and Nagasaki, respectively. ABCC became a collaborative endeavor of the U. S. National Academy of Sciences and the Japanese National Institute of Health (JNIH). The Commission collected data and published reports on

man but not the chronic lymphocytic form. An increase in leukemia rates has been observed at doses as low as 20 to 49 rads. Children under 10 years of age at the time of the bomb were more susceptible to leukemogenesis than were older persons. Those under 10 years when exposed also exhibited a substantially higher frequency than usual of other cancers when they reached the ages of 16 to 31 years, a possible portent of a still greater excess as the group enters the age for cancer.

Persons over 10 years of age when exposed exhibited an excess mortality from all cancers. Morbidity studies showed an overabundance of thyroid cancer.

In Britain and the United States, **in utero** exposures to diagnostic irradiation were reported to increase the relative risk of death from cancer before 10 years of age by about 50%. Alice Stewart (1906-) of England first called attention to the possible increased risk of leukemia following low-dose radiation exposure of the fetus.

Cytogenetic studies among atomic bomb survivors show complex chromosomal abnormalities in peripheral lymphocytes more than 25 years after radiation exposure. Long-persisting chromosomal abnormalities also were found among persons exposed **in utero**, even during the first trimester, but not among the next generation.

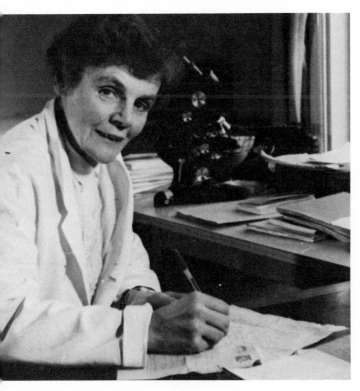

Alice Stewart

the health of atomic bomb survivors since 1948. In 1975 it became the Radiation Effects Research Foundation (RERF).

As the ABCC has matured, research productivity has increased, particularly with regard to radiogenic cancer. In consequence, it became known that radiation induces several forms of leukemia in

R. Keith Cannan. Contribution to the work of the Atomic Bomb Casualty Commission (ABCC). **Arch. Environ. Health** 21: 263-66, 1970.

R. W. Miller. Delayed radiation effects in atomic-bomb survivors. **Science** 166: 569-74, 1966.

Alice Stewart, J. Webb and D. Hewett. A survey of childhood malignancies. **Brit. Med. J.** 1: 1495-1508, 1958.

Alice Stewart. Low dose radiation cancers in man. **Adv. Cancer Res.** 14: 359-90, 1971.

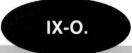

Cancer Epidemiology

IX-O-2. Tobacco and lung cancer: Wynder and others.

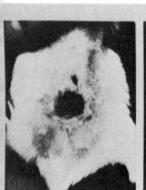 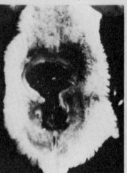 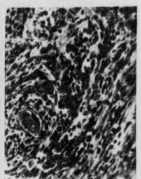

After 494 days   After 564 days   Photomicrograph of tumor (x 200)

Cancer in a mouse, at the site of cigarette tar paintings. (From Wynder et al., 1953).

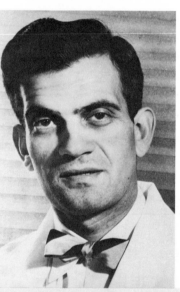

E. L. Wynder

PERCENTAGES FOR AMOUNT OF SMOKING AMONG 605 MALE PATIENTS WITH LUNG CANCER AND 780 MEN WITHOUT CANCER

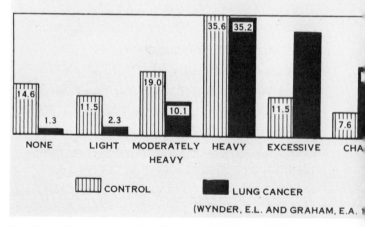

| NONE | LIGHT | MODERATELY HEAVY | HEAVY | EXCESSIVE | CHA |
| 14.6 / 1.3 | 11.5 / 2.3 | 19.0 / 10.1 | 35.6 / 35.2 | 11.5 | 7.6 |

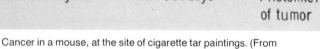

CONTROL   LUNG CANCER

(WYNDER, E.L. AND GRAHAM, E.A.

Smoking and lung cancer. (From Wynder and Graham, 1950).

The association of tobacco smoking and lung cancer gained visibility in 1950 by the publication of 4 retrospective case-control studies.

One of these was by a medical student and his professor of surgery.

Ernst L. Wynder was born in Germany in 1922. He received his B.A. degree from New York University in 1943 and his M.D. from Washington University in St. Louis in 1950. He began his initial interviews on lung cancer patients and controls as a sophomore medical student.

Evarts A. Graham (1883-1957) was the professor of surgery at Washington University School of Medicine. In 1933 he had performed the first successful pneumonectomy for lung cancer.

Wynder, Graham, and Adele B. Croninger recorded the induction by cigarette tar of skin cancer in mice and in rabbits. Wynder, with Dietrich Hoffmann, conducted extensive studies on tobacco products while on the staff of the Sloan-Kettering Institute and the Memorial Cancer Center, 1951-1969. He also carried out international epidemiological investigations on many of the major cancer sites of man.

In 1969 Wynder established and headed the American Health Foundation and published the journal, **Preventive Medicine**, in New York. In 1974 the Naylor Dana Institute for Disease Prevention was opened as part of the Foundation.

The other 3 reports on smoking and lung cancer were by Levin et al., Schreck et al. and Mills and Porter, as summarized in the eventual **Smoking and Health** report of the advisory committee to the Surgeon General of the Public Health Service, issued in 1964. The report by Levin et al. was printed immediately following the paper by Wynder and Graham.

E. L. Wynder and E. A. Graham. Tobacco smoking as a possible etiologic factor in bronchiogenic carcinoma. A study of six hundred and eighty-four proved cases. **J. Am. Med. Assn.** 143: 329-36, 1950.

E. L. Wynder, E. A. Graham, and A. B. Croninger. Experimental production of carcinoma with cigarette tar. **Cancer Res.** 13: 855-64, 1953 and 15: 445-8, 1955.

E. L. Wynder and D. Hoffmann. **Tobacco and Tobacco Smoke.** New York: Academic Press, 1967.

M. L. Levin, H. Goldstein and P. R. Gerhardt. Cancer and tobacco smoking. A preliminary report. **J. Am. Med. Assn.** 143: 336-8, 1950.

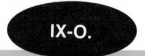

Cancer Epidemiology

IX-O-3. Tobacco hazards: Doll and Hill.

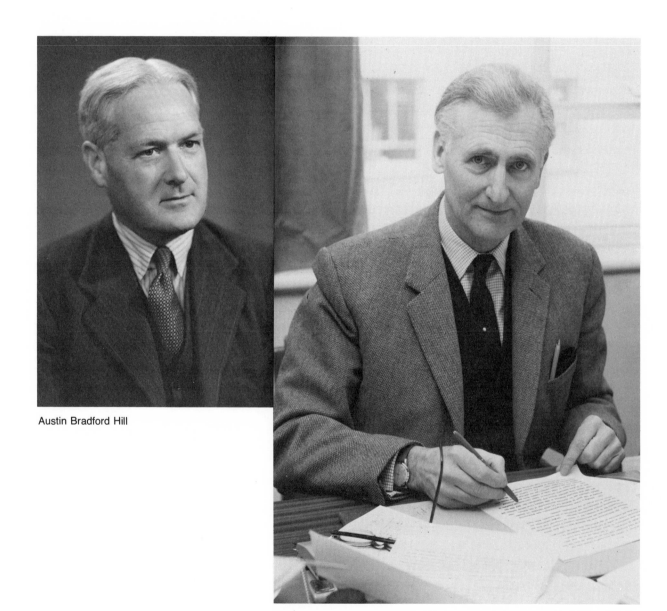

Austin Bradford Hill

Richard Doll

Signal contributions to cancer research and prevention of cancer have been made by epidemiologists and statisticians. Eminent among them have been two British colleagues, Austin Bradford Hill and Richard Doll. They collaborated in the pioneer prospective investigations on the relationship of smoking to lung cancer which with the preceding retrospective studies helped to establish the carcinogenic and other health hazards of tobacco smoking. It is noteworthy that the findings of all such studies were remarkably similar, presenting no conflicting evidence. The most important findings were that the total death rate from all causes combined is far higher among cigarette smokers than among pipe and cigar smokers and among nonsmokers, that the death rate increases in direct relation to the amount of cigarette smoking, and that the incidence of carcinoma of the lung would be reduced by 80 or 90% in the absence of smoking. Subsequent studies by Hill and Doll revealed that the agent in tobacco smoke might act as a cocarcinogen in the presence of another element in the environment, provided some additional evidence that lung carcinoma is more common in urban areas than in rural areas, that the greater mortality in cigarette smokers over pipe smokers is a function of method of smoking irrespective of amount, and that deaths from cancer in

sites other than the lung and upper respiratory and digestive tracts reveal little association between mortality and smoking.

Austin Bradford Hill (born in 1897 in London) was professor of medical statistics at the University of London and member of the British Committee on the Safety of Medicines and of the International Statistical Institute. He has written many papers on clinical trials of drugs, smoking and lung cancer, and experimental methods in preventive medicine, which are included in his book **Statistical Methods in Clinical and Preventive Medicine**.

William Richard Doll (born in 1912 in London) has since 1969 held the position of regius professor of medicine at the University of Oxford. Since 1936 he has written various articles on the etiology of cancer, many of which are summarized in his brilliant Carling Lectures of 1967, **Prevention of Cancer, Pointers from Epidemiology**. In this book he indicates ways in which epidemiological studies can contribute to the prevention of cancer, the most intensively used method being that of correlating differences in cancer incidence in various communities with differences in the prevalence of a potential etiological factor.

Hill and Doll have been knighted for their work.

Richard Doll and A. Bradford Hill. Smoking and carcinoma of the lung. **Brit. Med. J.** 2: 739-48, 1950.

Richard Doll and A. Bradford Hill. A study of the aetiology of carcinoma of the lung. **Brit. Med. J.** 2: 1271-86, 1952.

Richard Doll and A. Bradford Hill. Lung cancer and other causes of death in relation to smoking. **Brit. Med. J.** 2: 1071-81, 1956.

Richard Doll and A. Bradford Hill. Mortality in relation to smoking: ten years' observations of British doctors. **Brit. Med. J.** 1: 1399-1410, 1964.

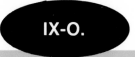

Cancer Epidemiology

IX-O-4. Smoking and health: Hammond, Horn and Dorn.

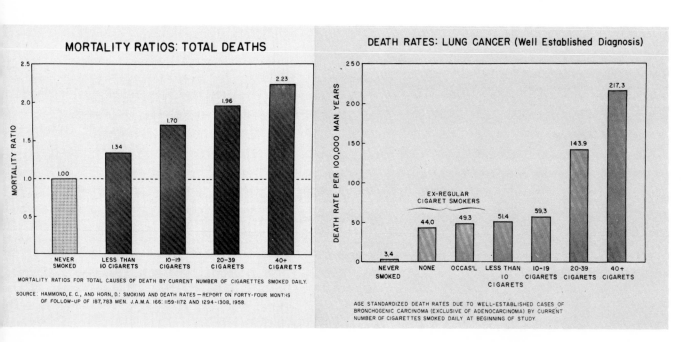

MORTALITY RATIOS: TOTAL DEATHS

MORTALITY RATIOS FOR TOTAL CAUSES OF DEATH BY CURRENT NUMBER OF CIGARETTES SMOKED DAILY.

SOURCE: HAMMOND, E. C., AND HORN, D.: SMOKING AND DEATH RATES — REPORT ON FORTY-FOUR MONTHS OF FOLLOW-UP OF 187,783 MEN. J.A.M.A. 166: 1159-1172 AND 1294-1308, 1958.

DEATH RATES: LUNG CANCER (Well Established Diagnosis)

AGE STANDARDIZED DEATH RATES DUE TO WELL-ESTABLISHED CASES OF BRONCHOGENIC CARCINOMA (EXCLUSIVE OF ADENOCARCINOMA) BY CURRENT NUMBER OF CIGARETTES SMOKED DAILY AT BEGINNING OF STUDY

The elucidation of tobacco smoking, especially in the form of cigarettes, as a major cause of lung cancer, and as a cause in other cancers of the oral cavity and urinary bladder, began with several retrospective studies in the 1950s. To the prospective study of British physicians by Doll and Hill was added one in the United States. It was organized by E. Cuyler Hammond and Daniel Horn of the American Cancer Society, and involved observations on 187,000 men identified by their smoking habits. The results were as definite as the results of other studies, the first being that smoking accelerated mortality from heart disease as well as being a carcinogenic hazard.

Harold Dorn also conducted a massive prospective study on 250,000 veterans of World War I, and obtained essentially identical data.

The evidence led to the examination of the subject by a committee appointed in 1959 to advise the Surgeon General of the U. S. Public Health Service. Their report appeared in 1964, and was similar to the report issued two years previously by the Royal College of Physicians of London.

E. Cuyler Hammond was born in 1912

Daniel Horn and E. Cuyler Hammond.

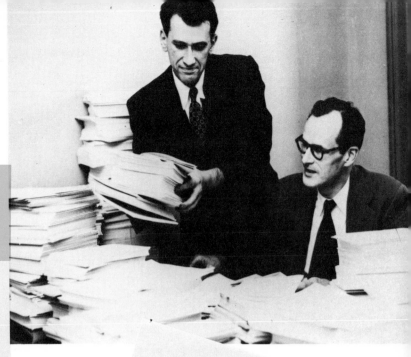

in Baltimore, Maryland, and received his doctorate from Johns Hopkins University in 1938. Since 1946 he has been with the American Cancer Society, as vice-

THE EFFECTS OF SMOKING: PRINCIPAL FINDINGS

igarette smoking is associated with a 70 percent increase in the age-
ific death rates of males. The total number of excess deaths causally
ed to cigarette smoking in the U.S. population cannot be accurately
nated. In view of the continuing and mounting evidence from many
ces, it is the judgment of the Committee that cigarette smoking con-
ates substantially to mortality from certain specific diseases and to the
all death rate.

Lung Cancer

igarette smoking is causally related to lung cancer in men; the magni-
of the effect of cigarette smoking far outweighs all other factors. The
for women, though les
he risk of developing l
the number of cigarett
inuing smoking. In
kers of cigarettes have a
cancer and heavy smoke
he risk of developing ca
kers, cigar smokers, an
smokers, but much less t
igarette smoking is muc
e causation of lung canc

SMOKING *and* HEALTH

REPORT OF THE ADVISORY COMMITTEE
TO THE SURGEON GENERAL
OF THE PUBLIC HEALTH SERVICE

Principal finding
on lung cancer
(from *Smoking
and Health*,
1964, p. 31).

U.S DEPARTMENT OF HEALTH, EDUCATION, AND WELFARE
Public Health Service

1964

THE
HEALTH CONSEQUENCES
OF SMOKING

JANUARY 1974

ask fr.

U.S. DEPARTMENT OF HEALTH, EDUCATION, AND WELFARE
Public Health Service

president for epidemiology and statistics. Daniel Horn was born in 1916, in Rochester, New York, and received his doctorate from Harvard in 1943. He was with the American Cancer Society from 1947 to 1962, when he moved to the U. S. Public Health Service, and became director of the Clearinghouse on Smoking and Health.

E. C. Hammond and D. Horn. Smoking and death rates—report of forty-four months of follow-up of 187,783 men. **J. Am. Med. Assn.** 166: 1159-72 and 1249-1308, 1958.

H. F. Dorn. Tobacco consumption and mortality from cancer and other diseases. **Pub. Health Repts** (USA) 74: 581-93, 1959.

Smoking and Health. Report of the Advisory Committee to the Surgeon General of the U.S. Public Health Service. U.S. Public Health Service Publication 1103, Washington, D.C.: U. S. Govt. Print. Off., 1964.

Smoking and Health. Summary and Report of the Royal College of Physicians of London on Smoking in Relation to Cancer of the Lung and Other Diseases. London: Pitman Publishing Co., 1962.

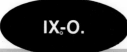

IX-O.

Cancer Epidemiology

IX-O-5. Burkitt's lymphoma: Burkitt and Burchenal.

The discovery of a variant of lymphoma primarily afflicting children in sub-Sahara Africa is a modern saga of epidemiology. It gained prominence following Denis Burkitt's field investigations of 1958. As is usual, retrospectively the disease was recorded in Africa as far back as 1904, and is now encountered throughout the world. The disease is manifested by aggressive tumors in the region of the jaw, a typical "starry-sky" microscopic appearance, and a high responsiveness to chemotherapy. It is associated with the presence of the Epstein-Barr virus, the exact role of which is not entirely clear. Burkitt's studies on the relation of the disease to temperature and humidity suggested the possibility of an insect vector in its occurrence. In 1960, Joseph Burchenal and Denis Burkitt initiated the treatment of the

lymphoma with alkylating agents and antifolates, in absence of other modalities, and encountered surprisingly satisfactory responses of long duration.

Denis Parons Burkitt was born in 1911 in North Ireland, and was a graduate in medicine from Dublin University in 1935. He went to Africa as a military physician in 1941, and joined the British Colonial Service in Uganda in 1946, remaining there as a senior consultant surgeon to the Ministry of Health until 1964, when he became a member of the Medical Research Council in London.

Joseph Holland Burchenal was born in 1912 in Delaware, and graduated in medicine from the University of Pennsylvania in 1937. He joined the Sloan-Kettering Institute for Cancer Research in 1946, and in 1964 became vice-president for clinical investigation.

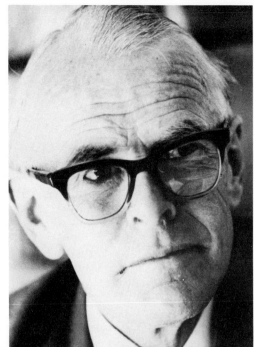

Denis Burkitt

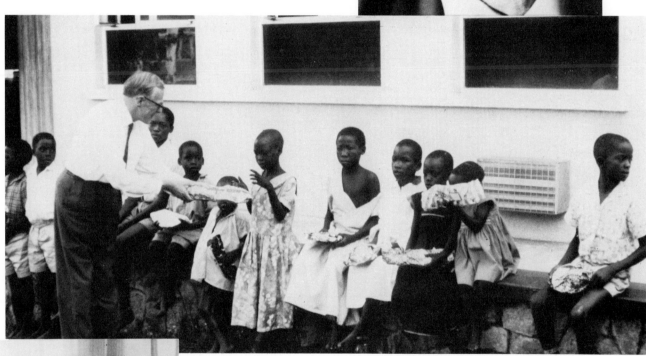

African children with Burkitt's lymphoma apparently cured by chemotherapy.

Bernard Glemser. **Mr. Burkitt and Africa.** New York: World Publishing Co., 1970.

D. P. Burkitt and D. H. Wright (eds). **Burkitt's Lymphoma.** Edinburgh: E. & S. Livingstone, 1970.

J. H. Burchenal and D. P. Burkitt. **Treatment of Burkitt's Tumour.** UICC Monograph 8. New York: Springer-Verlag, 1967.

Joseph H. Burchenal

437

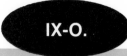

Cancer Epidemiology

IX-O-6. Early sex and cancer: Rotkin and MacMahon.

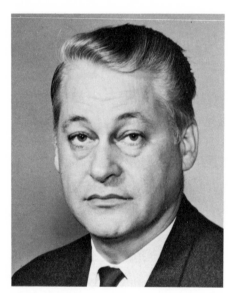

I.D. Rotkin

Clinical and pathological descriptions during the 19th Century suggested that cancer of the uterine cervix was related to pregnancies, and that it was rare among Jewish women. The relationships of sexual experience to cervical cancer was established by demographic and case-control studies. In one careful study conducted by I. D. Rotkin, not only were the relationships reiterated to low economic status, early first coitus and multiple sex partners, but an important determinant was revealed in adolescent coitus. The roles of carcinogens in smegma, and of herpes hominis infection remain to be clarified, but it seems established that the cervical epithelium is particularly susceptible before full maturity.

Breast cancer shows the obverse to cervical cancer: it is more frequent among unmarried women, as Rigoni-Stern knew by 1842. International epidemiological studies organized by

Brian MacMahon elicited more subtle information, that early complete pregnancy was related to a lower frequency of breast cancer. Thus, the breast epithelium is in some way protected by early "priming" for its mammalian functions.

Isadore David Rotkin was born in 1921 in Chicago, and obtained a doctorate in genetics at the University of California at Berkeley in 1954. The epidemiological studies on cervical cancer were started when he was a graduate student and continued while with the Kaiser Foundation. Since 1970 he has been professor of preventive medicine at the University of Illinois School of Medicine in Chicago.

Brian MacMahon was born in England in 1923, and educated at the University of Birmingham, where he obtained a Ph.D. in 1952 and an M.D. in 1955. After 3 years with the State University of New York, he became professor of epidemiology at the School of Public Health at Harvard University.

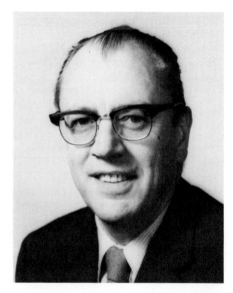

Brian MacMahon

I. D. Rotkin. Relation of adolescent coitus to cervical cancer risk. **J. Am. Med. Assn.** 179: 486-91, 1962.

Brian MacMahon, Philip Cole and James Brown. Etiology of human breast cancer: a review. **J. Natl. Cancer Inst.** 50: 21-42, 1973.

M. B. Shimkin. Some historical landmarks in cancer epidemiology. In D. Schottenfeld (ed). **Cancer Epidemiology and Prevention.** Springfield, Ill.: C. C. Thomas, 1975. (p. 60-75).

IX-O.

Cancer Epidemiology

IX-O-7. Malformations and cancer: Good, Miller and Fraumeni.

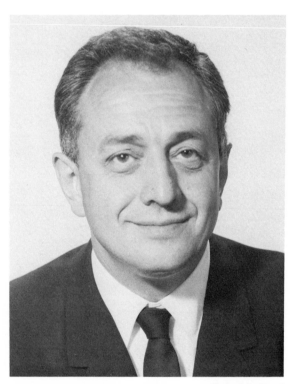

Robert A. Good

The simultaneous occurrence of leukemia and mongolism was established as an important association by William Krivit and Robert A. Good of Minnesota. Their first article, on 5 such cases, was followed by a nationwide survey. Case reports of congenital leukemia and mongolism appeared before this work, but its significance was not recognized.

Robert Alan Good was born in Minnesota in 1922, and obtained his doctorate from the University of Minnesota in 1947. He rose rapidly in three fields, pediatrics, microbiology and pathology, with special emphasis on research in immunology. In 1972 he became research director of the Sloan-Kettering Memorial Cancer Center in New York.

The association of congenital malformations and neoplastic disease was pursued by R. W. Miller and J. F. Fraumeni, Jr., of the National Cancer Institute. In 1964 they described the association of Wilms' tumor with aniridia and hemihypertrophy. They have performed critical studies on the genetic, familial and environmental determinants in human cancer.

Robert Warwick Miller was born in Brooklyn, New York in 1921, and obtained his doctorate at the University of Pennsylvania in 1946. He trained in pediatrics and served with the Atomic Bomb Casualty Commission in Japan. Since 1961 he has been chief of the epidemiology branch of the National Cancer Institute.

Joseph F. Fraumeni, Jr., was born in Boston in 1933 and graduated in medicine at Duke University in 1958. He trained in internal medicine, and came from the Sloan-Kettering Institute to the epidemiology branch of the National Cancer Institute in 1962.

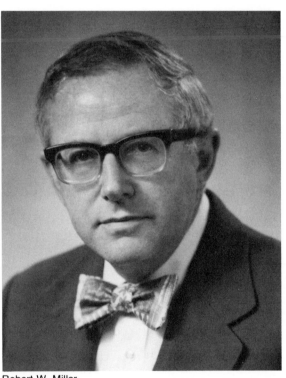

Robert W. Miller

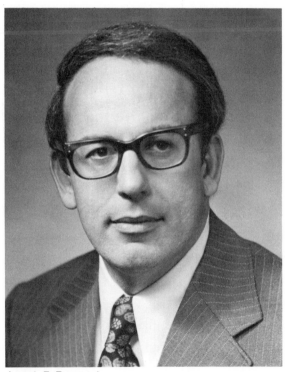

Joseph F. Fraumeni

William Krivit and Robert A. Good. The simultaneous occurrence of leukemia and mongolism. **Am. J. Dis. Child.** 91: 218-22, 1956 and 94: 289-93, 1957.

R. W. Miller, J. F. Fraumeni and M. D. Manning. Association of Wilms's tumor with aniridia, hemihypertrophy and other congenital malformations. **New Engl. J. Med.** 270: 922-27, 1964.

J. F. Fraumeni, Jr. Genetic factors. In J. F. Holland and E. Frei, III (eds). **Cancer Medicine.** Philadelphia: Lea and Febiger, 1973. p. 7-15.

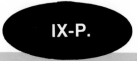

Molecular Biology

IX-P-1. Heredity and DNA: Avery, MacLeod and McCarty.

A milestone in molecular biology was the demonstration in 1944 that transformation of pneumococci from one type to another could be induced by desoxyribonucleic acid (DNA), thus establishing that DNA is the chemical material directing heredity.

The discovery was made at the Rockefeller Institute in New York by O.T. Avery and two young associates, C. M. MacLeod and M. McCarty. The work was based on earlier observations of pneumococcal transformation, by Fred Griffith.

Photograph of pneumococcal colonies, reproduced from the original article by Avery et al. shows, in figure 1, colonies of the attenuated, nonencapsulated R variant of pneumococcus Type II, on blood agar, magnified X3.5. Figure 2 shows colonies of the same cells after induction of transformation by addition of DNA isolated from Type III pneumococci. The smooth, glistening mucoid colonies are characteristic of the encapsulated, virulent (S) cells of pneumococcus Type III and readily distinguished from the small rough colonies of the parent R strain.

Oswald Theodore Avery (1877-1955) was born in Nova Scotia, attended Colgate University and obtained his M.D. at Columbia University in 1904. He joined Rockefeller Institute in 1913 and remained there until his retirement in 1947. A. F. Coburn has published an account of the pneumococcal work.

Colin Munro MacLeod (1909-1972) was born in Nova Scotia, and graduated with an M.D. from McGill University in 1932. He joined Rockefeller Institute in 1934, and in 1941 became chairman of the department of microbiology at New York University. He held posts at the University of Pennsylvania (1956-60), Office of Science and Technology, Executive Office of the White House (1963-66), Commonwealth Foundation (1966-70), and the Oklahoma Research Foundation (1970-72).

Maclyn McCarty (1911-   ) was born in Indiana, graduated from Stanford University in 1933 and obtained an M.D. from Johns Hopkins University in 1937. He joined the Rockefeller Institute in 1941 and in 1965 became vice-president of Rockefeller University and physician-in-chief of its hospital.

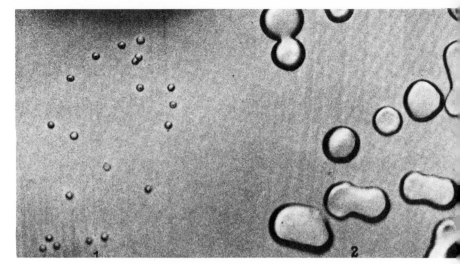

Transformation of pneumococci by exposure to DNA. **Left,** small colonies of R variant of pneumococcus Type II. **Right,** transformation following addition of DNA from Type III pneumococci. (From Avery *et al.,* 1944).

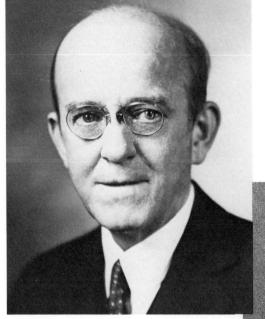

O.T. Avery

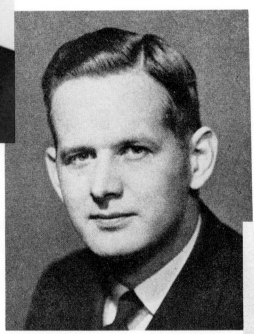

Maclyn McCarty

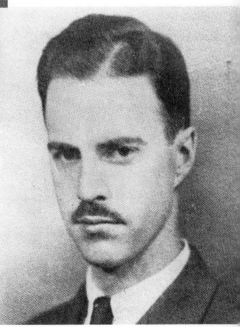

Colin M. MacLeod

O. T. Avery, C. M. MacLeod and M. McCarty. Studies on chemical nature of substance inducing transformation of pneumococcal types; induction of transformation by desoxyribonucleic acid fraction from pneumococcus type III. **J. Exper. Med.** 79: 137-58, 1944.

Fred Griffith. The significance of pneumococcal types. **J. Hyg.** 27: 113-59, 1928.

A. F. Coburn. Oswald Theodore Avery and DNA. **Perspect. Biol. and Med.** 12: 623-30, 1969.

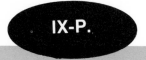

IX-P.

Molecular Biology

IX-P-2. Cell fractions and functions: Claude.

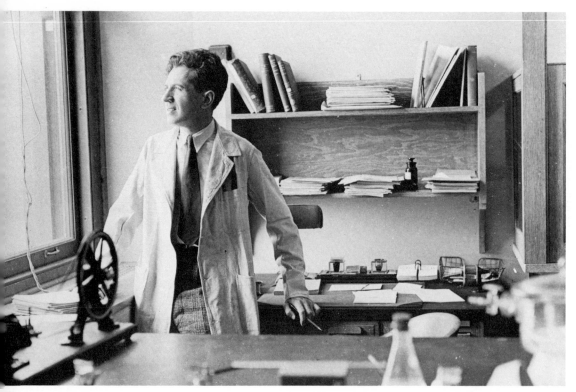

Albert Claude

Albert Claude (born 1899 in Belgium), Director of Jules Bordet Institute for Cancer Research in Brussels, worked at the Rockefeller Institute in New York, 1929-1949. He was a pioneer in fractionating cells by differential centrifugation, correlating the fractions to chemical constituents and biochemical functions. Studies on isolated mitochondria, in collaboration with R. Hotchkiss,

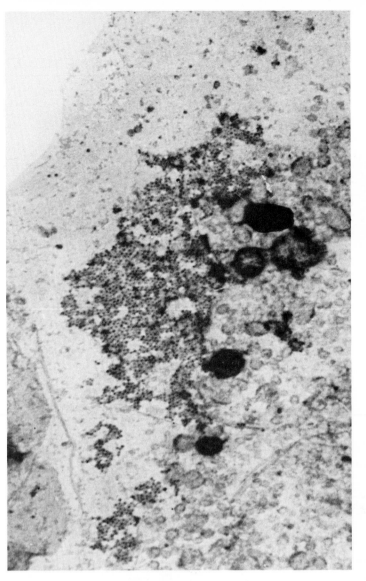

Rous chicken tumor virus particles

G. Hogeboom, and W. Schneider, clarified the role of mitochondria as cellular "power plants."

Concentration and isolation of the Rous chicken sarcoma agent was achieved by fractionation, by adsorption and elution with alumina gels, and by differential centrifugation. The agent was shown by 1939 to be a nucleic acid of the ribose type. Electron microscopy studies, in collaboration with K. R. Potter and E. G. Pickels, showed the Rous agent particles within tumor cells, proving that the agent was a virus.

Claude received the Nobel Prize in medicine or physiology in 1974 for his studies.

Upper electron micrograph shows colonies of Rous chicken tumor 10 virus in a 13-day-old tumor in a Plymouth Rock pullet. The lower micrograph shows Rous virus in a 5-day-old tumor explant on an embryonated egg. The virus is 70 to 85 mμ in diameter, and "budding" can be seen at the cell surface.

Albert Claude. Studies on cells: morphology, chemical constitution and distribution of biochemical functions. **Harvey Lectures** 43: 121-64, 1947-48.

A. Claude, K. R. Porter and E. G. Pickles. Electron microscope study of chicken tumor cells. **Cancer Res.** 7: 421-30, 1947.

A. Claude. The coming of age of the cell. (Nobel lecture) **Science** 189: 433-35, 1975.

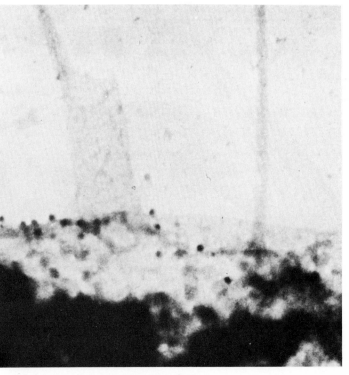

Budding of virus particles at cell surface

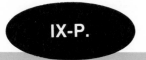

IX-P.

Molecular Biology

IX-P-3. DNA repair: Cleaver and Ames.

Xeroderma pigmentosum is a rare hereditary disease, caused by an autosomal recessive gene, in which the skin is extremely sensitive to ultraviolet radiation and soon develops multiple cancers.

In 1968 James E. Cleaver at the University of California Medical Center in San Francisco performed experiments with skin fibroblasts cultured from normal individuals and 3 patients with xeroderma pigmentosum. Normal skin fibroblasts can repair ultraviolet radiation damage to DNA by inserting new bases into DNA in the form of small patches. Cells from patients with xeroderma pigmentosum carry a mutation such that replication of DNA is either absent or much reduced in comparison to normal fibroblasts.

This abnormal DNA repair defect in xeroderma pigmentosum attracted wide interest and application to many related problems. Carcinogenesis may be postulated as the result of somatic mutations caused by unrepaired damage. Carcinogens can be classified according to how xeroderma pigmentosum cells respond to them. The metabolic basis of an inherited neoplastic condition reached the level of DNA repair, with hopes that the findings can be applicable to other neoplastic transformations.

James E. Cleaver was born in England in 1938 and obtained his education in radiobiology and medicine at Cambridge. He trained in neurosurgery at Massachusetts General Hospital and has been with the University of California in San Francisco since 1966. Much of his work was supported by the U. S. Atomic Energy Commission.

DNA repair in **Salmonella** histidine mutants following exposure to chemicals, including liver homogenates to effect metabolic conversion, was elaborated as a test for mutagenic and carcinogenic activity.

Bruce Nathan Ames has pioneered in the development of the procedures. Ames was born in 1928 in New York City, and obtained his doctorate in biochemical genetics from the California Institute of Technology in 1953. He became professor of biochemistry at the University of California at Berkeley in 1968.

J. E. Cleaver. Defective repair replication of DNA in xeroderma pigmentosum. **Nature** 218: 652-56, 1968.

J. E. Cleaver. DNA repair with purines and pyrimidines in radiation- and carcinogen-damaged normal and xeroderma pigmentosum human cells. **Cancer Res.** 33: 362-69, 1973.

B. N. Ames, W. E. Durston, E. Yamasaki and F. D. Lee.

Carcinogens as mutagens: a simple test system combining liver homogenates for activation and bacteria for detection. **Proc. Natl. Acad. Sci.** USA 70: 2281-85, 1973.

J. McCann, E. Choi, E. Yamasaki and B. N. Ames. Detection of carcinogens as mutagens in the *Salmonella*/microsome test: Assay of 300 chemicals. **Proc. Natl. Acad. Sci.** USA 72: 5135-39, 1975.

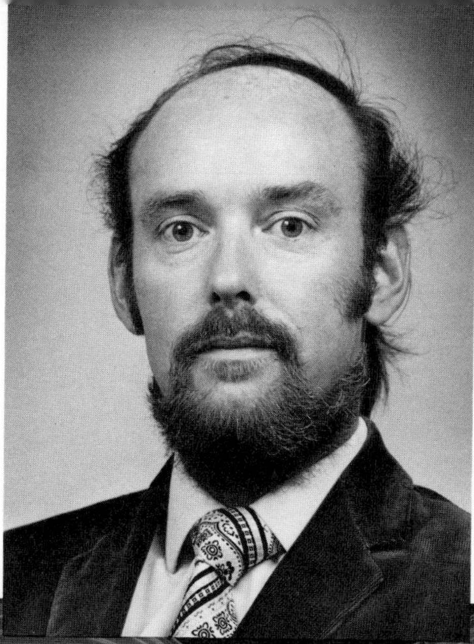

James E. Cleaver

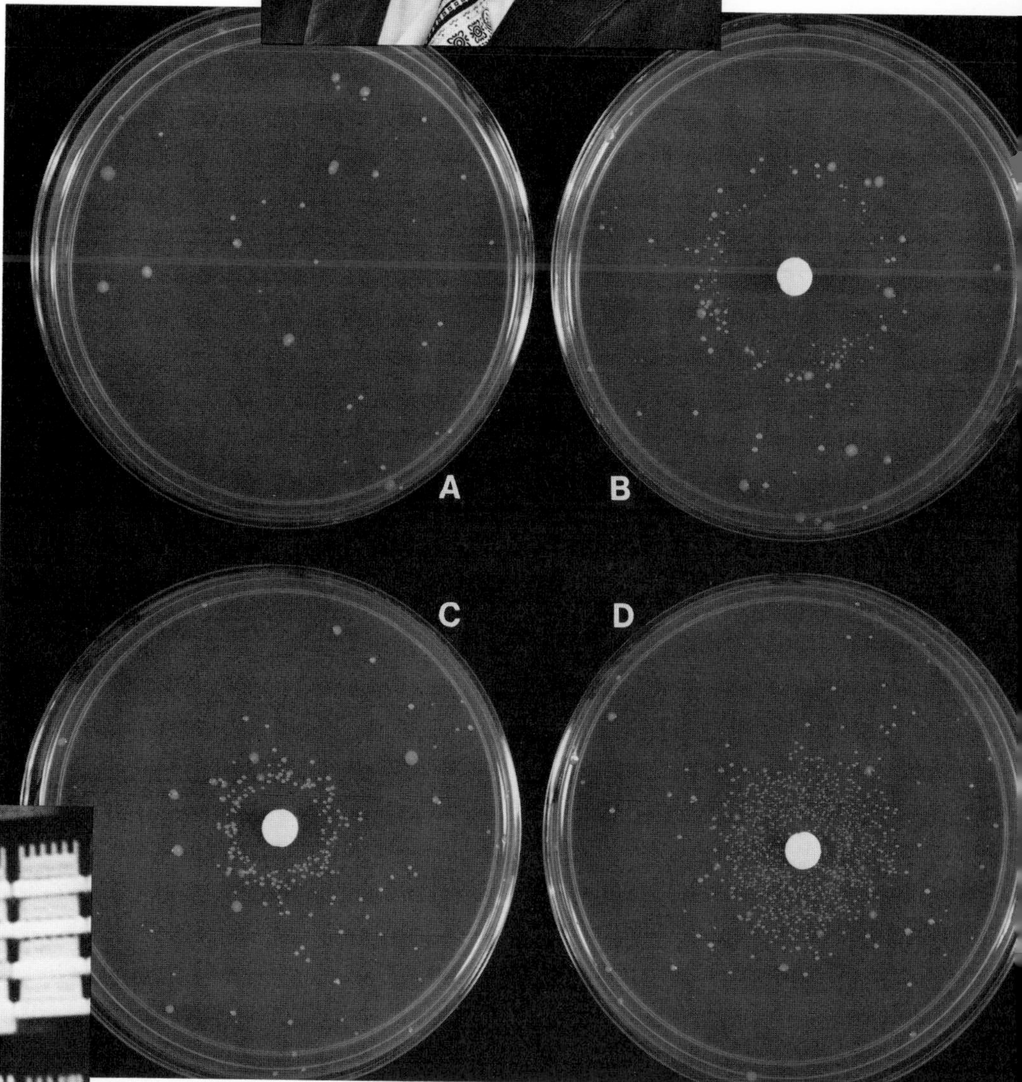

Carcinogenesis and mutagenesis: Salmonella strain TA98 and liver microsomal activation system, with test materials on central paper discs. A, spontaneous revertants; B, furylfuramide (AF-2), 1 μg; C, aflatoxin B$_1$, 1 μg; D, 2-aminofluroene, l0 μg. Mutagen induced revertants appear as a ring of colonies around each disc. (from B.N. Ames, J. McCann and E. Yamasaki, Methods for detecting carcinogens and mutagens with Salmonella/microsome mutagenicity test. Mutation Res. 1975).

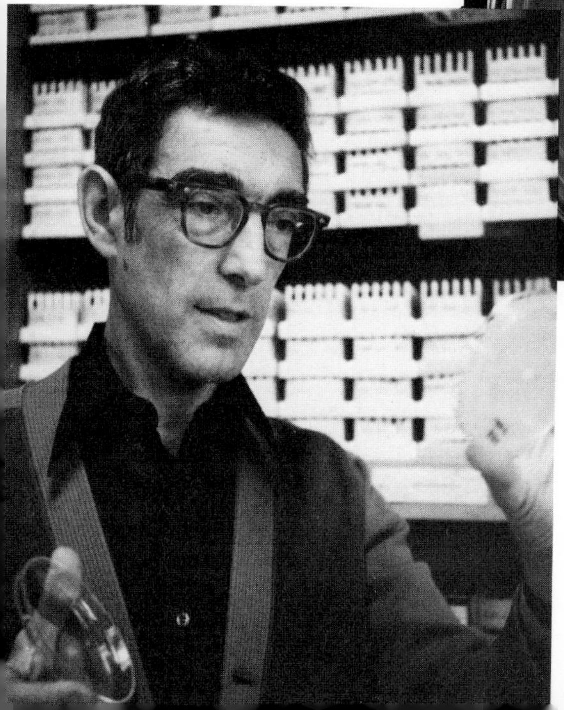

Bruce N. Ames

IX-P.

Molecular Biology

IX-P-4. Cell-virus interaction: Dulbecco, Temin and Baltimore.

The 1975 Nobel Prize for physiology or medicine was awarded for discoveries on the mechanisms of "the interaction between tumor viruses and the genetic material of the cell."

Renato Dulbecco, born in 1914 in Italy and a medical graduate from the University of Turin in 1936, turned his attention to the problem of cell-virus interaction while on the staff of the Salk Institute in La Jolla, California. His Harvey Lecture of 1967 indicated approaches to the problem of oncogenic conversion by viruses.

Discovery of RNA-directed DNA polymerase, or reverse transcriptase, was reported simultaneously in 1970, by David Baltimore and Howard M. Temin and Satoshi Mizutani, in back-to-back articles in **Nature**. The work was conducted with Rous sarcoma and Rauscher murine leukemia viruses. It helped to elucidate the mechanism by which RNA viruses can convert their genetic informa-tion into DNA and it suggested that information in biological systems can flow into as well as out of DNA.

David Baltimore was born in New York in 1938, and received his doctorate from the Rockefeller University, New York, in 1946. He has been with the Massachusetts Institute of Technology, Cambridge, Mass., since 1968, as professor of biology.

Howard M. Temin was born in Philadelphia in 1934, and received his doctorate at the California Institute of Technology in 1959. He has been with the University of Wisconsin's McArdle Laboratory since 1960, as professor of oncology. Satoshi Mizutani was born in Yokohama in 1937, and received his doctorate in microbiology at the University of Kansas. He was on a Fullbright scholarship while Temin's coworker, and continues at the University of Wisconsin as assistant scientist.

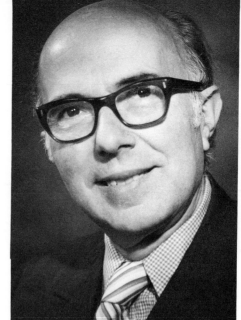

Renato Dulbecco

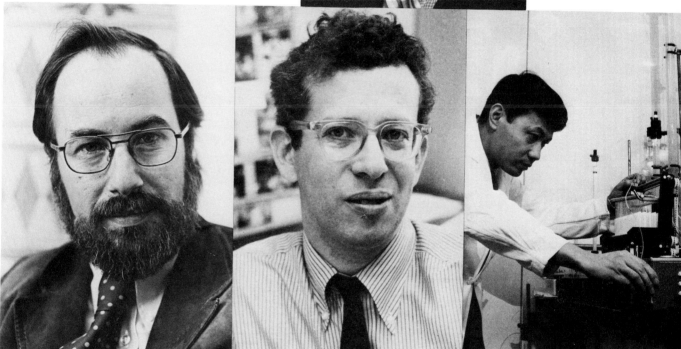

David Baltimore

Howard M. Temin

Satoshi Mizutani

Renato Dulbecco. Cell transformation by the small DNA-containing viruses. **Harvey Lectures** 63: 33-46, 1967-68.

David Baltimore. RNA-dependent DNA polymerase in various of RNA tumour viruses. **Nature** 226: 1209-11, 1970.

H. M. Temin and S. Mizutani. RNA-dependent DNA polymerase in virions of Rous sarcoma virus. **Nature** 226: 1211-13, 1970.

H. Temin. The protovirus hypothesis: speculations on the significance of RNA-directed DNA synthesis for normal development and for carcinogenesis. **J. Natl. Cancer Inst.** 46: iii-vii, 1971.

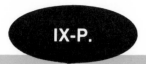

Molecular Biology

IX-P-5. Nucleotide sequences: Spiegelman.

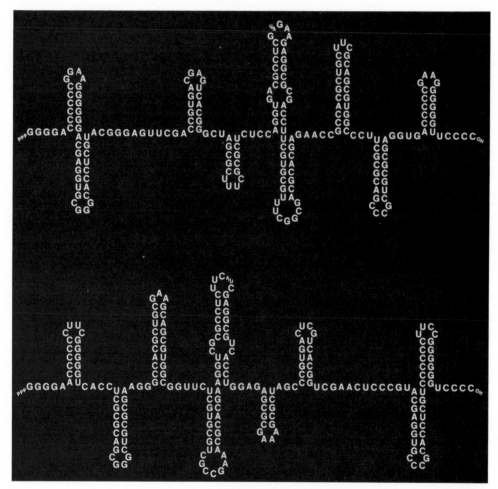

Complete nucleotide sequence of a replicating RNA molecule
(from D.R. Mills, F.R. Kramer and S. Spiegelman, Science
180:916-27, 1973).

Francis Delafield Hospital, New York

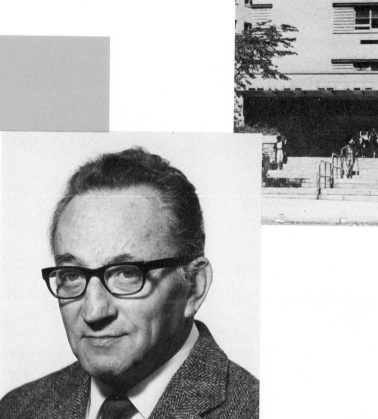

Sol Spiegelman

Spiegelman and his associates succeeded in synthesizing infectious viral nucleic acid and demonstrated that faithful copies of molecules containing genetic information could be synthesized in the laboratory. Studies on molecular hybridization showed that this technique could be utilized to detect the presence and operation of specific genes, including viral genes, within cells. These approaches may permit a definitive conclusion on the role of viruses in human cancer.

Sol Spiegelman was born in New York City in 1914 and received his doctorate in biochemistry from Washington University in St. Louis in 1944. He was on the faculty of the University of Illinois between 1949 and 1969, when he moved to the directorship of the Institute of Cancer Research of the College of Physicians and Surgeons, Columbia University in New York.

S. Spiegelman. The development and use of an extracellular RNA replicating system. **Harvey Lectures** 64: 1-68, 1968-69.

S. Spiegelman, D. Kufe, R. Hehlmann and W. P. Peters. Evidence for RNA tumor viruses in human lymphomas including Burkitt's disease. **Cancer Res.** 33: 1515-26, 1973.

D. R. Mills, F. R. Kramer and S. Spiegelman. Complete nucleotide sequence of a replicating RNA molecule. **Science** 180: 916-27, 1973.

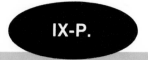

Molecular Biology

IX-P-6. Oncogene theory: Huebner and Todaro.

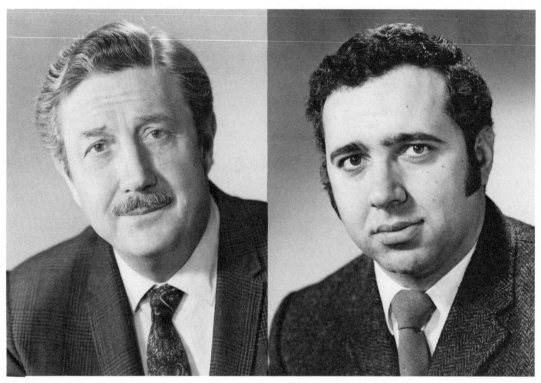

Robert J. Huebner   George J. Todaro

At the last quarter of the century, there are two preeminent general theories on the cause and nature of cancer. These are the protovirus theory of Temin, and the oncogene concept of Huebner and Todaro. The theories, in a way, are restatements of the earlier postulations of virus infestation proposed by Borrel, and of chromosomal changes suggested by Boveri in 1907.

The oncogene concept suggests that in the course of evolution a type RNA virus became incorporated in the genome, and exists there as a silent infection prior to birth. The oncogene can be activated by the myriad exogenous causes of cancer. Evidence from sero-epidemiological and cell culture studies lend credence to the view that cells of many vertebrates contain information for producing C-type viruses.

Robert J. Huebner was born in Ohio in 1914, and received an M.D. degree from St. Louis University School of Medicine in 1942. He joined the U.S. Public Health Service, and had a distinguished career in the study of viral and rickettsial diseases from 1944 to 1968, when he be-

came chief of the viral carcinogenesis branch of the National Cancer Institute.

George J. Todaro was born in New York City in 1937, and graduated with an M.D. degree from the New York University School of Medicine in 1963. After training in pathology, he joined the National Cancer Institute in 1967.

The protovirus and the oncogene theories appear to overlap at the level of molecular biology. Perhaps, as Wallace Rowe expressed it, neoplasia may represent a virus-cell relationship that can be described as a genetic infection.

Robert J. Huebner and George J. Todaro. Oncogenes of RNA tumor viruses as determinants of cancer. **Proc. Natl. Acad. of Sciences** (USA) 64: 1087-94, 1969.

Wallace P. Rowe. Genetic factors in the natural history of murine leukemia virus infection. **Cancer Res.** 33: 3061-68, 1973.

IX-Q.

Cancer Institutes and Services.

The post-World War II period for biomedical research and related activities was one of reconstruction in Europe and expansion in the United States.

In the United States, the larger, older institutions such as those in New York and in Buffalo were enlarged and their research and service components broadened. Vigorous new institutions devoted to cancer arose in Houston, Texas, and in Madison, Wisconsin. Programs of cancer research were reorganized or initiated at several Universities, such as Columbia, Pennsylvania, Minnesota, and California.

In Europe and Japan, some cancer institutions with histories going back to before World War I were restituted, and new ones were added.

Systematic regionalization of clinical services to patients with cancer became a feature in several European countries, notably France and the Soviet Union.

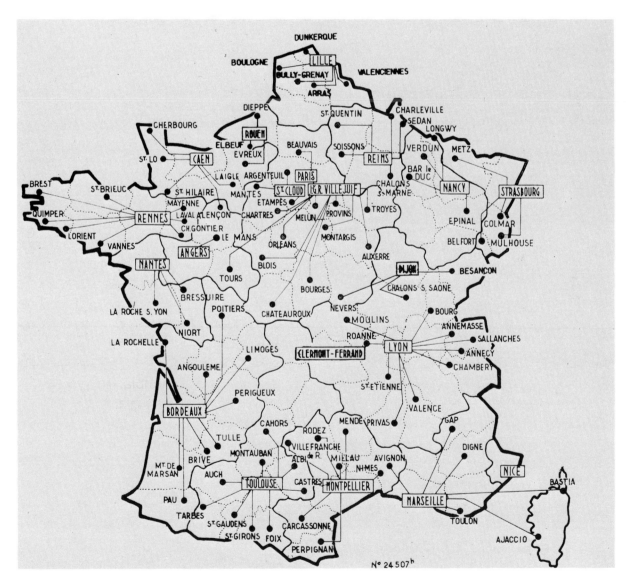

Anti-cancer clinical center network of France (from Denoix, 1974).

Pierre Denoix. **Clefs pour la Cancérologie.** Paris: Seghers, 1974.

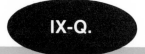

Cancer Institutes and Services.

IX-Q-1. M. D. Anderson Hospital and Tumor Institute: Clark.

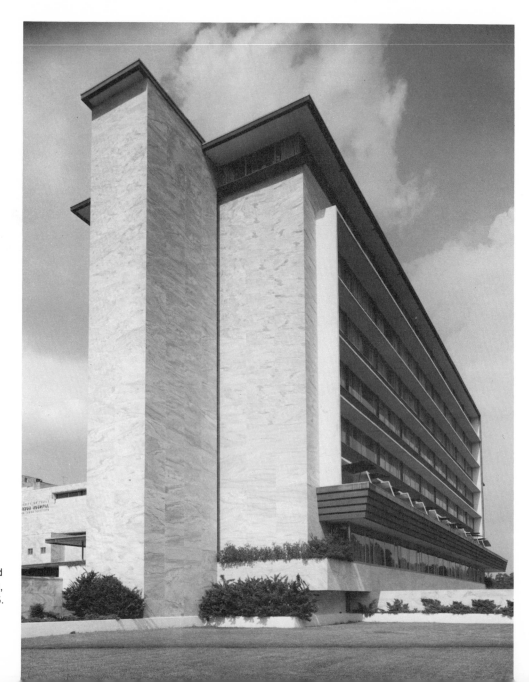

M. D. Anderson Hospital and
Tumor Institute, Houston, Texas,
1965.

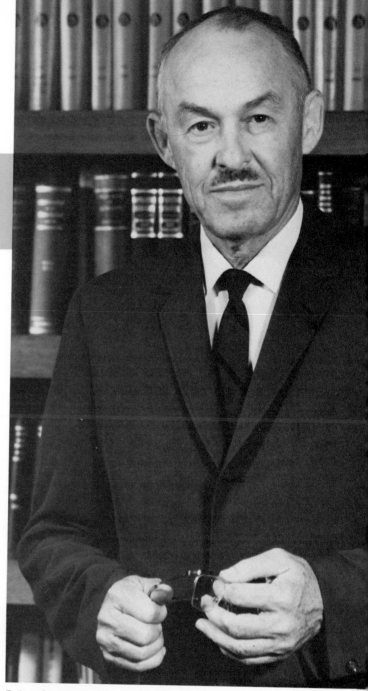

R. Lee Clark

The State Legislature of Texas, in 1941, appropriated $500,000 for a cancer hospital and division of cancer research to be affiliated with the University of Texas at Houston. The same year an additional $500,000 was made available by the M. D. Anderson Foundation, a trust established in 1936 by Monroe D. Anderson (1873-1939), of Houston, to advance medical and educational philanthropies in his native city.

Between 1942 and 1954, the first clinical and laboratory sections were established on the James A. Baker estate, Houston, and were named the M. D. Anderson Hospital for Cancer Research of the University of Texas. Ernest W. Bertner (1889-1950), was appointed acting director in 1942; he was succeeded in 1946 by Randolph Lee Clark (1906-   ). Clark, a native of Texas and a surgeon, has steadily expanded the size and scope of the institution, now the hub of the University of Texas Cancer Center. His national and international influence in cancer activities is manifested by his membership on the 3-man National Cancer Board, and the hosting of the Ninth International Cancer Congress in Houston in 1968.

In 1954, a modern hospital and research complex were opened at the Texas Medical Center in downtown Houston. To designate its expanded scope to a full range of cancer services and studies, the institute was renamed The University of Texas M. D. Anderson Hospital and Tumor Institute. It is now the comprehensive Cancer Center of the University of Texas system.

The First Twenty Years of the University of Texas M. D. Anderson Hospital and Tumor Institute. Houston, Texas: M. D. Anderson Institute, 1964.

IX-Q.

Cancer Institutes and Services.

IX-Q-2. McArdle Cancer Institute: Rusch.

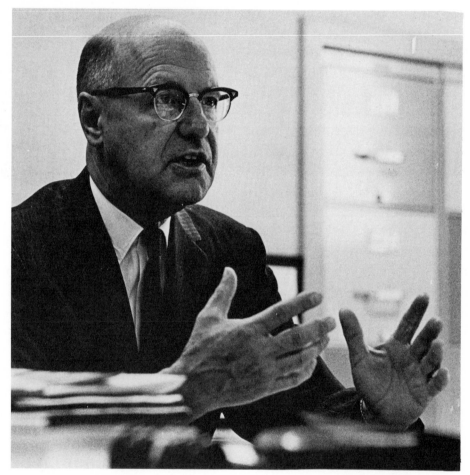

Harold P. Rusch

McArdle Institute for Cancer Research, Madison, Wisconsin, 1965.

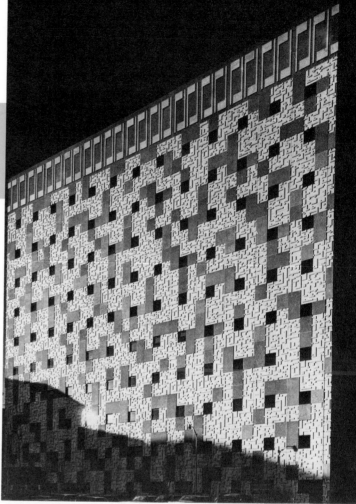

In 1934 the Chicago industrialist, Michael W. McArdle, bequeathed a sum of money to the University of Wisconsin for cancer research. This bequest, together with matching funds from the Public Works Administration, was used to construct a building for this purpose in 1940 at the Medical School on the Madison campus—the McArdle Laboratory for Cancer Research.

Harold P. Rusch (1908-   ) was the first director and chairman of the Medical School's Department of Oncology. The Laboratory became an Institute, and, more recently, the hub of the University of Wisconsin Cancer Center. Rusch was editor of **Cancer Research** during the years 1950-1964 and was president of the American Association for Cancer Research 1953-1954.

In 1961 the National Institutes of Health awarded a grant to the University of Wisconsin for the construction of an 11-story building, the new McArdle Institute for Cancer Research. The move to the new building was made in 1964.

The McArdle Laboratory accommodates a staff of thirteen senior investigators, as well as numerous graduate students, postdoctoral fellows, and supporting personnel. The research is concerned with fundamental aspects of the cancer problem, such as the mechanisms involved in carcinogenesis by chemicals and by viruses; the biochemical processes and control mechanisms associated with growth and differentiation; and studies on antitumor agents. In 1957 the potent antimetabolite, 5-fluorouracil (5-FU), was developed at the McArdle Laboratory.

Harold P. Rusch. The first 40 years of the McArdle laboratories. **Wisconsin Med. Alumni Quart.** 13: 4:2-6, Fall, 1973.

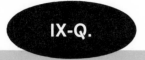

Cancer Institutes and Services.

IX-Q-3. Institute for Cancer Research, Philadelphia: Reimann.

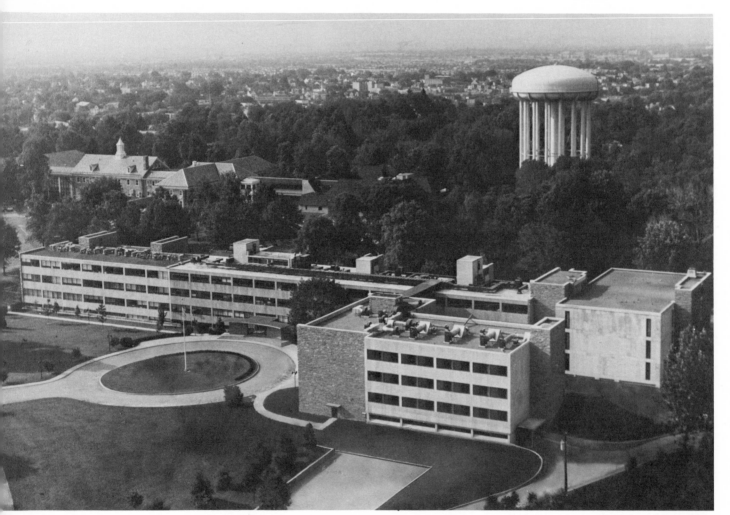

Institute for Cancer Research, Philadelphia, Pa., 1970.

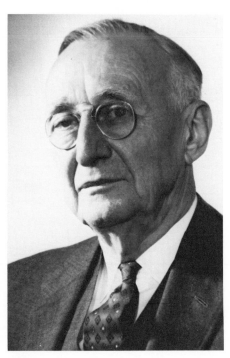

Stanley P. Reimann

The Institute for Cancer Research, Philadelphia, has its origins in the Lankenau Hospital Research Institute founded by Stanley P. Reimann (1891-1968), chief pathologist of the Lankenau Hospital. Reimann was a native Philadelphian, and received his M.D. from the University of Pennsylvania in 1913. His career was in pathology and in cancer research. Funds donated by Rodman Wanamaker permitted the construction of a laboratory building on the hospital grounds (1925), and in 1927, Frederick S. Hammett, a physiological chemist, was appointed scientific director.

In 1949, the Lankenau Hospital Research Institute and The Institute for Cancer Research, both under the direction of Reimann, took possession of an enlarged facility adjacent to the Jeanes Hospital. At the time of Reimann's retirement in 1957, the two institutes were amalgamated into The Institute for Cancer Research, under the direction of Timothy R. Talbot, Jr. In 1961, an affiliation was established with the Jeanes Hospital, and two years later with The American Oncological Hospital which, in 1967, entered a new building adjacent to both the Jeanes Hospital and The Institute for Cancer Research. These units now comprise The Fox Chase Center for Cancer and Medical Sciences. The Institute has maintained an affiliation with the University of Pennsylvania since 1962. A clinical division, added to the Institute in 1964, operates a unit at Jeanes Hospital for the study of inherited variability in selected groups of patients and its bearing on susceptibility to disease, particularly to neoplasia.

IX-Q.

Cancer Institutes and Services.

IX-Q-4. Institut du Cancer de Montréal: Simard.

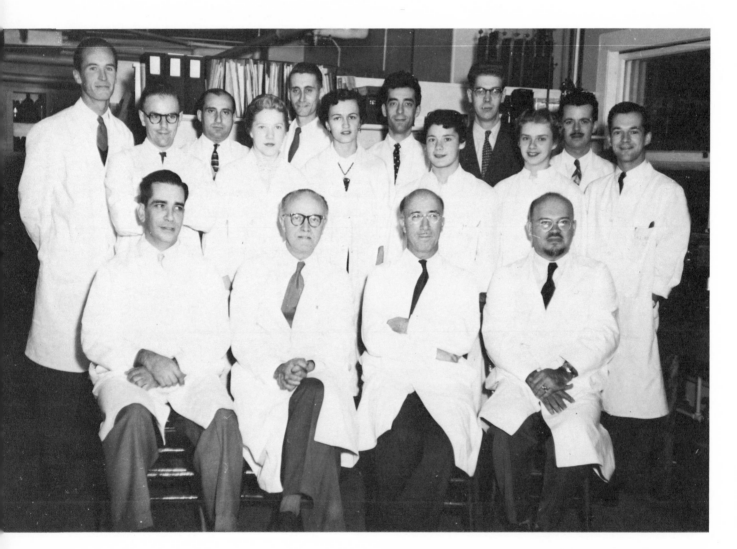

The research team in 1952. **First row:** Dr. H.C. Da Costa, Dr. L.C. Simard, Dr. A. Cantero, Dr. H. Faria. **Second row:** Dr. G. De Lamirande, Miss L. Gagnon, Miss D. Plante, Miss M. Garneau, Miss C. Laurendeau, Dr. R. Daoust. **Third row:** Dr. C. Allard, Dr. G. Weber, Dr. B. Messier, Mr. R. Lemay, Dr. J. Vallée, Dr. R. Mathieu.

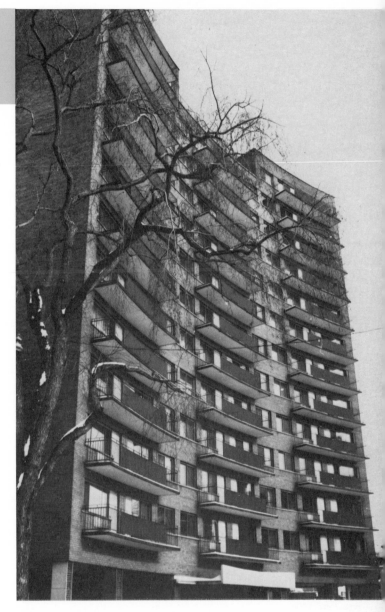

Institute du Cancer de Montréal, Montreal, Canada, 1975.

Louis-Charles Simard (1900-1970), professor of Pathological Anatomy at the Université de Montréal, and head of the Pathology Department of the Hôpital Notre-Dame, organized an anti-cancer center at this hospital in 1942, and founded the Institut du Cancer de Montréal in 1947 to promote the different aspects of the fight against cancer in the Montreal area. He remained the president and executive director of the Institut until his death in 1970. He also participated extensively in the activities of the Canadian Cancer Society and was an early president of the National Cancer Institute of Canada. The Hôpital Notre-Dame paid a tribute to Simard by giving his name to a newly acquired building which houses part of the activities of the Institut. A view is illustrated of this Pavillon Louis-Charles Simard adjacent to the hospital.

A. Cantero (1902-   ), was pursuing cancer research at the Université de Montréal in 1950. He developed an active group engaged mainly in problems of chemical carcinogenesis. Under his directorship, the Montreal group made several contributions related to changes in cell populations and cell metabolism in preneoplastic rat liver. Original methods were developed by members of the team and new avenues were opened by their studies on the neoplastic transformation. Cantero retired as director of the research laboratories in 1967 but remained a member of the Institut and still participates in its activities. The present director is Roger Daoust.

IX-Q.

Cancer Institutes and Services.

IX-Q-5. German Cancer Research Center: Bauer.

The Deutsches Krebsforschungszentrum Heidelberg (German Cancer Research Center) has a predecessor in one of the first cancer institutes not only on German soil but in the world. This was the Institut für experimentelle Krebsforschung of the University of Heidelberg, founded in 1906, together with a clinical facility, the "Samariterhaus," by Vincenz Czerny (1842-1916), professor of surgery at the University of Heidelberg. The Heidelberg Institute pioneered in the development of radiation therapy for cancer, and its clinical facility came to be known as the Czerny-Krankenhaus für Strahlenbehandlung.

In the late 1940s the "Hinterzartener Kreis" of German cancer research workers, headed by A. F. J. Butenandt and sponsored by the Deutsche Forschungsgemeinschaft, proposed establishing a national German Cancer Research Institute. Through efforts led by Professor K. H. Bauer, surgeon and oncologist of the University of Heidelberg, this was achieved in 1964.

One of the reasons for selecting Heidelberg—an ancient seat of learning—as the site for the Cancer Center was the prior existence of the above-mentioned Institut für experimentelle Krebsforschung and the Institute of Virus Research of the Community of the Federal States (Prof. Dr. K. Munk, Director). These institutes, still located within the old city of Heidelberg, were incorporated into the Center in 1966. The five other institutes, i.e., the Institute of Experimental Toxicology and Chemotherapy (Prof. Dr. D. Schmähl, Director), the Institute of Experimental Pathology (Prof. Dr. Kl. Goerttler, Director), the Institute of Biochemistry (Prof. Dr. E. Hecker, Director), the Institute of Documentation, Information and Statistics (Prof. Dr. G. Wagner, Director), and the Institute of Nuclear Medicine (Prof. Dr. K. H. Scheer, Director), are located in provisional buildings within the new university campus north of the Neckar River. All seven institutes are devoted primarily to basic cancer research.

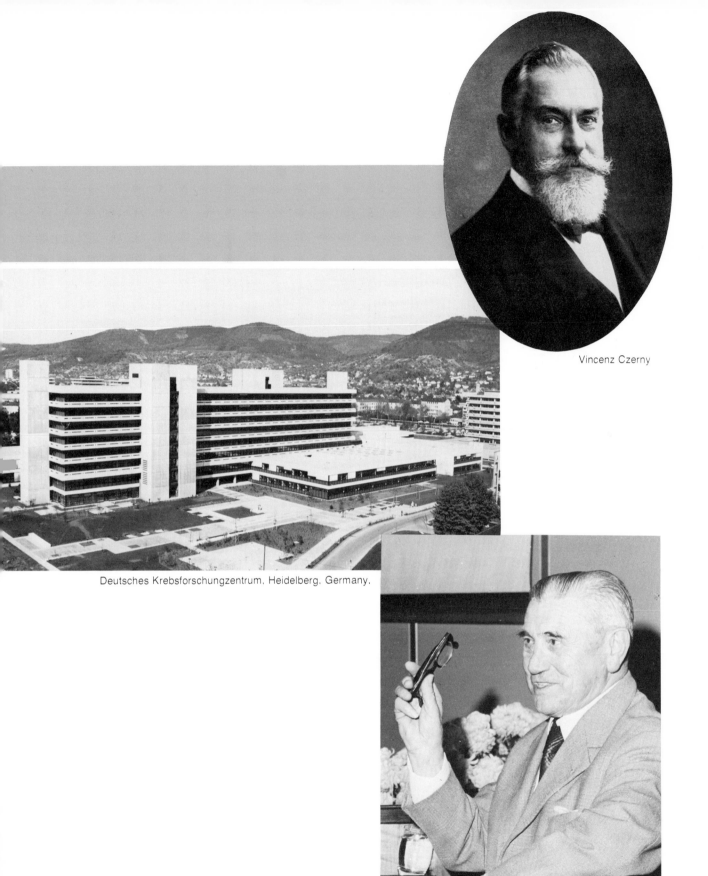

Vincenz Czerny

Deutsches Krebsforschungzentrum. Heidelberg. Germany.

K.H. Bauer

Cancer Institutes and Services.

IX-Q-6. Chester Beatty Research Institute: Haddow.

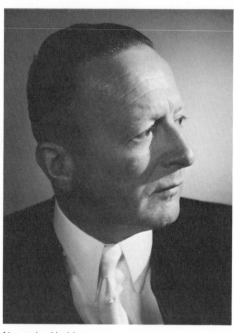

Alexander Haddow

The Chester Beatty Research Institute is descended from the Free Cancer (Royal Marsden) Hospital, founded by William Marsden, in 1851, for the purposes of treatment and research. Cancer investigations were begun here in 1856: at the turn of the century, a Cancer Research and Pathology Department was established under Alexander Paine. In 1909 the department was reconstituted as the Cancer Hospital Research Institute, which was removed to a separate building two years later. The Institute of Cancer Research of the Royal Cancer Hospital was again enlarged in 1939 when new quarters were provided at Fulham Road (S.W.3). This facility became known as the Chester Beatty Research Institute in honor of its benefactor and patron, Sir Alfred Chester Beatty.

Alexander Haddow (1907-1976) was appointed fourth director of the Chester Beatty Institute in 1946. Classic contributions from the Institute include Leitch's work on the latency of tumor induction through coal tar applications to mouse skin and the carcinogenic effect of shale oil ("mule spinners' cancer"). The

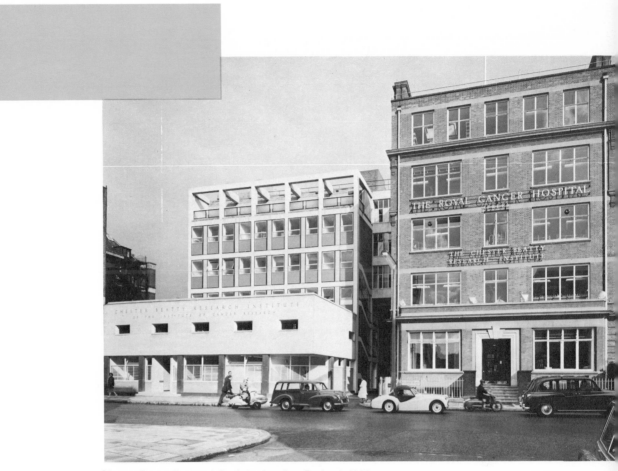

Chester Beatty Research Institute, London, England, 1968.

pioneer studies on hydrocarbon carcinogenesis by Ernest Kennaway, third director, and his coworkers took place here. Under Haddow, the Institute undertook fundamental explorations on the mechanisms of carcinogenesis, aimed at "a kind of synthetic comprehension of the carcinogenic process in general," and has been in the forefront of investigations on the chemotherapy of cancer.

D. A. Brunning and C. E. Dukes. The origin and early history of the Institute of Cancer Research of the Royal Cancer Hospital. **Proc. Roy. Soc. Med.** 58: 33-6, 1965.

A. Haddow. An autobiographical essay. **Cancer Res.** 34: 3159-64, 1964.

IX-Q.

Cancer Institutes and Services.

IX-Q-7. Institut Gustave-Roussy.

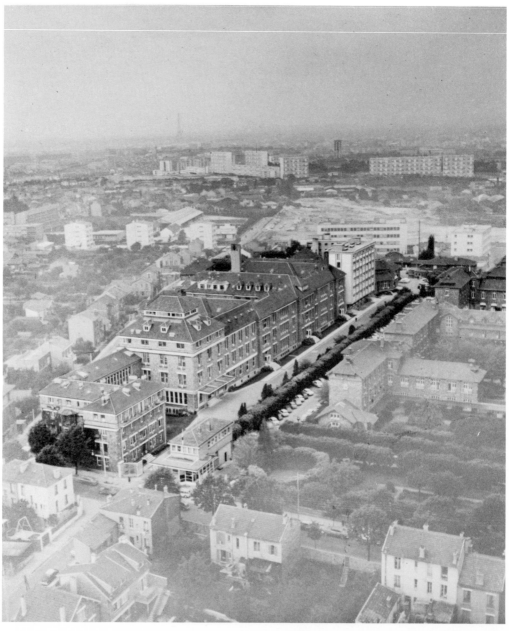

Institut Gustave-Roussy, Villejuif, France, 1968.

The premier cancer center of France, Institut Gustave-Roussy, memorializes Gustave Roussy (1874-1948), Professor of Pathological Anatomy and Dean of the Faculty of Medicine at Paris. In 1921 Roussy created the nucleus of the present facility, Le Fondation de l'Institut du Cancer, at Villejuif, a suburb of Paris. This organization was to operate "under a single authority capable of maintaining its cohesion and averting the causes of divisiveness between clinicians and laboratory workers." A laboratory division and a clinical department were fully established at the Institut in 1930 and 1934 respectively.

Each section remained under separate administrations responsible to Roussy until 1945, at which time the Institut was incorporated into a network of anti-cancer centers under the authority of the French Republic.

The same year Roussy was succeeded by two appointees, François Haguenin as director of the hospital division and Charles Oberling as director of research laboratories. Successive decrees of the French government, in 1950 and 1963, affixed the permanent title, "Institut Gustave-Roussy," to commemorate its founder, and inaugurated a progressive design for the center, which now operates under the Ministry of Public Health. The Institut is composed of 12 divisions—clinical, experimental, and administrative—under a single directorate. The director since 1963 has been Pierre Denoix.

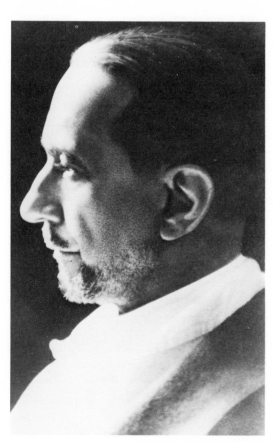

Gustave Roussy

IX-Q.

Cancer Institutes and Services.

IX-Q-8. Institut Jules Bordet

The Institut Jules Bordet, Centre Anticancereaux de l'Université Libre de Bruxelles, is a foremost cancer research and treatment center of Belgium. It commemorates the eminent Belgian bacteriologist Jules Bordet (1870-1961), founder and director, until 1940, of the Institut Pasteur of Brussels. Bordet, who also occupied (since 1907) the Chair of Bacteriology in the Faculty of Medicine at the Free University (Brussels), was noted for his fundamental discoveries in immunology, blood coagulation phenomena, and bacteriophage research.

Various honors were accorded to this gifted scientist, including the Nobel Prize in 1919 for his studies on immunity. The centennial anniversary of his birth was celebrated in 1970 in Belgium.

The Bordet Institut was founded in 1925, the result of an agreement between the Faculty of Medicine in Brussels and the Brussels Commission of Public Assistance to inaugurate a cancer facility. Its scope has included therapeutic, research, and teaching activities. In collaboration with the Belgian National Anit-Cancer League, the Institut, since its inception, has treated over 30,000 cancer patients with the most advanced tools of radiotherapy and has maintained close follow-up surveillance on these cases. Moreover, its laboratories conduct basic research on a wide range of problems, such as electron microscopy of normal and neoplastic cells, cancer biochemistry, the cytogenetics of leukemia, and experimental chemotherapy, among others. This center has also played a prominent part in organizing international cooperation in the field of cancer research.

The Institut is supervised by the College of the Chiefs of Service. They designate an executive officer in conjunction with the University. Albert Claude and Henri J. Tagnon are on its staff.

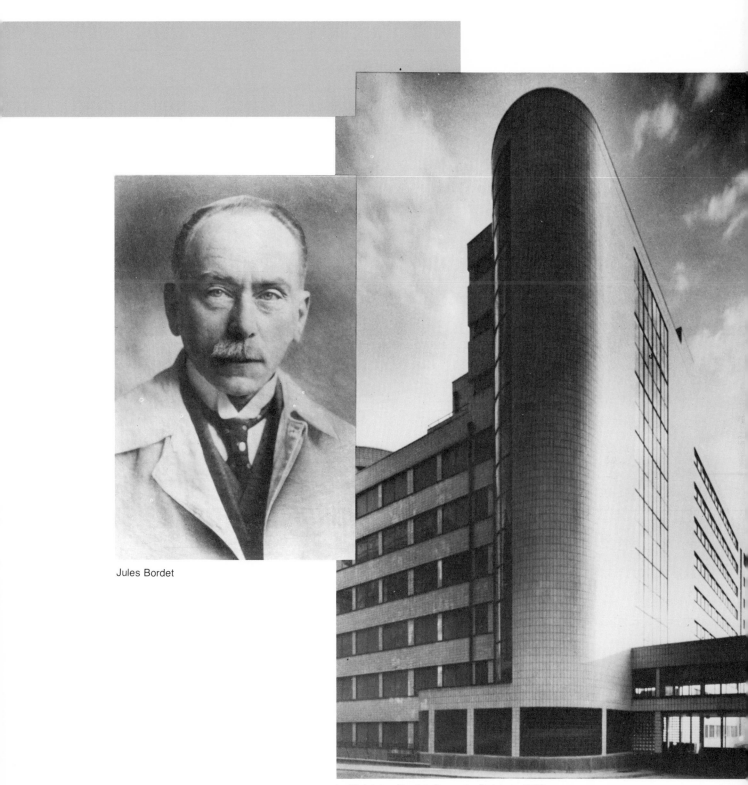

Jules Bordet

Institut Jules Bordet, Brussels, Belgium, 1970.

J. Beumer. Jules Bordet, 1870-1961. **J. Gen. Microbiol.**
29: 1-13, 1962.

IX-Q.

Cancer Institutes and Services.

IX-Q-9. Leningrad Institute of Oncology: Petrov.

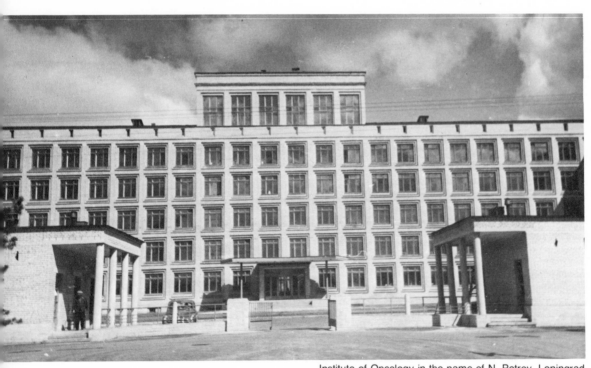

Institute of Oncology in the name of N. Petrov, Leningrad,
U.S.S.R., 1968.

Nikolai Nikolaevich Petrov (1876-1964), of Leningrad, was an outstanding clinical and experimental oncologist of the Soviet Union, and the doyen of Russian oncology. Among his contributions to cancer research were the induction of carcinoma of the gall baldder and the induction of osteogenic sarcoma in monkeys.

The Leningrad Institute of Oncology was founded by Petrov in 1926, and now memorializes his name. Since 1964 it

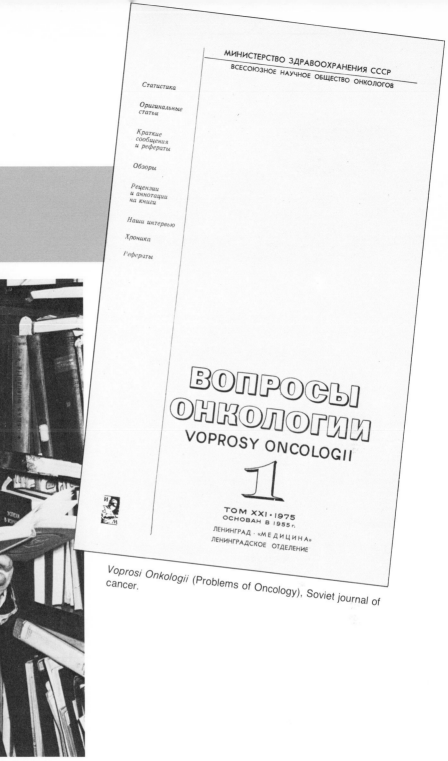

МИНИСТЕРСТВО ЗДРАВООХРАНЕНИЯ СССР
ВСЕСОЮЗНОЕ НАУЧНОЕ ОБЩЕСТВО ОНКОЛОГОВ

Статистика

*Оригинальные
статьи*

*Краткие
сообщения
и рефераты*

Обзоры

*Рецензии
и аннотации
на книги*

Наши интервью

Хроника

Рефераты

ВОПРОСЫ
ОНКОЛОГИИ
VOPROSY ONCOLOGII

1

ТОМ XXI · 1975
ОСНОВАН В 1955 г.
ЛЕНИНГРАД · «МЕДИЦИНА»
ЛЕНИНГРАДСКОЕ ОТДЕЛЕНИЕ

Voprosi Onkologii (Problems of Oncology), Soviet journal of cancer.

Nikolai N. Petrov

has occupied a complex of 14 buildings 20 kilometers from the city (Pesochnaya Station). The Institute has clinical facilities and has admitted over 55,000 patients between 1926 and 1965. The radiotherapy unit includes a linear ac-celerator and betatron. There are also some 12 laboratories, including experimental therapy, biophysics, biochemistry, carcinogenic agents, immunology of tumors, virology, and endocrinology.

Sorok Let Deyatelnosti Leningradskovo Instituta Onkologii, 1926-1966. (Forty Years' Activity of the Leningrad Institute of Oncology.) Leningrad: Meditsina, 1966.

IX-Q.

Cancer Institutes and Services.

IX-Q-10. Institute of Experimental and Clinical Oncology: Blokhin and Shabad.

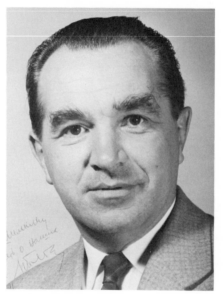

Nikolai N. Blokhin

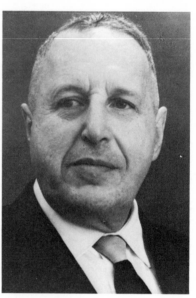

L. M. Shabad

The Institute of Experimental and Clinical Oncology of the Academy of Medical Sciences of the USSR is located on Kashirskoye Chausse in Moscow. It was founded in 1951 and is the largest center in the USSR for laboratory and clinical research on cancer.

Nikolai Nikolaevich Blokhin (born in 1912 in Lukoyanov) has been director of the Institute since its opening. He was graduated from Gorky State Medical In-

stitute in 1934 and in the same year founded the Institute of Restorative Surgery, Orthopedics, and Traumatology where he was director of general surgery from 1950 to 1952. He was president of the Academy of Medical Sciences of the USSR (1960-1968) and president of the International Union Against Cancer (1966-1970). The author of over 50 works, Dr. Blokhin has contributed to the literature on cancer control, plastic sur-

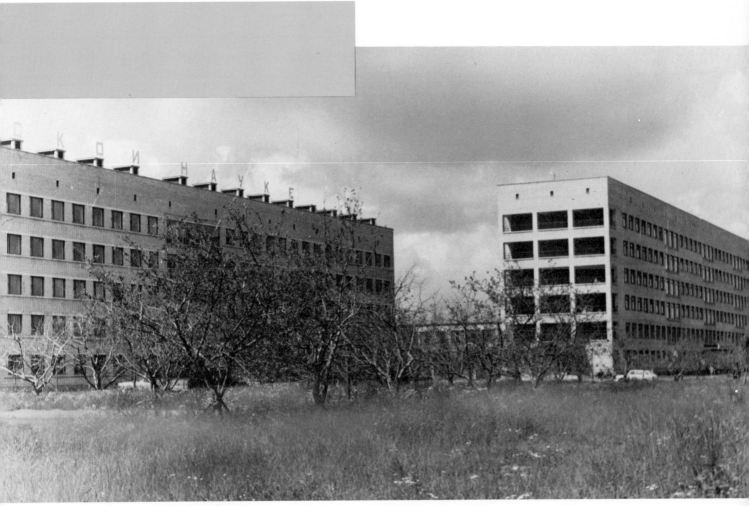

Institute of Experimental and Clinical Oncology, Moscow, U.S.S.R., 1970.

gery, and chemotherapy of cancer.

Leon Manusovich Shabad (born in 1902 in Minsk) is a pathologist who is chief of the Department of Carcinogenic Agents at the Institute. He was graduated from the Leningrad Medical Institute in 1924, and in 1925 began working in the field of experimental oncology. Shabad is a member of the Academy of Medical Sciences of the USSR. He is world renowned for his work on environmental carcinogenesis, for which he was awarded a prize by the United Nations in 1962. His numerous publications include books on pathology and oncology. He continues to be a frequent contributor to the cancer literature in English as well as in the Russian language.

L. M. Shabad. Studies in the USSR on the distribution, circulation, and fate of carcinogenic hydrocarbons in the human environment and the role of their disposition in tissues in carcinogenesis: a review. **Cancer Res.** 27: 1132-37, 1967.

IX-Q.

Cancer Institutes and Services.

IX-Q-11. National Cancer Institute of Japan: Nagayo and Nakahara.

The Japanese Foundation for Cancer Research, a forerunner of Japan's National Cancer Institute, was established in April 1908. In May 1934 the Foundation opened a cancer institute in Tokyo known as the Laboratories and Koraku Hospital of the Japanese Foundation for Cancer Research. Until World War II most of the financial aid for cancer investigations in Japan was provided by the Foundation. Mataro Nagayo (1878-1941) was the director from 1929 until his death.

The hospital and institute buildings were destroyed by an air-raid fire in 1945. Hospital activities were resumed in 1946 and research in 1953. In February 1962 the present National Cancer Center Research Institute was opened on premises formerly occupied by the Imperial Japanese Navy, which disbanded its facilities at the close of World War II. The former Naval Medical College and Hospital buildings were converted into the first units of the National Cancer Center Research Institute and Hospital. The Japanese Cancer Center includes 12 divisions in the basic biomedical, clinical, and epidemiological sciences.

Waro Nakahara (1896-1976), whose training in cancer research included work at the Rockefeller Institute in New York under James P. Murphy, was the director from 1953 to 1974. He has contributed his reminiscences of his long career.

W. Nakahara. A pilgrim's progress in cancer research, 1918 to 1974: autobiographical essay. **Cancer Res.** 34: 1767-74, 1974.

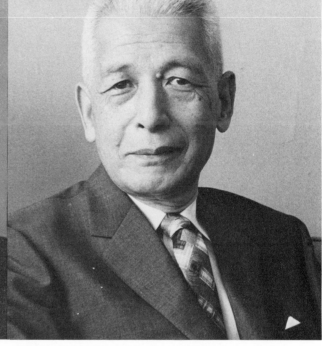

Waro Nakahara

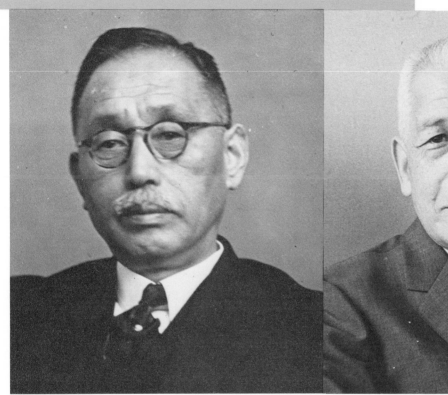

Mataro Nagayo

National Cancer Center Research Institute, Tokyo, Japan,
1960.

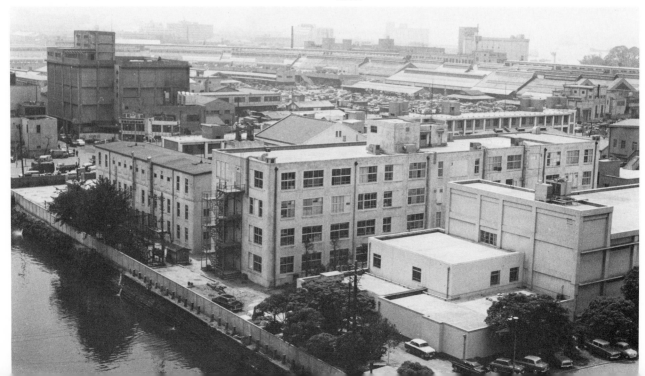

IX-Q.

Cancer Institutes and Services.

IX-Q-12. Tata Memorial Hospital.

The establishment of the Tata Memorial Hospital in Bombay in 1941 was a landmark step in cancer activities in India. The Hospital was established by the Trustees of the Drabji Tata Trust. In 1957 its management was transferred to the Ministry of Health, and in 1962 to the Atomic Energy Department of the Government of India.

The primary mission of the Hospital is the treatment of cancer, by surgery and by radiation. Approximately 12,000 new patients are seen annually, of which 8,000 are proved cancer cases. The Hospital and the Indian Cancer Society also operate outreach detection centers.

The staff of the Hospital also conducts epidemiologic and other research, especially on cancers of the mouth and throat that are particularly prevalent in the area.

The Tata Memorial Hospital was named for Lady Tata, and its first director was Jamshedji Duggan.

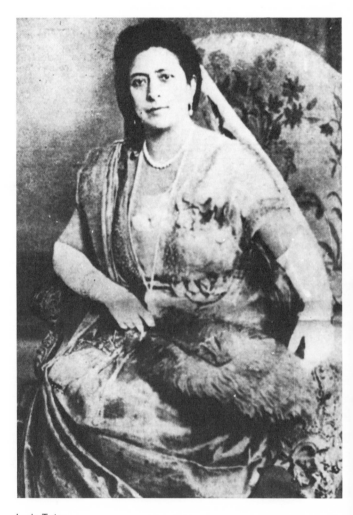

Lady Tata

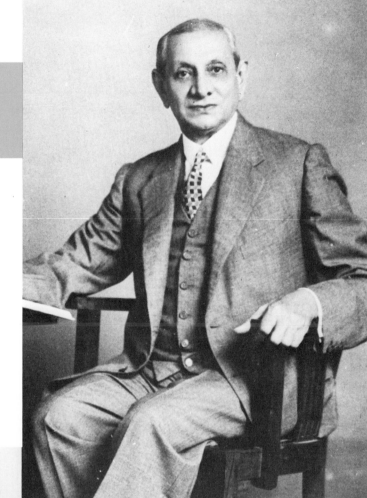

J. C. Paymaster. Cancer and its distribution in India.
Cancer 17: 1026-34, 1964.

D. J. Jussawalla *et al*. Cancer incidence in greater Bombay:
assessment of the cancer risk by age. **Brit. J. Cancer** 22:
623-36, 1968.

Jamshedji Duggan

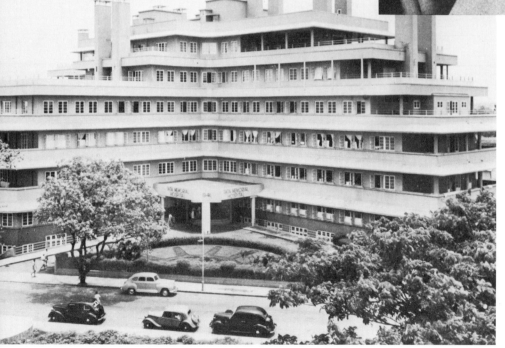

Lady Tata Memorial Hospital, Bombay, India, 1970.

IX-R.

Cancer Organizations

IX-R-1. Professional societies.

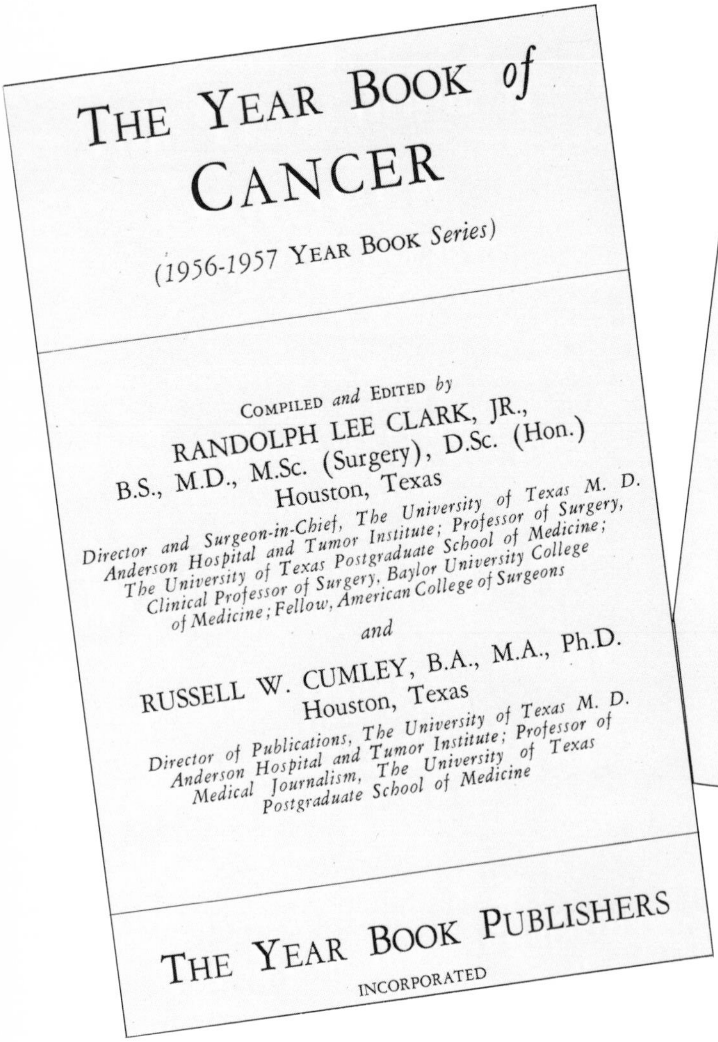

THE YEAR BOOK *of* CANCER

(1956-1957 YEAR BOOK *Series*)

COMPILED *and* EDITED *by*

RANDOLPH LEE CLARK, JR.,
B.S., M.D., M.Sc. (Surgery), D.Sc. (Hon.)
Houston, Texas

Director and Surgeon-in-Chief, The University of Texas M. D. Anderson Hospital and Tumor Institute; Professor of Surgery, The University of Texas Postgraduate School of Medicine; Clinical Professor of Surgery, Baylor University College of Medicine; Fellow, American College of Surgeons

and

RUSSELL W. CUMLEY, B.A., M.A., Ph.D.
Houston, Texas

Director of Publications, The University of Texas M. D. Anderson Hospital and Tumor Institute; Professor of Medical Journalism, The University of Texas Postgraduate School of Medicine

THE YEAR BOOK PUBLISHERS
INCORPORATED

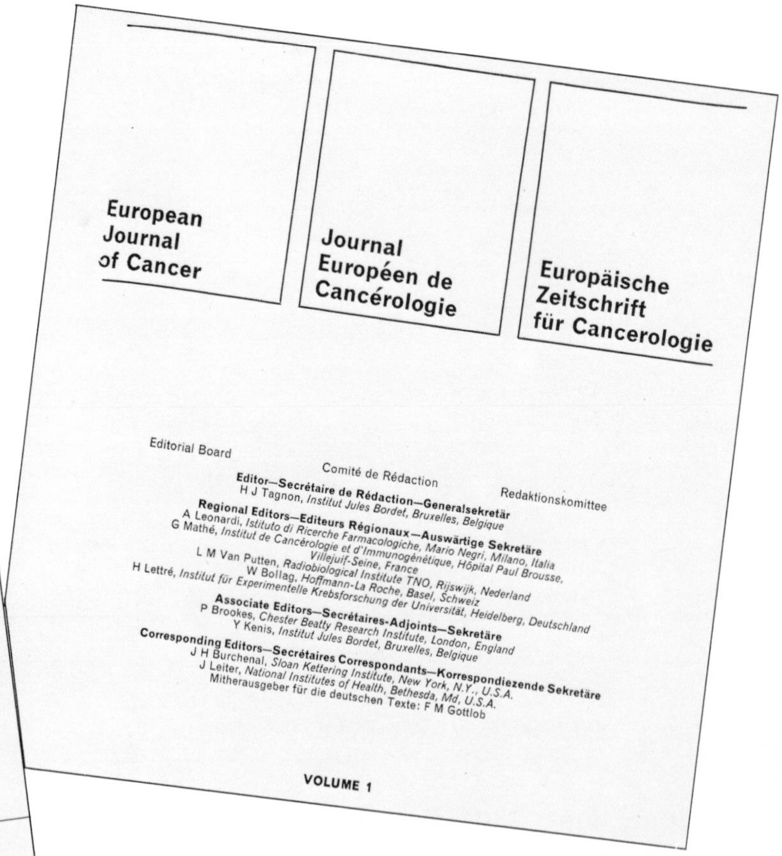

European Journal of Cancer

Journal Européen de Cancérologie

Europäische Zeitschrift für Cancerologie

Editorial Board

Comité de Rédaction

Redaktionskomittee

Editor—Secrétaire de Rédaction—Generalsekretär
H J Tagnon, *Institut Jules Bordet, Bruxelles, Belgique*

Regional Editors—Editeurs Régionaux—Auswärtige Sekretäre
A Leonardi, *Istituto di Ricerche Farmacologiche, Mario Negri, Milano, Italia*
G Mathé, *Institut de Cancérologie et d'Immunogénétique, Hôpital Paul Brousse, Villejuif-Seine, France*
L M Van Putten, *Radiobiological Institute TNO, Rijswijk, Nederland*
W Bollag, *Hoffmann-La Roche, Basel, Schweiz*
H Lettré, *Institut für Experimentelle Krebsforschung der Universität, Heidelberg, Deutschland*

Associate Editors—Secrétaires-Adjoints—Sekretäre
P Brookes, *Chester Beatty Research Institute, London, England*
Y Kenis, *Institut Jules Bordet, Bruxelles, Belgique*

Corresponding Editors—Secrétaires Correspondants—Korrespondiezende Sekretäre
J H Burchenal, *Sloan Kettering Institute, New York, N.Y., U.S.A.*
J Leiter, *National Institutes of Health, Bethesda, Md, U.S.A.*
Mitherausgeber für die deutschen Texte: F M Gottlob

VOLUME 1

The expanded activities in cancer led to the creation of more professional societies, now dealing with various specialties with interests in the neoplastic disease.

The American Society of Clinical Oncology (ASCO) was founded in 1964, and became an increasingly important forum in the new specialty of medical oncology, leading to official board certification.

The European Cancer Society was organized in 1964, and the **European Journal of Cancer**, with Henri Tagnon as editor, began publication in 1965.

By 1970 there were in the United States 7 professional societies in clinical oncology which included the American Association for Cancer Education, cal Oncology in 1969, **Cancer Treatment Reviews** in 1974, and **Cancer Biochemistry-Biophysics, Medical and Pediatric Oncology**, and **Radiation Oncology** in 1975. Several survey an-

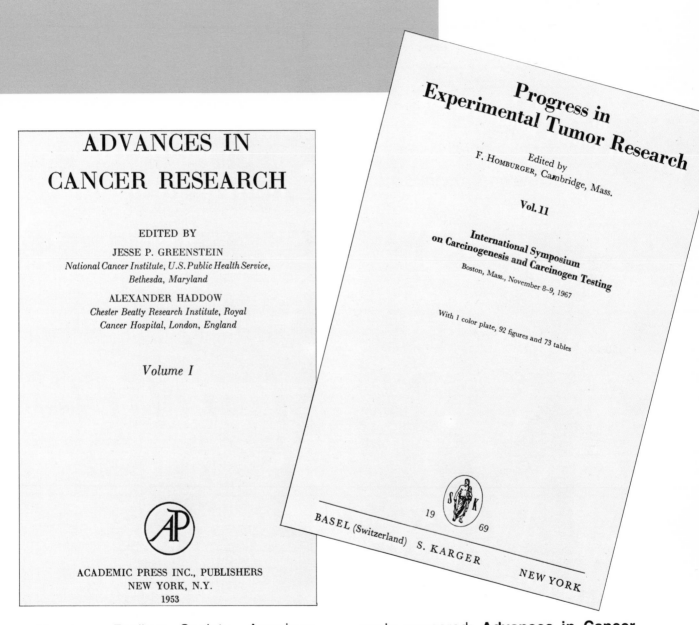

ADVANCES IN
CANCER RESEARCH

EDITED BY

JESSE P. GREENSTEIN
National Cancer Institute, U.S. Public Health Service,
Bethesda, Maryland

ALEXANDER HADDOW
Chester Beatty Research Institute, Royal
Cancer Hospital, London, England

Volume I

ACADEMIC PRESS INC., PUBLISHERS
NEW YORK, N.Y.
1953

Progress in
Experimental Tumor Research

Edited by
F. HOMBURGER, Cambridge, Mass.

Vol. 11

International Symposium
on Carcinogenesis and Carcinogen Testing
Boston, Mass., November 8–9, 1967

With 1 color plate, 92 figures and 73 tables

19 69

BASEL (Switzerland) S. KARGER   NEW YORK

American Radium Society, American Society of Clinical Oncology, American Society of Therapeutic Radiologists, James Ewing Society, Society of Gynecologic Oncologists and the Society of Head and Neck Surgeons. These organizations in 1972 agreed to form the American Federation of Clinical Oncologic Societies.

There was a proliferation of periodicals in cancer, such as the **Journal of Surgi-** nuals appeared: **Advances in Cancer Research, Recent Progress in Experimental Tumor Research**, and the **Yearbook of Cancer**.

The number of meetings and symposia grew proportionately, so that communication steadily became a problem unto itself.

IX-R.

Cancer Organizations

IX-R-2. American Cancer Society.

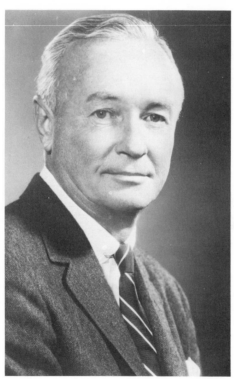

Charles S. Cameron

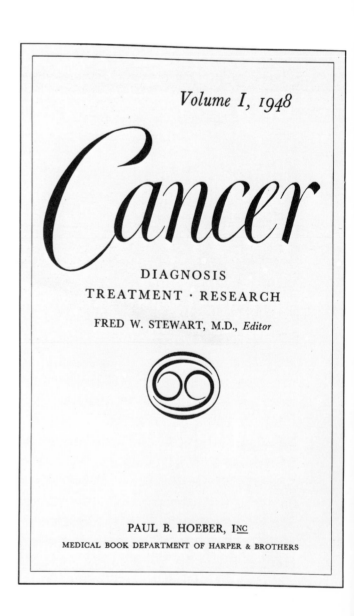

Volume I, *1948*

Cancer

DIAGNOSIS
TREATMENT · RESEARCH

FRED W. STEWART, M.D., *Editor*

PAUL B. HOEBER, INC
MEDICAL BOOK DEPARTMENT OF HARPER & BROTHERS

In 1944 the American Society for the Control of Cancer expanded on a national basis as the American Cancer Society (ACS). Its programs were broadened, and one-third of the funds derived from its annual campaign was allocated to research. The ACS requested the National Research Council to advise it on the award of grants. This was done through the Committee on Growth, which from 1945 to 1956 recommended $25 million in support of grants and fellowships. ACS also administered funds for international cancer fellowships.

ade 1946-1956, was instrumental in these enterprises.

Education of the public about cancer was conducted directly and through public media. Pat McGrady of the ACS organized annual seminars for science writers, which improved and accelerated information on cancer. The list grew of pamphlets and books on cancer written for the public.

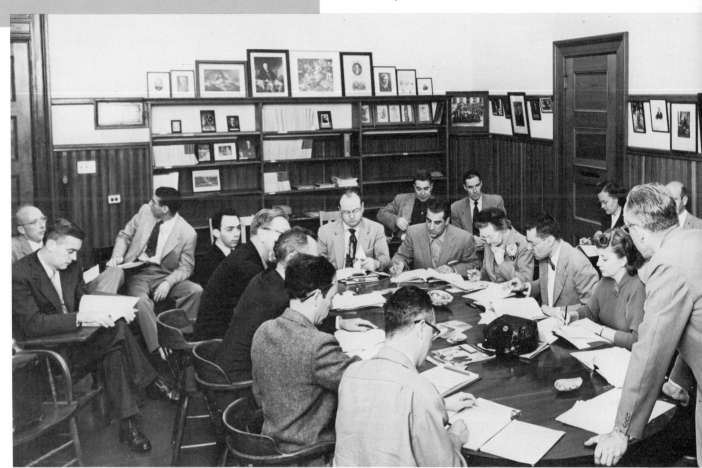

American Cancer Society Science Writers' tour at Stanford University in 1953. Pat McGrady is in the right rear corner, in a dark shirt.

Public and professional education were expanded. National Cancer Conferences, jointly supported by the National Cancer Institute, were convened every four years, and there was formal participation in the international congresses assembled by the International Union Against Cancer. **Cancer**, a new periodical with emphasis on clinical oncology, was started in 1948, and an abstract journal, **Ca**, was sent to all physicians. Charles S. Cameron, medical and scientific director during the dec-

Charles Cameron. **The Truth About Cancer.** Engelwood Cliffs, N.J.: Prentice-Hall, 1956.

Pat McGrady. **The Savage Cell.** New York: Basic Books, 1964.

M. B. Shimkin. **Science and Cancer.** U.S. Public Health Serv. Publ. 1162. Washington, D.C.: U.S. Govt. Printing Ofc., 1964. Revised, 1973.

Victor Richards. **Cancer. The Wayward Cell.** Berkeley: Univ. of Calif. Press, 1972.

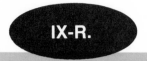

IX-R.

Cancer Organizations

IX-R-3. Support for cancer research.

Research on cancer requires funds and facilities. Since research is not a self-sustaining activity, support for it must come from private and public sources. This is the place to acknowledge a few of the individuals who contributed financially to the developments.

Samuel Whitbread, a brewer of London, in 1791 endowed the cancer facility at the Middlesex Hospital, probably the first cancer institute in the world. The name of the donor was unknown for many years.

William Marsden (1796-1867) in 1851 founded the Royal Free and Cancer Hospital in London.

In the United States, John Jacob Astor in 1888 donated $145,000 to the New York Cancer Hospital for a pavilion for male patients, in memory of his wife. At the turn of the century, Mrs. Collis P. Huntington set up foundations at Harvard and at Memorial Hospital that allowed the beginnings of cancer research in those two institutions. George Crocker in 1909 endowed the Crocker Research Fund at Columbia University that funded its Institute for Cancer Research.

During the 20th Century, up to World War II, there were two major philanthropic endowments for cancer research. One was the International Cancer Research Foundation, later renamed the Donner Foundation, established by William Henry Donner (1864-1953) of Philadelphia. The other was the Jane Coffin Childs Memorial Fund for Medical Research established in 1937 at Yale University.

The interests and funds from Monroe D. Anderson in Houston, Texas, and Michael W. McArdle in Wisconsin supported the cancer institutions there bearing their names. Alfred P. Sloan, Jr. and Charles F. Kettering joined in funding the Sloan-Kettering Institute in New York.

The private funds supplemented and stimulated the ever-growing governmental allocations for cancer research. Public-spirited citizens, especially Mary Lasker of New York, worked closely with the United States Congress in justifying funds. Particularly understanding members of Congress were Lister Hill, Senator from Alabama, and John E. Fogarty (1913-1967), Representative from Rhode Island.

Board of Scientific Advisors of the Jane Coffin Childs Fund, 1941. **From left to right:** Rudolph J. Anderson (1879-1961), professor of chemistry; Milton C. Winternitz (1885-1959), professor of pathology; Ross G. Harrison (1870-1959), professor of biology, all at Yale; the chairman, Stanhope Bayne-Jones (1888-1970), dean of Yale University School of Medicine; Peyton Rous (1879-1970), of the Rockefeller Institute for Medical Research; John J. Morton (1886-   ), professor of surgery, Rochester University School of Medicine; George Milton Smith (1879-1951).

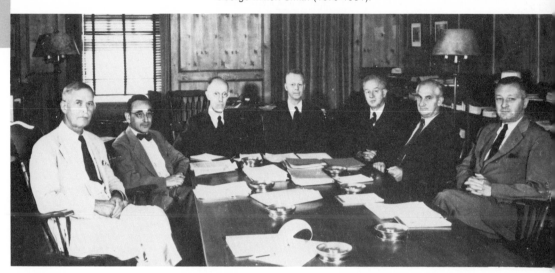

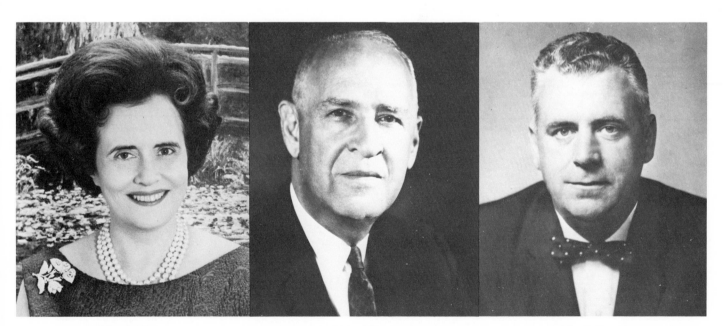

Mary Lasker   Lister Hill   John E. Fogarty

American Association for Cancer Research Honorary Memberships and Certificates of Award for 1967. **Cancer Res.** 27: 2241-44, 1967.

Stanhope Bayne-Jones. Aspects of cancer research in the United States of America: a tribute to George Milton Smith (1879-1951). **Texas Repts. Biol. & Med.** 10: 1084-98, 1952.

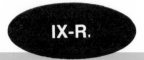

Cancer Organizations

IX-R-4. International Agency for Research on Cancer: Higginson.

The International Agency for Research on Cancer (IARC) was established in 1965 as an autonomous body within the World Health Organization (WHO), representing on a modest scale the implementation of the proposal by a group of French intellectuals that the industrial nations should expand their collaborative efforts in cancer research. The budget is provided by ten states: Australia, Belgium, Federal Republic of Germany, France, Italy, Japan, Netherlands, Union of Soviet Socialist Republics, United Kingdom and United States of America.

The IARC commenced operations in Lyon in 1967 in rented quarters and moved into a new building donated by the French authorities in the autumn of 1972.

The Agency has approximately 70 on-going programs in different geographic areas. Its overall scientific objectives are to identify potential toxic factors in the human environment, whether chemical or biological, that may cause cancer in man, and to evaluate the hazards of compounds suspected as a result of animal studies. While research is mainly epidemiologically oriented, every attempt is made to integrate laboratory and field investigations in order to exploit the ideas of all disciplines and to apply more sophisticated techniques to epidemiological investigations. Specific attention is being paid to the role of environmental pollution in industrial states, and also to the possibilities of developing monitoring systems for cancer. Programs include studies on esophageal cancer in Iran, liver cancer, aflatoxin and hepatitis in Africa, and the role of viruses in Burkitt's lymphoma and nasopharyngeal cancer.

The Agency has established Research Centers in Teheran, Nairobi and Singapore to permit more extensive investigations into local cancer patterns and the environment. Other investigations include pesticides and transplacental carcinogenesis. A monograph series on the **Evaluation of the Carcinogenic Risk of Chemicals to Man** has been commenced (IARC Monograph Series, Vol-

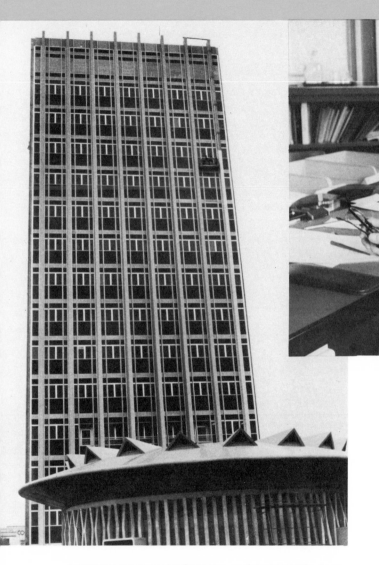

John Higginson

International Agency for Research on Cancer (IARC), Lyon, France, 1975.

ume 1, Lyon, 1972). Close contacts are maintained with national institutes through research contracts and joint programs. The Agency also supports a Fellowships program.

The Agency employs approximately 120 people, including scientists from Australia, Belgium, Colombia, Denmark, France, Holland, Hungary, Iceland, Italy, Yugoslavia, Switzerland, USSR, United Kingdom and USA.

John Higginson, M.D., born in 1922 in Belfast, and formerly American Cancer Society Career Professor of Geographical Pathology, University of Kansas, was the first and remains the present director.

IX-S.

The National Cancer Plan:

IX-S. The National Cancer Plan Schmidt and Rauscher.

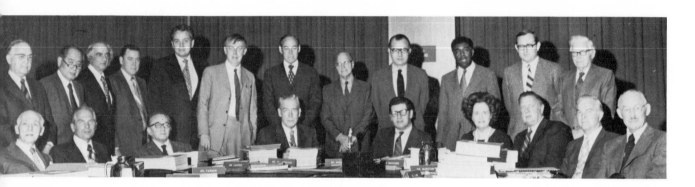

Cancer Panel and National Cancer Advisory Board, U.S.A., 1972. **From left to right, seated are:** Sidney Farber, M.D. (deceased 1973), Children's Cancer Research Foundation, Boston, Mass. (now the Sidney Farber Institute); Frank J. Dixon, M.D., Scripps Clinic and Research Foundation, La Jolla, Calif.; Sol Spiegelman, Ph.D., Institute of Cancer Research, College of Physicians and Surgeons, Columbia University, New York, N.Y.; Jonathan E. Rhoads, M.D., School of Medicine, University of Pennsylvania, Philadelphia, Pa. (chairman of board); Frank J. Rauscher, Jr., Ph.D.; Mary Lasker, Albert and Mary Lasker Foundation, New York, N.Y.; Benno C. Schmidt, LL.B., J.H. Whitney and Co., New York, N.Y. (chairman of Panel); Robert Q. Marston, M.D., Director, National Institutes of Health, Bethesda, Md., (ex-officio); R. Lee Clark, M.D., M.D. Anderson Hospital and Tumor Institute, Houston, Texas (member of Panel). **From left to right, standing are:** D. Murray Angevine, M.D., Armed Forces Institute of Pathology, Washington, D.C. (ex-officio); Joseph H. Oguar, M.D., School of Medicine, Washington University, St. Louis, Mo.; Philippe Shubik, M.D., The Eppley Institute for Research in Cancer, University of Nebraska, Omaha, Neb.; Kenneth R. Krabbenhoft, M.D., School of Medicine, Wayne State University, Detroit, Mich.; John R. Hogness, M.D., Institute of Medicine, National Academy of Sciences, Washington, D.C.; James D. Watson, M.D., Cold Spring Harbor, N.Y.; William W. Shingleton, M.D., Duke University Medical Center, Durham, N.C.; Harold P. Rusch, M.D., University of Wisconsin Medical Center, Madison, Wisc.; Arnold L. Brown, M.D., Mayo Clinic, Rochester, Minn.; Harold Amos, Ph.D., Harvard Medical School, Boston, Mass.; Gerald P. Murphy, M.D., Roswell Park Memorial Institute, Buffalo, N.Y.; Donald E. Johnson, Advertiser's Press, Flint, Mich. Eleven other members of the Board and one other member of the Panel, as well as three ex-officio members, were absent.

The United States has made the solution of the cancer problem a national goal, and has expressed the goal in two laws: the National Cancer Institute Act of 1937, and the National Cancer Act of 1971.

The National Cancer Act of 1971 expanded the activities to include not only a programmed research attack, but the application of research findings through cancer control, a network of cancer centers, and an international cancer data bank. The initial annual budget was over $500 million.

The Act established a three-man President's Cancer Panel with direct access to the President, as well as an expanded National Cancer Advisory Board. The

The National Cancer Program Strategy Hierarchy, developed for the National Cancer Plan.

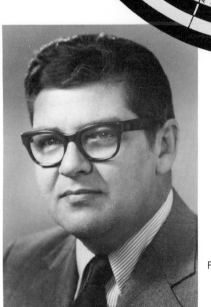

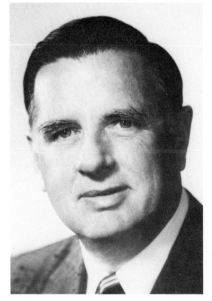

Benno C. Schmidt

Frank J. Rauscher, Jr.

chairman of the Panel was Benno C. Schmidt, a business executive from New York, who was born in Texas in 1913. The two members were R. Lee Clark and Robert A. Good.

Frank Joseph Rauscher, Jr., in 1972 became director of the National Cancer Institute and the National Cancer Plan. He was born in Hellertown, Pennsylvania, in 1931, graduated from Moravian College in 1953, and obtained his Ph.D. in microbiology from Rutgers University in 1957. He joined the National Cancer Institute in Bethesda, Maryland, in 1959, continuing research in viral aspects of cancer, which included the identification of a murine leukemia virus known by his name.

The National Cancer Act of 1971. **J. Nat. Cancer Inst.**, 48: 577-84, 1972.
Frank J. Rauscher, Jr. Budget and the National Cancer Program (NCP). **Cancer Res.** 34: 1743-48, 1974.

X. Afterwords

The last quarter before the Twenty-First Century marks:

- 200 years since the first description of an occupational cancer
- 140 years since the first histologic studies of cancer
- 100 years since the advent of modern surgical approaches to cancer therapy
- 100 years since the first successful transplantation of cancer in animals

It has been less than 100 years since radium and X-rays were discovered, and since cancers were induced in animals with viruses and chemicals. And the modern period of cancer chemotherapy is only 35 years old.

Cancer research is research aimed at a specific goal: the acquisition of knowledge that can be applied to the prevention and cure of cancer. There has been a steady accumulation of such knowledge for several centuries, but especially during the twentieth century.

At the beginning of the last quarter of the twentieth century, knowledge regarding cancer can be summarized as follows:

- Cancer is a great group of diseases characterized by changes in somatic cells that are transmissible to daughter cells.
- The basic cellular change that eventually leads to the clinical manifestations of cancer involves the genetic component, the desoxyribosenucleic acid moiety, of the nucleus.
- The cancerous change can be triggered by a wide variety of environmental stimuli, physical, chemical, or viral.
- The cancerous process in most instances is manifested after prolonged, repeated exposures to the carcinogenic stimulus, and evolves through several stages.
- The cancerous process is influenced by many host factors, including heredity, nutrition, and immunologic status.
- In regard to **prevention**, hundreds of environmental hazards have been defined. Tobacco smoking, industrial exposure to carcinogenic chemicals, and ionizing radiation are important man-made carcinogenic hazards, which also include natural products such as aflatoxin. Avoidance or termination of such exposures would prevent a significant proportion of cancer occurrences.
- In regard to **diagnosis**, pathology remains supreme, with the biopsy being the basis and microscopic designation of histogenesis, staging and grading leading to determination of prognosis as well as to diagnosis.
- In **treatment**, surgery remains the most definitive and widely used approach, aiming at a total excision of the tumor and its extensions. Radiotherapy is another curative method, if the tumor is

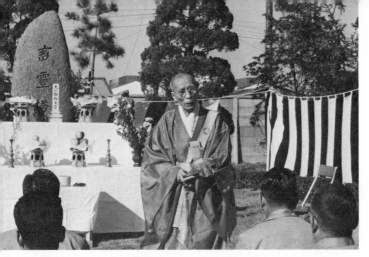

Memorial services for experimental animals.

responsive at host-tolerated doses and if it can be encompassed by the beam. Chemotherapy is curative in a proportion of patients with some rapidly-proliferating tumors but its total contribution to the results remains small. Combinations of all three modalities are of increasing importance.

• The salvage rate of all patients with cancer is approximately 40 percent at five years after treatment. The improvements in the salvage rates for patients with some cancers are not sufficient to reverse the still-rising mortality rate from neoplastic diseases. Thus, the real victory over cancer as a disease is still in the future, requiring not only better application of available knowledge but the discovery of new therapeutic methods through research.

Biomedical research during the twentieth century can be divided into periods of physiology, biochemistry, and molecular biology. Physiology with its electrocardiographs occupied the medical research stage for the first two decades, and biochemistry with its conquest of diabetes and pernicious anemia was the star actor up to World War II. Cancer is **the** disease of the molecular biology era, in which the constituents of DNA, and their interactions with the bits of DNA or RNA we call viruses, are at the heart of the problem.

The tactics of how best to approach the problem involve the relative role and support of basic biomedical research and of more applied cancer research. On this point Pasteur wrote a century ago: ". . . there does not exist a category of science to which one can give the name applied science. There are science and the applications of science, bound together as the fruit to the tree which bears it."

The panorama of cancer research provides many portents that significant advances are inevitable. Indeed, victory over cancer may well be in the process of being spelled out by virology, immunology and chemotherapy. If history implies prediction as well as recall, the twenty-first century will see the taming of the malignant crab so that it no longer is contrary to nature.

When that happy day comes, the efforts of all persons mentioned in this compilation, and many more who were not, will fit into place. Most of the contributions will sink into obscurity, placing into sharper relief the crucial events attributed to a few. That is the way science advances, and a review of its processes should have heuristic value.

Man claims an anthropocentric position in this world, but shares the environment with innumerable species of flora and fauna upon which he is totally dependent. Biological research would be impossible without the use of animals and plants. The Japanese hold memorial services for their experimental animals. The monument at which such services are held at the Takeda Research Laboratories is inscribed with words written by a Buddhist priest: "Born as animals, they have offered their bodies for revelation of medical science. A memorial is here set up to honor their souls."

And, perhaps, man's acquisition of Knowledge will become increasingly translated into Wisdom . . .

Louis Pasteur. **Oeuvres de Pasteur.** VII: 215. Paris: Masson et cie 1922-30.

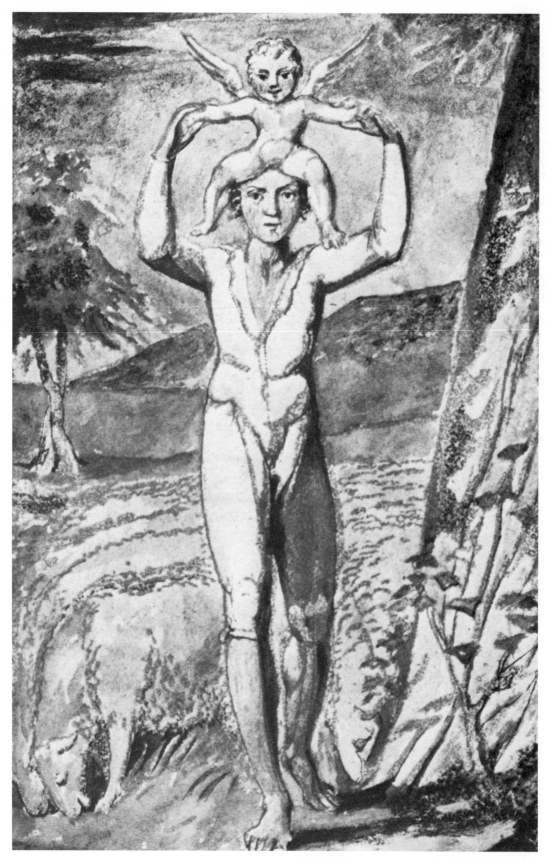

. . . . wisdom begins at the end. Frontispiece of William Blake's "Songs of Experience," 1794.

"The disease of cancer will be banished from life by calm, unhurrying, persistent men and women, working with every shiver of feeling controlled and suppressed, in hospitals and laboratories, and the motive that will conquer cancer will not be pity nor horror; it will be curiosity to know how and why."
—H.G. Wells, "Meanwhile,"
New York: J. H. Doran, 1927.

Things won are done: joy's soul lies in the doing.
—William Shakespeare,
Troilus and Cressida, Act I, scene ii,
line 313, 1603.

INDEX

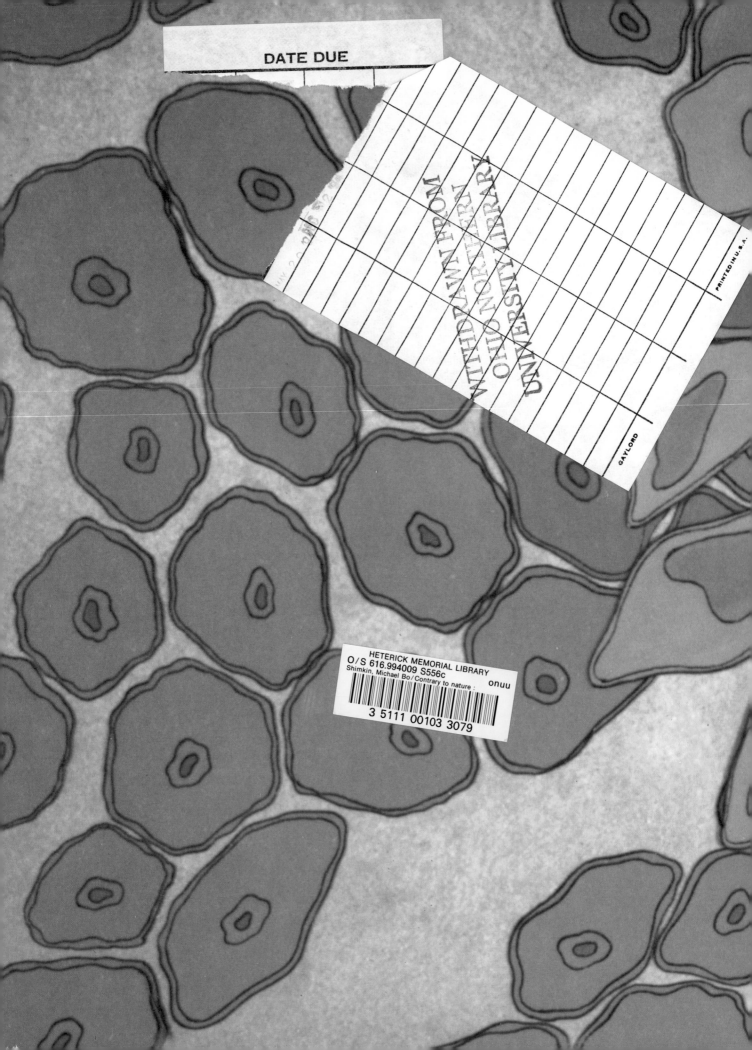